The Biology of *Trypanosoma* and *Leishmania*, Parasites of Man and Domestic Animals

D. H. Molyneux

Professor of Biology,
University of Salford

and

R. W. Ashford

Senior Lecturer,
Department of Parasitology,
Liverpool School of Tropical Medicine

Taylor and Francis
London
1983

First published 1983 by Taylor & Francis Ltd,
4 John Street, London WC1N 2ET.

Phototypesetting by Georgia Origination, Liverpool
Printed and bound in the United Kingdom by
Taylor and Francis (Printers) Ltd, Rankine Road,
Basingstoke, Hampshire RG24 0PR

British Library Cataloguing in Publication Data

Molyneux, D. H.
The biology of Trypanosoma and Leishmania, parasites of man and domestic animals.
1. Trypanosomiasis 2. Leishmaniasis
I. Title II. Ashford, R. W.
616.9′363 RC186.T82

ISBN 0-85066-242-7

Contents

Acknowledgements

We are grateful to very many colleagues who have taken considerable trouble to help in the task of preparing this book. We wish to record our gratitude to Drs Michael Chance, Bill Crewe, Simon Croft, Tony Jordan, Peter Dukes, Chris Schofield, Lee Ryan, Leo Jenni, Peter Heywood, Richard Ward, Mervyn Turner, Rick Stokes, Walter Petana, Michael Miles, Mr Ken Tiezsen and Miss Janet East; in particular to Professor George Nelson who valiantly scrutinized the whole of the final manuscript. Any errors are our own responsibility; that there are not many more is due to the diligence of those mentioned above. We have also been considerably aided by colleagues who provided photographic material so willingly and gave us permission to publish hitherto unpublished photographs; they are Drs David Baldry, Walter Petana, Malcolm Coe, Brian Bertram, Nestor van Miervenne, Lee Ryan, Simon Croft, Ian Maudlin, Max Murray, Leo Jenni, Y. A. Dubrovsky and Professor Keith Vickerman and the Liverpool School of Tropical Medicine, Ms Heather Brown, Joe Brady, Ken Jones and Mike Whiting all gave their time and advice on photographic problems and produced prints without complaint virtually instantaneously. We thank the Editors of *Acta Tropica, Annals of Tropical Medicine and Parasitology, Proceedings of the Royal Society* and *Annales de la Société belge de Médecine tropical,* and *Academic Press* and George Allen & Unwin for permission to reproduce material. We also wish to record our sincere thanks to Mrs D. Steedman and particularly Mrs Kay Smith for their tolerance during the typing of innumerable drafts and interpreting our own scribbles and those of colleagues. Without their help this task would have been infinitely more difficult.

Finally our thanks to our wives and families to whom this book is dedicated for their tolerance of our interests and our frequent absences.

D. H. M.
R. W. A.
August 1982

Introduction

The trypanosomiases and leishmaniases are widespread and economically important parasitic infections of man and his domestic animals. Over recent years there has been increasing interest shown in these infections, because they restrain the development of the livestock potential of Africa and cause important diseases in man. The medical importance of the trypanosomiases and leishmaniases is emphasized by the inclusion of African and South American trypanosomiasis and the leishmaniases as two target diseases of the World Health Organisation Programme for the Research and Training in Tropical Diseases (TDR) sponsored by the World Bank and the United Nations Development Programme. The diseases attract the interest of many scientists throughout the developing and developed world; in addition, many medical, paramedical and entomological workers at various levels are employed in their control.

The parasites have been extensively investigated because of unusual characteristics, such as antigenic variation in trypanosomes and, in *Leishmania*, their ability to survive and multiply in macrophages, the very cells which are responsible for the destruction of foreign organisms. These phenomena have interested scientists in countries remote from the field problems, as an understanding of these processes could lead to the elucidation of wider biological problems. For these reasons *Trypanosoma* and *Leishmania* are being extensively used as biological models by cell and molecular biologists.

We have written this book because we believe that an attempt should be made to present a summary of knowledge of the biology of what we have called the 'haemoflagellates', and their vectors, at such a level that it is comprehensible for the non-specialist reader. We consider the subject encompasses such wide fields of biology that researchers and students interested in these organisms and the diseases they cause cannot easily obtain a background in their biology. There are several notable research texts which provide a wealth of information on aspects of the biology of these parasites and their vectors and it is not our intention to provide an additional review. We aim to bridge the gap between what appears in textbooks and the appropriate research texts. Reference to the appropriate reviews are given at the end of the book and this should enable any student to gain immediate access to the relevant literature in his field of specific interest, be it vector ecology or parasite immunology. We have refrained from including references in the text.

We are particularly interested in whole animal (be it parasite, vector or host) biology, ecology and control. To some extent this may be reflected in the text. We have felt it inappropriate to consider physiology, biochemistry and immunology in great detail and we have tried to summarize recent views on pathogenesis and treatment as they apply to practical considerations. We have also attempted to achieve a balance between the biological and medical disciplines represented in the topics we have covered. Part of the great attraction of these diseases for the biologist is the diversity of interests which are represented in original papers published on the organisms and the diseases. It is hoped this text will enlighten the specialists and students who desire an understanding of aspects of the biology of these organisms and their vectors outside their specific interest, whether it be molecular biology or *Glossina* control.

There can be little doubt of the social and economic importance of these diseases: international and bilateral agencies as well as national governments allocate enormous resources to research and control activities. Development in Africa has been hindered by animal trypanosomiasis; human trypanosomiases in the Old and New Worlds continue to take their toll (sometimes spectacularly in large epidemics in Africa). The leishmaniases persist insidiously throughout the Old and New Worlds. For both diseases vector control is either very expensive or impractical, drugs are either toxic or unavailable; almost no new chemotherapeutics have been marketed for two decades and pharmaceutical companies have turned their backs on these diseases as potential sources of revenue, hence R & D has almost ceased to be financed by industry.

Against this background we hope that in some way we can contribute to a broader understanding of these organisms, the diseases they cause, their natural history and control. If we succeed in enthusing some readers with a desire to become involved with these extraordinarily diverse and successful organisms we will have gone some way to achieving our goals.

To Anita and Kay
and the Children

PART I

INTRODUCTION TO THE TRYPANOSOMATIDAE AND THEIR VECTORS

Chapter 1. The Parasites

CLASSIFICATION

Taxonomic position

The organisms considered in this book represent some of the most primitive and specialized in the animal kingdom. The most recent classification of the Protozoa compiled by a Committee of the Society of Protozoologists has designated the Protozoa a subkingdom rather than a phylum and raised the former class Mastigophora to the subphylum level (see table 1).

The current taxonomic position of the organisms which form the subject of this book is the following:

Kingdom	Protista	
Subkingdom	Protozoa	
Phylum	Sarcomastigophora	Honigberg & Balamuth, 1963
Subphylum	Mastigophora	Diesing, 1866
Class	Zoomastigophorea	Calkins, 1909
Order	Kinetoplastida	Honigberg, 1963 *emend* Vickerman, 1976
Suborder	Trypanosomatina	Kent, 1880
Family	Trypanosomatidae	Doflein, 1901 *emend* Grobben, 1905

The Order Kinetoplastida, Honigberg, 1963 *emend* Vickerman, 1976 is diagnosed as follows.

Flagellates with one or two flagella typically arising from a flagellar pocket or pit. (Flagella typically with paraxial rod in addition to axoneme.) There is a single mitochondrion typically extending the length of the body either as a simple tube, a hoop or a network of branched tubes and usually containing a conspicuous Feulgen-positive (DNA containing) nucleoid or kinetoplast close to the flagellar basal bodies; basal bodies inserted on (or close to) the mitochondrial envelope;

Table 1. Classification of Kinetoplastida.

Kingdom	Protista
Subkingdom	Protozoa
Phylum	Apicomplexa, Sarcomastigophora, Microspora, Ciliophora
Subphylum	Opalinata, Mastigophora, Sarcodina
Class	Phytomastigophorea, Zoomastigophorea
Order	Kinetoplastida
Suborder	Bodonina, Trypanosomatina
Family	Trypanosomatidae
Genus	*Crithidia*, *Leptomonas*, *Herpetomonas*, *Blastocrithidia*, *Trypanosoma*, *Phytomonas*, *Leishmania*, *Endotrypanum*, *Rhynchoidomonas*

supporting microtubular elements of body largely peripheral (pellicular); microtubule surrounded cytopharynx present in many species, presumably secondarily lost by many saprozoic forms; pseudopodia absent; single vesicular nucleus with prominent endosome; no plastids; Golgi apparatus typically in region of the flagellar pocket but not connected to basal bodies and flagella; contractile vacuole, if present, emptying into flagellar pocket. Parasitic (majority of known species) or free living.

The order Kinetoplastida, Honigberg, 1963 *emend* Vickerman, 1976 has two suborders: the largely free living Bodonina and the exclusively parasitic Trypanosomatina. It is the second of these suborders which occupies our interest. There is only one family in this suborder — the Trypanosomatidae. The diagnosis of this family is as follows.

Kinetoplastid flagellates with a single locomotory flagellum either free or attached to pellicle as an undulating membrane; second flagellum represented by a barren basal body only; kinetoplast relatively small and compact with DNA fibrils arranged in marked anisotropic fashion. All members of the Family Trypanosomatidae are parasitic in either invertebrate or vertebrate hosts contrasting with other Kinetoplastida which can be free living.

This work concentrates on the genera *Leishmania* and *Trypanosoma* as these are the most studied genera and are of greatest economic importance (tables 2 and 3). However, studies of the other genera have contributed considerably to our understanding of trypanosomes and *Leishmania* and this text would not be complete without some mention of the biology of these genera, as they are zoologically close and provide insight into the diversity of the family. The following genera make up the family Trypanosomatidae (see tables 1, 2, 3): *Crithidia, Blastocrithidia, Leptomonas, Herpetomonas, Endotrypanum, Phytomonas, Leishmania, Trypanosoma* and *Rhynchoidomonas*. *Trypanosoma, Leishmania* and *Endotrypanum* have both vertebrate and invertebrate hosts, although one member of the genus *Trypanosoma* has become adapted secondarily to coital transmission (*T. equiperdum*). The genera *Leptomonas, Herpetomonas, Crithidia, Blastocrithidia* and *Rhynchoidomonas* are monoxenous and are almost exclusively parasites of insects, although there are some records from arachnids, nematodes and acanthocephalan worms. The genus *Phytomonas* are plant parasites living in sap and are transmitted between plants by plant-sucking insects.

Trypanosomatid parasites change their configuration during their life cycles, particularly when they change hosts from vertebrate to invertebrate and vice versa; and because monoxenous flagellates such as *Blastocrithidia* and *Leptomonas* can parasitize the same insects such as *Triatoma* and various Siphonaptera (fleas) at the same time, there are considerable difficulties in recognition. This has led at times to misunderstandings in nomenclature and identification. Originally, each morphological type was referred to by the genus in which it mainly occurred. Thus the 'crithidial' form occurred mainly in the genus *Crithidia* and 'leishmanial' forms were found mainly in *Leishmania*. Confusion arose when referring for example, to the 'leishmanial' form of *Trypanosoma cruzi*. Sometimes it was not clear whether two

Table 2. Classification of the genus *Trypanosoma*.

	Trypanosoma						
Section	Stercoraria			Salivaria			
Subgenus	*Megatrypanum*	*Herpetosoma*	*Schizotrypanum*	*Duttonella*	*Nannomonas*	*Trypanozoon*	*Pycnomonas*
Representative species	*T.(M.) theileri*	*T.(H.) lewisi* *T.(H.) musculi* *T.(H.) rangeli*	*T.(S.) cruzi*	*T.(D.) uniforme* *T.(D.) vivax*	*T.(N.) congolense* *T.(N.) simiae*	*T.(T.) brucei* *T.(T.) b. brucei* *T.(T.) b. rhodesiense* *T.(T.) b. gambiense* *T.(T.) equiperdum* *T.(T.) evansi*	*T.(P.) suis*

Table 3. Classification of the Genus *Leishmania*.

	Leishmania		
Section	Hypopylaria (Parasites of reptiles)*	Peripylaria (parasites of reptiles* and mammals)	Suprapylaria (Parasites of mammals)
Representative species	"*L. agamae*" "*L. ceramodactyli*"	"*L. adleri*" *L. braziliensis* *L. peruviana* "*L. tarentolae*"	*L. aethiopica* *L. donovani* *L. major* *L. mexicana* *L. tropica*

*Recent studies on reptile trypanosomes question the validity of lizard *Leishmania* morphological types in a given host belonged to a single species or two. Hoare and Wallace introduced a rational nomenclature, replacing the old names with new ones describing the morphology rather than relating to generic names. This forms the basis of modern nomenclature. It refers to the arrangement of the flagellum: its starting point, its course either inside or outside the body of the parasite and its point of emergence to the exterior of the organism (see figure 1). These characteristics are important in classification and identification. This terminology relies on the Greek-based suffix mastigote (literally 'whip-like'). The prefixes used refer to the position of the flagellum in the organism. These terms are used as nouns or adjectives.

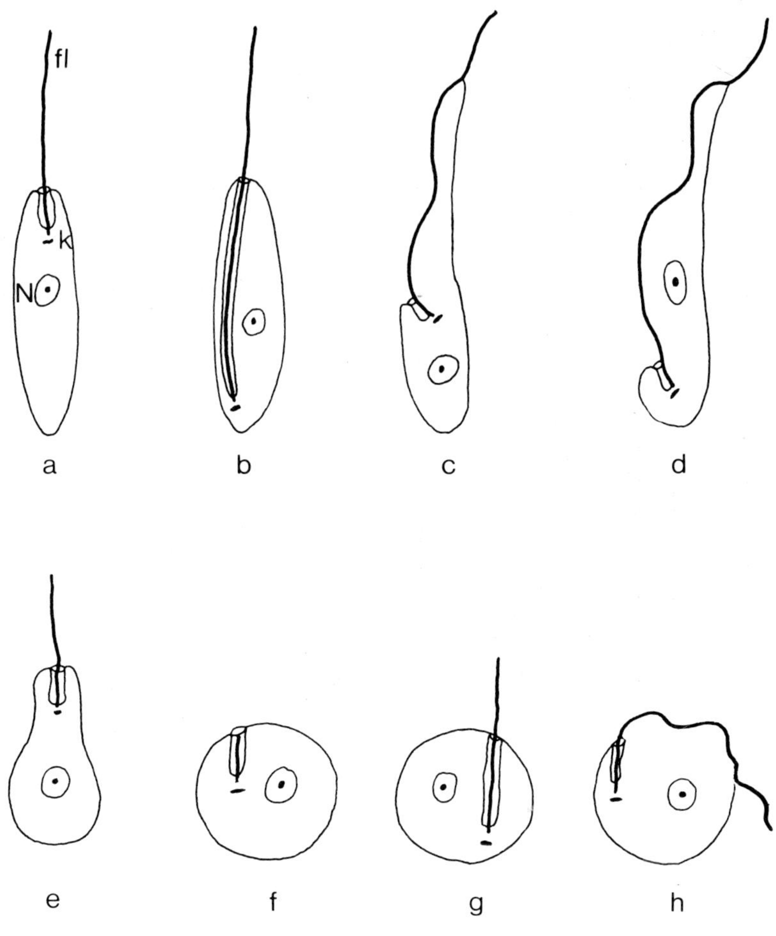

Figure 1. Diagrammatic configuration of morphological types of Trypanosomatidae (× 1300). a, Promastigote. b, Opisthomastigote. c, Epimastigote. d, Trypomastigote. e, Choanomastigote. f, Amastigote. g, Paramastigote. h, Sphaeromastigote.

Abbreviations: fl = flagellum; N = nucleus; k = kinetoplast.

The following descriptions and definitions of the configurations of trypanosomatid flagellates are currently in use and are generally accepted.

(*a*) Promastigote: elongated form with antenuclear kinetoplast with flagellum arising near it and emerging from the anterior end of the body.

(*b*) Opisthomastigote: elongated form with postnuclear kinetoplast; flagellum arising near kinetoplast and passing through the body and emerging from the anterior end.

(*c*) Epimastigote: elongated form with juxtanuclear kinetoplast.

(*d*) Trypomastigote: elongated form with postnuclear kinetoplast; flagellum arising near it and emerging from the side of the body to run along the surface to form an undulating membrane.

(*e*) Choanomastigote: 'barley corn' form with antenuclear kinetoplast; the flagellum arises from a wide funnel-shaped reservoir and emerges anteriorly.

(*f*) Amastigote: round, oval, or elongated form devoid of flagellum.

(*g*) Paramastigote: form with kinetoplast close to nucleus; intermediate between Pro- and Opisthomastigote; flagellum emerges from anterior end and reservoir extends through body to point where flagellum and kinetoplast are close.

(*h*) Sphaeromastigote: rounded form with a free flagellum, which represents a transitional stage between an amastigote and mastigote form.

Table 4. Occurrence of -mastigotes in genera of Trypanosomatidae.

	Pro-	Opistho-	Epi-	Trypo-	Choano-	A-	Para-	Sphaero-
Leptomonas	*					*		
Crithidia					*	*		
Herpetomonas	*	*					*	
Blastocrithidia	*		*			*		
Rhynchoidomonas				*				
Endotrypanum	*		*	*		*		
Phytomonas	*							
Trypanosoma	*		*	*		*		*
Leishmania	*					*	*	

The organization of the organelles and their relative position is shown in figure 1.

Genera of Trypanosomatidae

The diagnostic characteristics, biology, hosts and life cycles of the genera referred to above are briefly discussed below. There is no significance in the order in which the genera are mentioned. The monoxenous genera are sometimes referred to as the 'Lower Trypanosomatidae'.

Genus Leptomonas

Leptomonas flagellates are most commonly found as monogenetic parasites in several orders of insects (Hemiptera, Diptera, Hymenoptera and Siphonaptera), where they usually parasitize the gut and less frequently the haemocoele and salivary glands. *L. ctenocephali* is a parasite of dog fleas and *L. oncopelti* is found in bugs (*Oncopeltus*). *Leptomonas* species have also been reported as parasites of nematodes and even in the macronucleus of *Paramecium*.

Promastigote and amastigote forms occur. Promastigotes usually range from around 10–40 μm in body length; the flagellum, when present, may be modified for attachment to the insect gut, and some authors describe flagella of *Leptomonas* having a brush at the tip. Free-swimming forms have flagella about the same length as the body. Some *Leptomonas* species can be extremely long, up to 200 μm, and the body may be twisted in a regular helix. Transmission from host to host is by contamination by amastigote cysts, which are small bodies referred to as strap-hangers because they are produced by an unequal division of the parent organisms and attach to the flagellum. *Leptomonas* species are transmitted from adult to larval flea by the larval flea feeding on faeces deposited by adults. The larval flea's habit of feeding on freshly deposited or dried blood from adult fleas ensures completion of the life cycle.

Genus Crithidia

This genus comprises monoxenous parasites of insects; the orders Diptera and Hemiptera are the most frequently parasitized. The genus has been recently revised and is defined by the presence of the choanomastigote or 'barley corn'-like forms with a free flagellum. Extensive studies have been carried out on the nutritional requirement of *Crithidia* and its biochemistry. Some species or stocks of the genus have bacterial endosymbionts which provide essential vitamins or co-factors. *C. fasciculata* is found in *Anopheles* and *Culex* mosquitoes throughout the world and, because of its ease of cultivation, this is one of the most studied flagellates. The parasites are usually localized in the mid- and hindgut of insects. Mosquito *Crithidia* have a free-living stage in water and thus pass between larvae resulting in later infection of adults. The length of *Crithidia* species is usually around 4–13 μm with the flagellum 7–14 μm.

Genus Herpetomonas

This genus has promastigotes, paramastigotes and opisthomastigotes at various stages of the life cycle. Paramastigotes are transitional forms between pro- and opisthomastigotes. Promastigotes are the commonest morphological forms found and hence this genus can be confused with *Leptomonas.* Transformation from promastigotes to opisthomastigotes is partly controlled by temperature. When the rate of multiplication in cultures decreases the proportion of opisthomastigotes rises, perhaps due to nutritional stress. Rapid division of promastigotes results in the frequent appearance of bi-flagellate stages. *Herpetomonas* species are found in Diptera (e.g., *H. muscarum* is found in the housefly *Musca domestica*; *H. ampelophilae* in *Drosphila*), in some reduviid bugs (e.g., *H. samuelpessoai* in *Zelus* spp.), and Hymenoptera (*H. swainei* in *Neodiprion swainei*). Infections are found in the mid- and hindgut and less frequently in the malpighian tubules and the haemocoele. Cysts have not been reported from *Herpetomonas* and recent studies suggest that free-living stages permit adult Diptera to acquire the infection. Infection can also be acquired by larval Diptera and retained through the pupae to adults. *Herpetomonas* can be maintained in culture. The size of *Herpetomonas* promastigotes is 6–30 μm with the flagellum up to 20 μm but usually around 10 μm in length. Opisthomastigotes are generally shorter, being 6–10 μm long.

Genus Blastocrithidia

This genus includes monoxenous epimastigote trypanosomatids; they can be confused with epimastigotes of the genus *Trypanosoma*. Cultivation is difficult, but recently *B. triatomae* has grown in insect cell cultures. Hosts of *Blastocrithidia* are mosquitoes and bugs. *B. culicis* is a mosquito parasite which possesses a dumb-bell shaped endosymbiont; *B. triatomae* is found in the mid- and hindgut of *Triatoma infestans* and could be confused with stages of *T. cruzi* in this vector; *B. triatomae* forms highly resistant cysts when deposited in faeces, which when dry are transmitted between bugs by coprophagy or contamination of mouthparts. *Blastocrithidia* species parasitize the mid- and hindgut of their insect hosts. Endosymbionts of *B. culicis* have been 'cured' by the antibiotic chloramphenicol. *B. gerridis* is a parasite found in the gut of water striders of the genus *Gerris*. *Blastocrithidia* species are about 10–70 μm long; the free flagellum is also variable in length at 5–12 μm. A species from a tick, *B. hyalommae,* is reported to be transmitted by transovarial transmission.

Genus Rhynchoidomonas

Very little is known about this genus which is characterized by monoxenous trypomastigotes without a free flagellum. They are parasitic in the gut of Diptera (Calliphoridae and Drosophilidae) and vary in size between 10 and 50 μm. They have most frequently been reported as parasites of the malpighian tubules.

Genus Endotrypanum

This is a genus of digenetic trypanosomatids found in erythrocytes of sloths (Edentata) in Central and South America. *Endotrypanum* is the only known intra-erythrocytic kinetoplastid and is transmitted by sandflies of the genus *Lutzomyia*. The infection in sandflies develops in the hindgut with profuse invasion of the malpighian tubules. Two species are recognized: *E. schaudinni* and *E. monterogei*. The former has intraerythrocytic epimastigotes, the latter trypomastigotes. Recently, however, several zymodemes of *Endotrypanum* have been characterized. Both species can be grown in culture where they form promastigotes, in which curious inclusions are seen resembling the virus-like particles in *Leishmania hertigi* (see p. 20).

Genus Phytomonas

This genus, as the name suggests, is parasitic in plants; the families of plants most frequently found infected are the lactiferous families Euphorbiaceae and Asclepiadaceae. Other families too may harbour flagellates.

Phytomonas is transmitted between plants by plant-sucking hemipterans, usually of the family Lygaeidae, for example, *Oncopeltus*. The parasites are transmitted by bite after invading the salivary glands from the haemocoele and the midgut. *Phytomonas* species parasitize lactiferous tubules of Asclepiadaceae; in non-lactiferous coffee plants (*Coffea*) and palms (*Cocos*) the parasites are found in sieve tubes. It is believed that a *Phytomonas* species is the agent responsible for a wilt disease in coffee and for hartrot in coconut palms. Recent reports suggest that thousands of economically valuable palms have been killed in Suriname. The disease has very similar symptoms to lethal yellowing of palms caused by a *Mycoplasma*-like organism. *Phytomonas* has a promastigote configuration and is structurally very similar to *Leptomonas*, but cannot be cultured. In plants the flagellates are around 20 μm in length with a free flagellum of around 7–10 μm.

Genus Trypanosoma

The genus is characterized by its parasitic mode of life. Trypanosomes are very variable in size from 10 μm to over 1200 μm (an enormous bat trypanosome), but generally these spindle-shaped organisms are 15–100 μm depending on species and subgenus (figures 2 and 3). The characteristic morphological forms are trypomastigotes, typically found in the blood and tissues of vertebrate hosts, and the epimastigote forms which are found in the invertebrate vector. However, other configurations of morphological forms are found, such as amastigotes and, more rarely, promastigotes. The infective forms which are produced in the vector are known as metacyclic and they are trypomastigote in configuration.

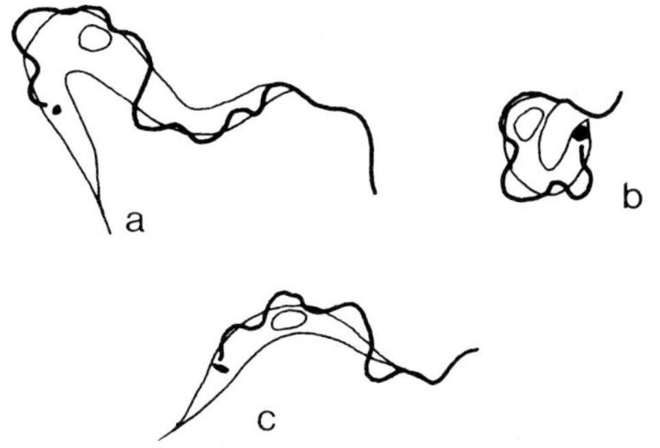

Figure 2. Trypanosomes of different subgenera (× 1300). a, Subgenus *Megatrypanum*, e.g., *T. theileri*. b, Subgenus *Schizotrypanum*, e.g., *T. cruzi*. c, Subgenus *Herpetosoma*, e.g., *T. lewisi*.

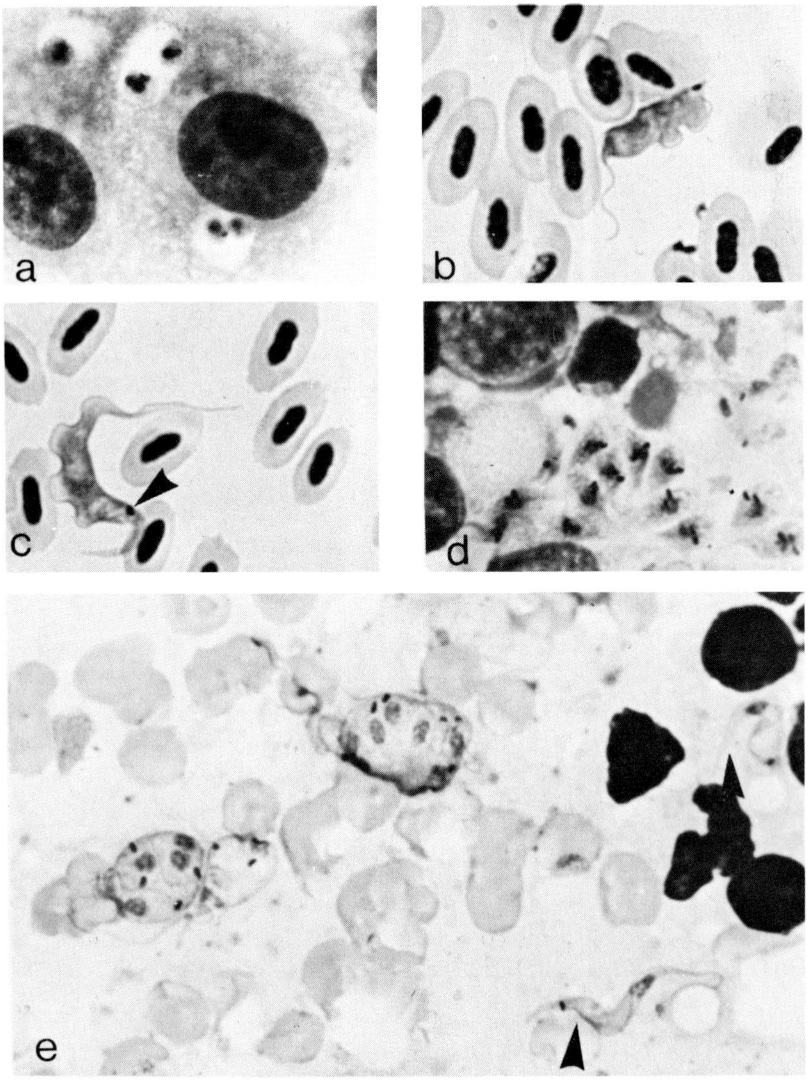

Figure 3. a, Amastigotes of *Leishmania* in dog sarcoma cells (× 1600). b, An avian trypanosome (*T. everetti*); this parasite is leaf or kite shaped in contrast to the more classical spindle shape shown in c and e (× 1200). c, A spindle shaped avian trypanosome; note the well developed undulating membrane and large kinetoplast (arrowed) (× 1200). d, Tissue form of the rat trypanosome *T. lewisi* showing amastigotes in an impression smear of kidney medulla (× 1600). e, Tissue impression smear of rat kidney medulla showing multinucleate division form of *T. lewisi* and non-dividing forms (arrowed) (× 1600).

Transmission to the vertebrate hosts is by the bite of a vector or by contamination of the skin or mucous membranes by faecal material containing infective metacyclic trypanosomes. The vectors are haematophagous arthropods (insects and arachnids), but leeches (Hirudinea: Annelida) act as vectors of some fish and amphibian trypanosomes.

In the vertebrate host parasites are found in the blood, but also localize in a variety of tissues. Reproduction in the vertebrate host is by a variety of different methods of cell division; no sexual processes are thought to occur in the vertebrate but recent studies using isoenzymes suggest that trypanosomes are diploid and exchange of genetic information does occur in the vector. Much work is required to elucidate the mechanism and extent of this process.

Genus Leishmania

The mammalian stages of the genus *Leishmania* are intracellular amastigotes (see figure 3a); the promastigote and paramastigote forms are found in the vector sandflies *Phlebotomus* and *Lutzomyia*. Among vertebrates, only mammals and reptiles are infected with *Leishmania*, and sandflies are the only known effective vectors.

The amastigote stages are intracellular parasites of macrophages and it is only in more restricted and rare conditions that other cells are invaded. Visceral and cutaneous manifestations of leishmaniasis occur, but in wild reservoir hosts few if any symptoms are seen.

The amastigotes taken up by sandflies rapidly transform through elongation into promastigotes, the typical form in the vector. Promastigotes are the infective form inoculated when infected sandflies bite their hosts (figure 79, p. 190)

Transmission of mammalian *Leishmania* is by the bite of an infected sandfly after development in the midgut, and occasionally hindgut, cibarium and pharynx (see figure 13, p. 32).

MORPHOLOGY

Light Microscope

The diagnostic feature of the Order Kinetoplastida is the possession of an organelle, the kinetoplast, which contains deoxyribonucleic acid, DNA. In *Trypanosoma* and *Leishmania* this is usually a rod shaped structure (Figure 3c) when stained with Giemsa or Leishman stains, but with the electron microscope it can be seen that it is a modified mitochondrion containing a rod of DNA in one part of it.

The parasites in stained smears vary considerably in shape and size (see figure 3). However, the densely staining kinetoplast and a less densely staining nucleus and, in all forms except amastigote, the presence of a flagellum are characteristic. The size of trypanosomatids varies from *L. donovani* amastigotes with a diameter of around 2–3 μm to a bizarre bat trypanosome with a length of over 1200 μm. However, trypanosomes generally range in length from 15 to 100μm and *Leishmania* amastigotes from 2 to 10 μm in diameter (see figure 3).

Trypomastigotes are normally elongated spindle shaped (fusiform). However, they may be leaf-like (figure 3b), or even almost spherical, as in some parasites of frogs and reptiles. The other morphological types are usually straight and, again, spindle shaped to spherical. Various inclusions may be seen which sometimes obscure the characteristic nucleus and flagellum. Where the flagellum enters the body the flagellar pocket or reservoir is clearly visible in some forms.

Preparations from blood, cerebrospinal fluid, lymph gland juice or material dissected from insects are frequently made to detect the presence of parasites. All stages exhibit some motility except the intracellular amastigotes.

Promastigotes normally appear to have a fixed body shape, movement being restricted to the flagellum. In forms with a relatively large flagellum and small body both flagellum and body may appear to vibrate. In epimastigotes, the anterior end appears to taper gradually into the flagellum, and thus undulates with the flagellum. The flagellar undulations of trypomastigotes are transmitted to the body via the undulating membrane and the whole organism moves rapidly. Normally, the flagellum is directed anteriorly during forward movement. Various forms of movement depend on the requirements of the parasites, such as penetration of tissues or free-swimming in capillaries, and the availability of energy. In preparations of blood infected with trypanosomes, parasites usually are initially detected as a result of the agitation of the erythrocytes (or, in lymph gland juice, lymphocytes) by the parasites' motility. Dark ground or phase contrast illumination of infected blood will enhance the chances of seeing the body of the parasite. The movement may be characteristic of a given species. For example, *T. vivax* is large and moves rapidly across the microscope field in a linear path, occasionally stopping briefly; *T. congolense* is frequently observed to be adherent to erythrocytes in wet film preparations and has sluggish activity. *T. brucei* is larger in size and highly active, but this movement is not progressive.

Parasites can thus be tentatively identified in fresh preparations after haematocrit centrifugation.

Stages in insects can be detected in preparations of the gut or salivary glands after dissection; parasites in such sites may be difficult to see in intact guts and may only be seen if the gut is ruptured and free parasites escape. Attached parasites are more difficult to detect as they are less motile and line the gut wall and may only occasionally twitch.

Cell structure and function

The electron microscope structure of kinetoplastid parasites in vertebrate (particularly mammalian) hosts has been intensively studied. Comparatively less attention has been paid to forms found in insects, partly due to the difficulties of keeping some of the vectors in laboratories (figures 4–10).

The plasma membrane (pellicle) and associated structures

The interface between parasite and host plays a vital role in any host–parasite relationship. The plasma membrane or plasmalemma of *Trypanosoma* and *Leishmania* is a typical unit membrane, similar in appearance to that in other animal cells. The plasma membrane is approximately 2–4 nm in total width and consists of outer dense osmiophilic layers separated by a clear layer (figure 4).

Beneath the plasma membrane is found a series of pellicular microtubules, present some 10 nm below the inner leaflet of the plasma membrane and having an external diameter of 20–22 nm; they are separated by distances varying from 10 to 25 nm. The subpellicular microtubules are believed to be cytoskeletal in function and are present in vertebrate and invertebrate forms of both *Trypanosoma* and *Leishmania*. Their regular distribution beneath the plasma membrane, usually in a single row arranged spirally around the body, only varies occasionally (figure 4). Examples are attached forms of *Crithidia* in mosquitoes or cyst-like forms of *Leptomonas* in fleas: here the microtubules are displaced further into the cytoplasm.

At points of attachment of the flagellum to the parasite body there is a gap in the continuity of the subpellicular microtubule ring. In those flagellates which have an undulating membrane the flagellar membrane is attached to the surface of the plasma membrane by desmosome-like structures which anchor the flagellum to the body in a manner which can be compared with a rivet passing between the two opposed plasma membranes. In promastigotes similar plaques attach the flagellum to the plasma membrane of the reservoir at the point of emergence. Three microtubules are present in the region of the flagellar pocket or reservoir, but microtubules do not line the reservoir plasma membrane. The base of the reservoir is the area where the membrane covering the axoneme of the flagellum (flagellar membrane) joins the plasma membrane of the body of the organism itself (figures 5 and 6). There is no recognizable difference in the structure of the flagellar and plasma membranes. In invertebrate hosts the flagellar membrane is capable of great modification when forms of the parasite attach to host tissues. In the gut of invertebrates the flagellum becomes shorter and an area of flagellar membrane comes into contact with the cuticular lining of either the insect foregut (stomodaeum) or hindgut (proctodaeum). Associated with this there is an increase in area of the flagellar membrane applied to the host cuticle, and within the flagellum electron dense material is formed which is termed a hemidesmosome (figure 7 and figures 60 and 61, pp. 18 and 137). Filaments are found associated with this structure orientated parallel to a shorter axoneme. These structures attach flagella to host surfaces. Flagellar contact with hemidesmosomes may occur without expansion of the flagellum, as in *Trypanozoon* species attached to *Glossina* salivary gland epithelium. Similar hemidesmosomal plaques have been found associated with flagella in the guts of leeches infected with amphibian trypanosomes. However, in the midguts of sandflies infected with *Leishmania* and sheepkeds *Melophagus ovinus* infected with *T. melophagium* the

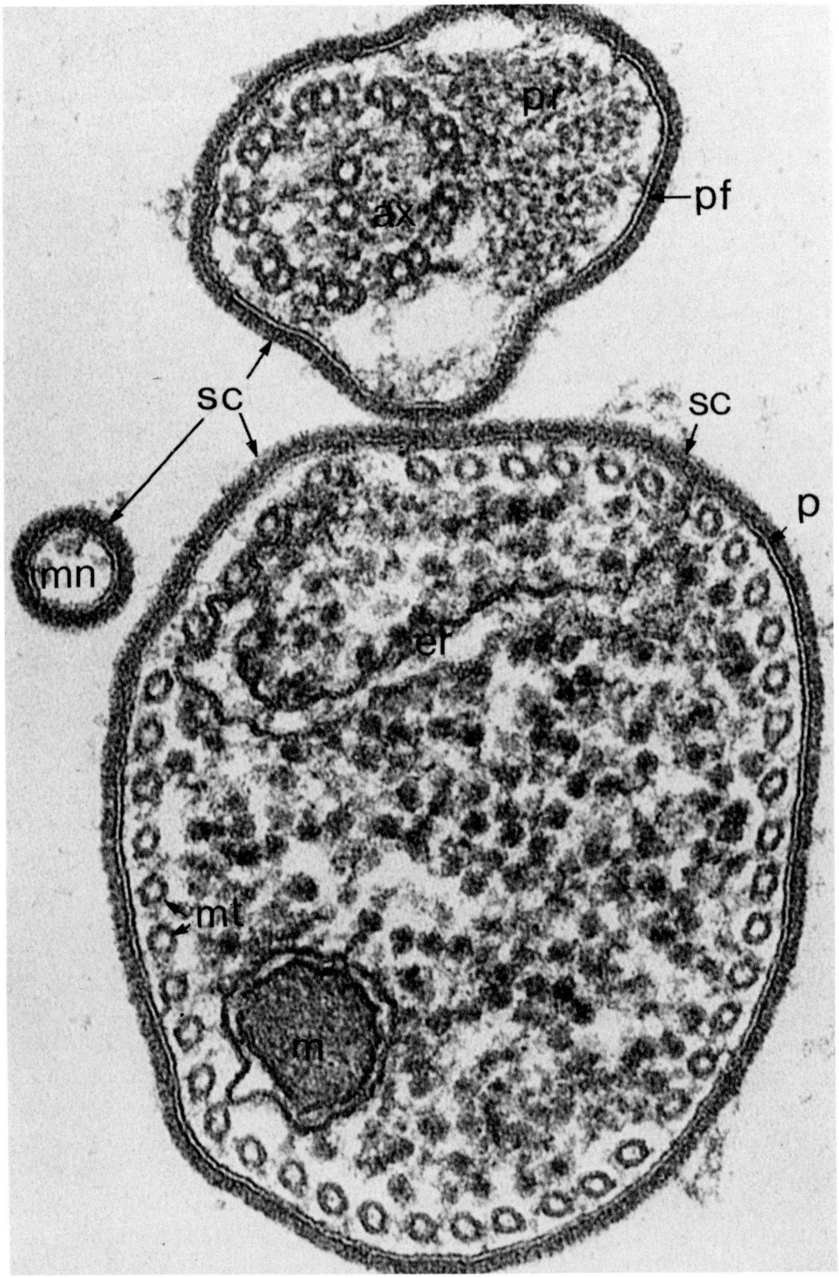

Figure 4. Electronmicrograph of *T. brucei* showing plasma membrane, p, plasma membrane of flagellum, pf, axoneme of flagellum, ax, paraxial rod, pr, surface coat, sc, microneme, mn and section through an acristate mitochondrion, m, microtubules, mt and endoplasmic reticulum, er (× 150 000).

Courtesy of Professor K. Vickerman.

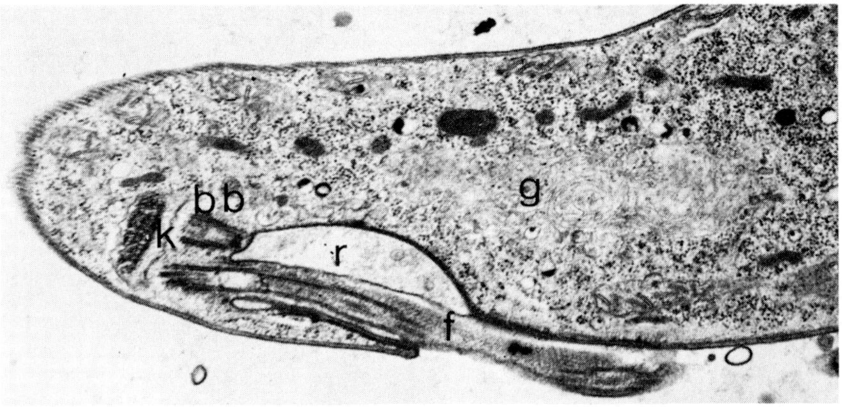

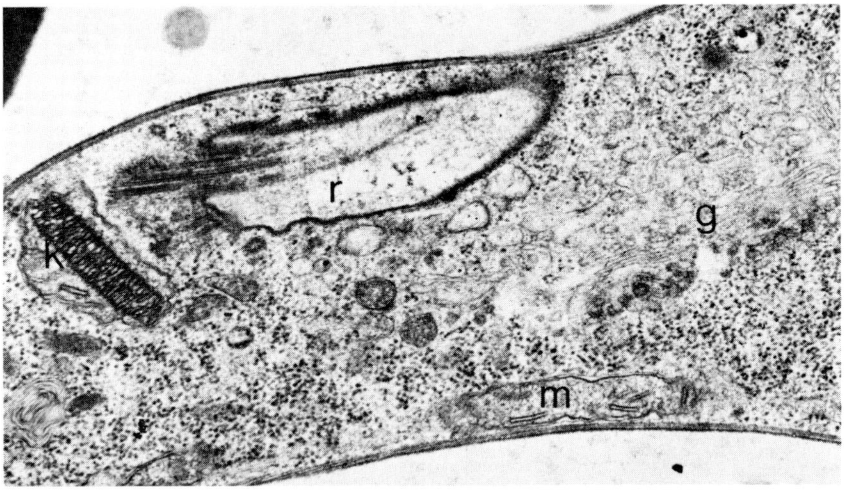

Figures 5 (top) and 6 (bottom). Electronmicrographs which show arrangement of flagellum, f, kinetoplast, k, basal body, bb, and reservoir, r of an avian trypanosome; note the other features, mitochondrion, m, and golgi apparatus, g (× 30 000).

flagellar membrane does not form hemidesmosomes with the microvilli of the midgut. When attached to insect cuticles the flagellar membranes have vesicles associated with them.

In the blood stream of vertebrates the plasma membrane of trypanosomes may have an exterior surface coat. This was first described in the subgenus *Trypanozoon*, some members of which cause sleeping sickness in man (figure 4). This surface coat has the appearance of a uniform layer of electron dense material over the whole surface of the parasite plasma and flagellar membranes. The coat is 10–15 nm wide in the *Trypanozoon* parasites which have been most closely studied, but it is less distinct in other subgenera, for example, *Herpetosoma (T. lewisi), Duttonella (T. vivax)* and *Nannomonas (T. congolense),* and in bird and fish trypanosomes.

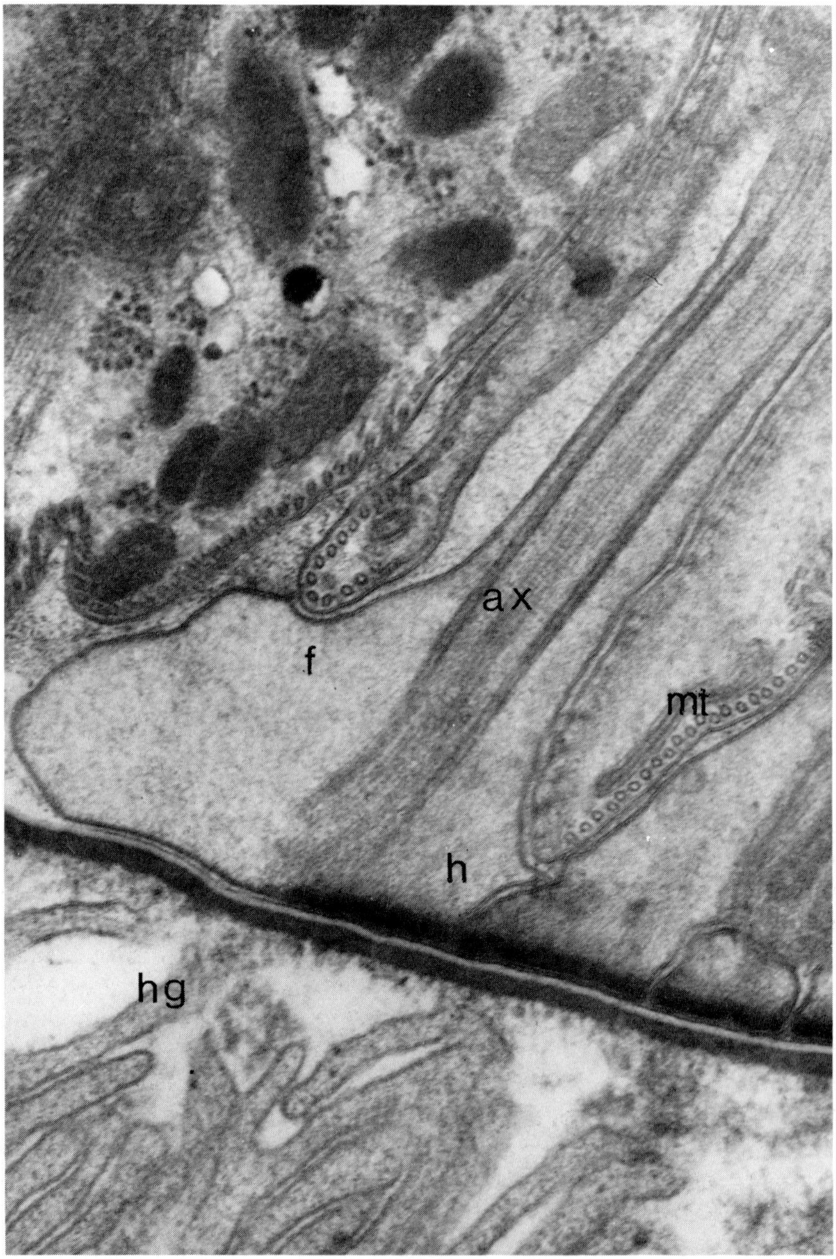

Figure 7. Electronmicrograph of an attached epimastigote flagellum of a trypanosome to an insect hindgut (× 66 000).

Abbreviations: h = hemidesmosome, ax = axoneme of flagellum, f = flagel um, hg = gut wall of host, mt = microtubules.

The surface coat has been shown to be the site of the variable antigen in *T. brucei*, which has been identified as a glycoprotein rich in the sugar galactose. In view of the importance of these glycoproteins in relation to possible vaccination, intense studies on the organization of the glycoprotein, its association with the plasma membrane and its assembly are being undertaken, and will be discussed in the section on antigenic variation (pp. 45–49).

The plasma membrane lining the flagellar pocket is modified for the intake of nutrient material; it is perhaps inappropriate to refer to this as a feeding process but the plasma membrane of the reservoir has been shown to be capable of pinocytosis. Small pinocytic or omega vesicles are observed to be formed in this specialized region and are subsequently pinched off and pass to the cytoplasm for digestion by lysosomal enzymes (figures 5 and 6). Lysosomal products are also discharged into the reservoir, as acid phosphatase has been detected cytochemically in the site.

In some species of *Trypanosoma* and *Crithidia* a distinct microtubule lined cytostome–cytopharynx apparatus has been observed associated with the plasma membrane of the reservoir. Cultured epimastigotes of *T. raiae,* a parasite of elasmobranch fish, have been shown to take nutrient into the body specifically through the cytostome area of the reservoir. The extent of the occurrence of this specialized structure in parasitic kinetoplastids is not sufficiently known.

The flagellum and basal body

In *Trypanosoma* in the vertebrate host the flagellum is responsible for movement, but in the invertebrate its role is a dual one of movement as well as attachment. The flagellum of *Leishmania* parasites in their mammalian host is markedly reduced — hence the term amastigote. This term implies the absence of a flagellum, but in fact in *Leishmania* amastigotes a flagellum is present, though it does not emerge from the periphery of the parasite and is entirely contained within the reservoir.

The axoneme of the flagellum of Trypanosomatidae has an internal structure similar to that observed in other groups in the animal kingdom (figure 4). It emerges from a basal body and has the typical 9 + 2 structure of nine outer microtubule doublets with arms and two inner but separate microtubules. This organization of the axoneme is common to all members of the group. The structure of the basal body is similar to the centrioles found in other animal cells. Occasionally a second basal body is observed adjacent to the one from which the flagellum emerges. The basal body is consistently found very close to the kinetoplast (figures 5, 6 and 9) and the distance between the two organelles remains the same throughout the life cycle of all species so far studied, indicating that during transformation the basal body and kinetoplast remain in some physical communication.

The region surrounding the axoneme has been called the intraflagellar region. In most species of *Trypanosoma* and *Leishmania* examined, a so-called paraxial rod runs parallel to the axoneme when it has emerged from the reservoir (figure 4).

The paraxial rod appears in transverse and longitudinal sections as a lattice work of filaments; no function has as yet been ascribed to it although it may play a role in flagellar contractility.

In flagellates attached in insect hosts this region becomes greatly expanded and contains filaments. Similarly, when rosettes of parasites form in the insect the intraflagellar region expands and desmosomes form between flagellar membranes of adjacent parasites. This is the mechanism by which parasites in rosettes adhere together.

Symbionts, micro-organisms and virus-like inclusions

It has been shown that symbionts and micro-organisms are present in *Crithidia* and in fish trypanosomes (*T. cobitis*). It is possible to 'cure' the *Crithidia* by the addition of chloramphenicol to the medium, which results in the destruction of the symbionts. However it has also been demonstrated that symbionts contribute to the metabolism of the parasites by supplying essential vitamins or enzyme co-factors.

Large arrays of virus-like particles (VLPs) measuring 55–60 nm have been found in cultured promastigotes of *Leishmania hertigi* from Panama and Brazil. This was the first demonstration of what are probably viral hyperparasites in *Leishmania*. If *L. hertigi* cultures are passed to macrophages and Dog Sarcoma cell lines and the temperature is increased to 35–37 °C then the parasites transform to amastigotes and the VLPs cannot be detected. Yet they are seen again after retransformation to promastigotes on reduction of temperature. When amastigote cultures are fed to sandflies in the laboratory, promastigotes containing VLPs are found in the midgut of the fly 3–5 days after the artificial feeding. Possible cytopathological changes are observed in VLP 'infected' promastigotes. Changes are seen in mitochondrial structure and in the synthesis of microtubules. The latter occur in the cytoplasm, where they are not usually found. Culture forms (promastigotes) of the intraerythrocytic parasite of sloths *Endotrypanum* have also been found to have inclusions which are not 'normal' cytoplasmic components of Trypanosomatidae.

The nucleus

The nucleus of kinetoplastids is surrounded by a nuclear envelope consisting of two membranes, punctured at varying intervals by the nuclear pores; the membranes are separated by 18–25 nm; the nuclear pores are 65–100 nm wide and physically link the cytoplasm with the nucleus. A feature of nuclear division in this group of organisms is the retention of the intact nuclear membranes (figures 8 and 9).

The ultrastructural appearance of the nucleus is similar in all the kinetoplastids studied to date. It is a spherical or slightly ovoid body approximately 1·5–2·5 μm in diameter. There is usually a thin layer of peripheral chromatin which lies close

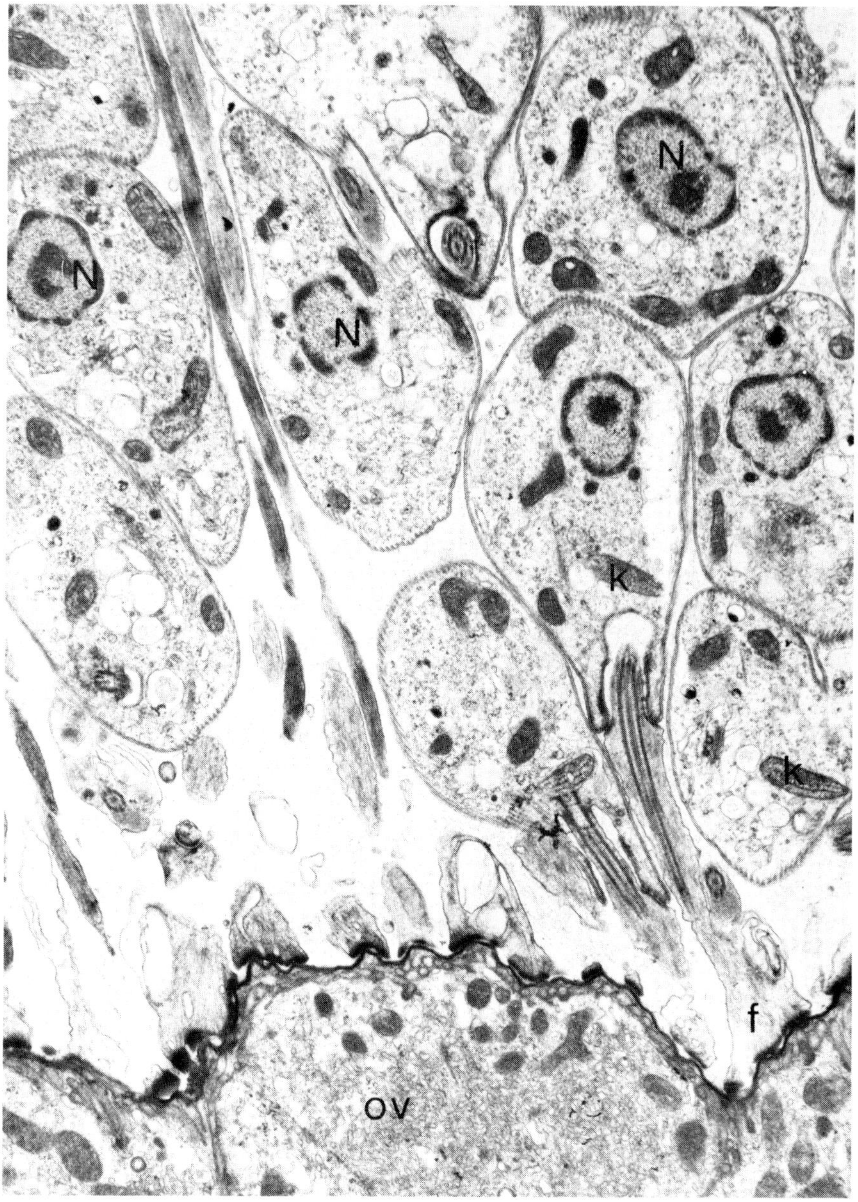

Figure 8. Electronmicrograph of attached promastigotes of *Leishmania mexicana amazonensis* to the oesophageal valve, ov, of a sandfly. Note the expanded flagellum, f, at the point of attachment (× 15 000).

Abbreviations: N = nucleus; k = kinetoplast.

Courtesy of Cambridge University Press and the Royal Society of London.

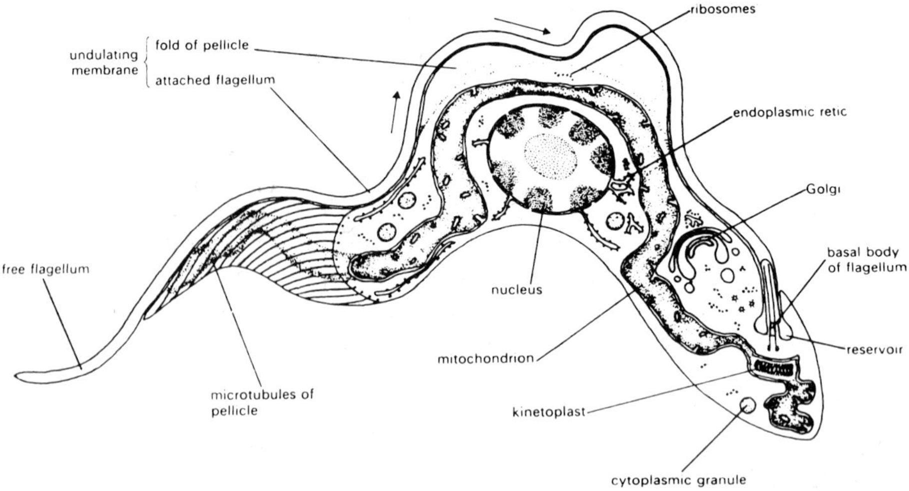

Figure 9. Diagram of the trypomastigote intermediate bloodstream form of *Trypanosoma b. rhodesiense* as seen at the level of the electron microscope. The arrows along the flagellum indicate the direction of travel of flagellar waves. Pellicular microtubules are shown only at the anterior end of the flagellate. Note the single mitochondrial canal.

Courtesy of George Allen & Unwin, Col. H.W. Mulligan and Prof. K. Vickerman.

to the inner nuclear membrane; the nucleolus is centrally placed and 0·5–1·0 μm in diameter; the peripheral chromatin and nucleolus, which have approximately the same electron density, are separated by a less electron-dense nucleoplasm (figures 8 and 9). In the dividing nucleus a microtubular spindle develops between the opposite poles of the elongating nucleus. The spindle microtubules have a similar diameter to the subpellicular microtubules.

There are no centrioles at the poles of the spindles. The nucleus divides by constriction of the nuclear membrane but the mechanism by which the genetic material is separated is not understood. Elongation of the nucleus during division is believed to be by elongation of spindle microtubules pushing apart future daughter nuclei.

The endoplasmic reticulum

The membrane systems which exist in eukaryotic cells and consist of flattened ramifying cisternae and tubules occur in *Trypanosoma* and *Leishmania*. Endoplasmic reticulum (ER) may be rough (granular), containing attached ribosomes, or smooth (agranular), without associated ribosomes. As in other eukaryotes the endoplasmic reticulum of kinetoplastids is continuous with the outer nuclear membrane and is most commonly concentrated around the nucleus and between the nucleus and the flagellar pocket. ER is also closely associated with the Golgi apparatus, subpellicular microtubules and the mitochondrial network. The endoplasmic reticulum is associated with subpellicular microtubules adjacent to the attachment zone linking the body of the parasite with the flagellum where it runs alongside the body (see figure 4). The ER closely associated with the Golgi stacks is smooth whereas the membrane facing away from the Golgi contains ribosomes. Ribosomes occur extensively throughout the cytoplasm of kinetoplastids as well as on the granular ER (figures 4, 5, 6 and 9). It is suggested that the ER of *Trypanosoma* and *Leishmania* functions in the same way as in other eukaryote cells and transports proteins which have been synthesized on ribosomes to the Golgi system where additional molecules are added and 'packaged'. A 'membrane lattice' of branched interconnected smooth membrane tubules 50 nm in diameter has been described in *Leptomonas collosoma* located near the plasma membrane and is associated in this species with a contractile vacuole.

The Golgi apparatus

The stacks of smooth flattened membranes and the vesicles which are budded off from the swollen ends are known as the Golgi apparatus or body and were called dictyosomes by earlier biologists. In trypanosomatids the Golgi apparatus is characteristically closely associated with the flagellar pocket and lies between the latter and the nucleus (figure 9).

The Golgi apparatus of phytoflagellates has been shown to package glycoprotein for structures such as scales and spines which are found on the surface of the cells, and the stages in their construction and synthesis have been followed through the Golgi system. It has been suggested that the surface coat of trypanosomes is produced by the Golgi apparatus in a similar way to these surface structures of phytoflagellates. The Golgi body also produces enzymes which are packaged in lysosomes; primary lysosomes are vesicular products of the Golgi membranes and have been identified by use of cytochemical tests for acid phosphatase. The lysosomal enzymes are secreted into the flagellar reservoir to begin digestion of material prior to pinocytosis by the flagellar pocket (reservoir) membrane or by the cytosome in those trypanosomatids possessing one (e.g., *T. raiae, T. cobitis* and *Crithidia fasciculata*). Further, intracellular digestion then occurs by the fusion of lysosomes with pinocytotic vesicles from the reservoir. The maintenance of the integrity of the lysosomal membrane is important to prevent autodigestion of the cell by its own enzymes.

Many vesicles and sacs, of undetermined function, lie alongside the Golgi apparatus. Examples of these are the so-called multivesiculate bodies and spiny coated vesicles or 'acanthosomes'; the likely function of the latter being the importation or exportation of protein.

The kinetoplast-mitochondrion complex

The characteristic feature of kinetoplastid flagellates is the possession of a kinetoplast. This organelle, with its intimate association with the mitochondrion, has attracted much attention over the past two decades with the improvement and standardization of electron microscope techniques. The kinetoplast is situated at

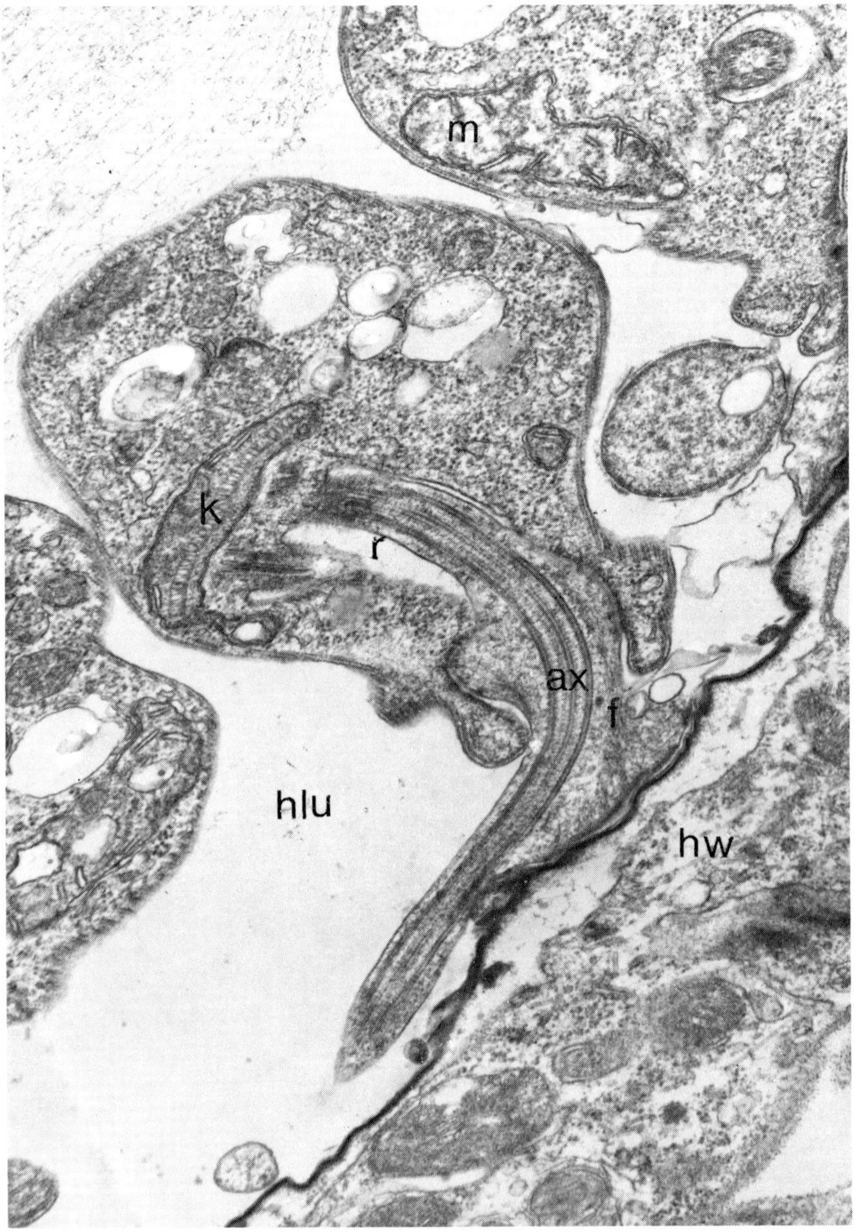

Figure 10. Electronmicrograph of *L. braziliensis* in the hindgut of a sandfly. Note the attachment to the hindgut wall, hw, by a flagellum, f; kinetoplast, k, and mitochondrion, m, are typical features of cytology of kinetoplastid parasites; hlu = hindgut lumen (× 25 000).

Courtesy of Cambridge University Press and the Royal Society of London.

the base of the flagellum within a short distance of the basal body from which the flagellum arises (figures 6, 9 and 10). There is a constant distance between the basal body and the membrane capsule surrounding the kinetoplast which remains the same throughout the life cycle of digenetic members of the Kinetoplastida. Clearly some physical connection must exist, for when cells are lysed the basal body and kinetoplast remain associated, but in many instances this connection is not demonstrable.

The capsule is continuous with the mitochondrial membrane. The central part contains the fibrous rod containing the kinetoplast DNA (figures 5 and 6). This has been shown to be composed of fibres densely packed in coils or figures of eight. From the inner membrane of the capsule cristae typical of the mitochondrial (chondriome) network are found extending into the matrix. Together with the frequently observed continuity of the kinetoplast capsule with the mitochondrion, this demonstrates that the kinetoplast is the specialized part of the mitochondrion.

Cytochemical and autoradiographic methods confirmed that the fibrous kinetoplast rod contains DNA. DNA-ase enzymes have been shown to digest the DNA. Sections show the kinetoplast to be a slightly concave disc. In *Trypanosoma* and *Leishmania* the disc of DNA (the nucleoid) is separated from the capsule by a variable amount of mitochondrial matrix. On the other hand, in the genera *Crithidia* and *Blastocrithidia* the nucleoid occupies the whole capsule. Isotropic fibrils connect the kinetoplast to the basal body face of the mitochondrial membrane and small satellite DNA puffs of diffuse fibrils are attached to the sides of the kinetoplast.

In the dyskinetoplastic (formerly termed akinetoplastic) flagellates, such as some stocks of *T. evansi* and "*T. equinum*", there is no fibroid rod in the mitochondrial envelope at right angles to the basal body–flagellar complex. However, both in dyskinetoplastic organisms induced by drugs (such as acridines, phenanthridines and diamidines) and in naturally occurring isolates there is a spherical electron-dense structure in the envelope of the mitochondrion. This structure is referred to as the kinetoplast remnant and, although it replicates at division and is attached to the mitochondrial membrane, its actual constitution is not fully known.

The structure of the k-DNA has been studied following its separation, isolation and purification; spreads of purified k-DNA when viewed with the electron microscope are found to be made up of 'minicircles' and linear molecules. The length of the k-DNA minicircles is very much less than that of the mammalian mitochondrial minicircular DNA (0·29–0·8 μm in kinetoplastids, compared with 4·4–5·0 μm in mammalian mitochondria). There is a relationship between half the circumference of the minicircle and the thickness of the nucleoid, and it is suggested that the figure of eight appearance of the nucleoid could correspond to a twisted minicircle. The DNA minicircles have a close resemblance to those of procaryotic organisms.

The mitochondrion itself is a prominent feature in sections of the cells. It is now believed that the mitochondrion is a single continuous unit which branches throughout the cytoplasm forming a network of canals lying close to the pellicle; evidence for this comes from cytochemical staining, from serial sections of parasites, and from high voltage electron microscopy which allows examination of whole organisms.

Functional morphology of the kinetoplast–mitochondrion complex

Of great interest in *Trypanosoma* and *Leishmania* are the changes observed in the mitochondrion during cyclical development related to the ability of the organism to switch rapidly from one type of respiratory pathway to another. This is best illustrated in *Trypanozoon* when the parasite is taken up by the tsetse fly and during the development of the infective forms in the salivary glands of the fly.

The slender bloodstream forms of the *T. brucei* group parasites have a simple unbranched mitochondrion with very few tubular cristae (figure 4). In the intermediate and stumpy forms there is an increase in the number of plate-like cristae, and an associated increase in the diameter of the mitochondrion. This process is continued in the *Glossina* midgut where the procyclic trypomastigotes contain a more branched mitochondrion with abundant cristae. On transformation to epimastigotes in the salivary glands there is a reduction of mitochondrial branches and a reversion to tubular cristae. Metacyclic forms show further reduction and possess tubular, bulbous cristae; they reacquire the surface coat in the salivary glands — a preadaptation to life in the bloodstream of mammals. These gross mitochondrial changes are associated with a respiratory switch which occurs in this group of trypanosomes. The mitochondrion is known to be the site of respiratory activity. The normal respiratory substrate, glucose, is used by bloodstream forms of *T. brucei* in large quantities, but pyruvate, the usual initial substrate for the Krebs cycle, is excreted. Hence it appears that only the initial pathway of glucose–pyruvate, which is a relatively inefficient producer of ATP, is functional and all the ATP of slender bloodstream trypanosomes of *T. brucei* is derived from glycolysis. This is confirmed by the insensitivity of the system to cyanide. A glycerophosphate oxidase system is located in microbodies in the cytoplasm rather than in the mitochondrion. The demand for energy is such that trypanosomes clearly require large amounts of glucose to fuel their activity in an environment — the mammalian blood stream — where oxygen supply is ample.

However, in the fly there is a switch to a more efficient utilization of available respiratory substrates such as amino acids by the synthesis or activation of Krebs-cycle enzymes enabling pyruvate to be oxidized, with the production of more ATP per glucose molecule. This switch is accompanied by structural changes such as the increase in cristae and expansion of the entire mitochondrion. The reverse changes occur in the lumen of the salivary glands where the mitochondrion and cristae of the metacyclic trypomastigotes regress.

The evidence for similar changes in respiratory pathways in the subgenera *Nannomonas* and *Duttonella* is less convincing, although it is known that there is an increase in size and in the number of plate-like cristae in the epimastigotes and that in trypomastigotes in the bloodstream there is a partially active mitochondrion with tubular cristae.

The Stercoraria subgenera *Herpetosoma* and *Schizotrypanum*, as exemplified by *T. lewisi* and *T. cruzi* respectively, have well developed cristae in the bloodstream forms and they also have cyanide-sensitive respiratory pathways which indicate a functional cytochrome system and Krebs cycle. In *T. lewisi*, however, it is believed that the dividing bloodstream forms found early in the infection are more dependent on glycolysis than the adult forms where the Krebs cycle plays a more dominant role.

In these subgenera the cristae are plate-like and there appears to be little difference in their structure between bloodstream, culture or vector forms.

The trypanosomes of lower vertebrates so far studied with the electron microscope do not show any evidence of respiratory switch in bloodstream forms. The mitochondrial system of the larger species of trypanosome is, however, extensive (figure 9). In avian species the mitochondrial branches are regularly distributed close to the periphery of the parasites and are the 'striae' or 'myonemes' observed in the light microscope; this distribution presumably reduces the distance for diffusion of oxygen from the bloodstream.

In *Leishmania* the cristae are present in mitochondria of amastigotes and there is mitochondrial proliferation during transformation to promastigotes both in culture and in sandflies. The elongation of the promastigotes seems to be due to mitochondrial extension. Although the mitochondrion is not extensive in the amastigotes the cristae are plate-like and cyanide-sensitive respiration occurs in both intracellular amastigotes and in promastigotes in culture. Tubular cristae found in bloodstream salivarian trypanosomes are not seen in *Leishmania* amastigotes.

Filopodia-like structures

The bloodstream forms of *Trypanozoon* have been shown to shed streamers ('micronemata' or 'filopodia') from the surface membrane at the extremities of the body. Such streamers are elongated structures which in transverse section show a small cytoplasmic core; micronemata (see figure 4) have a normal plasma membrane and surface coat. The function of such structures is as yet unknown, but it may be related to membrane flow over the parasite surface or shedding of antigens.

Scanning electron microscopy of parasites

Scanning electron microscopy has been used to demonstrate the appearance of trypanosomes and *Leishmania* parasites in three-dimensional view. It is a technique with limited application but can, when used in appropriate situations, reveal data on host–parasite interactions.

Studies on trypanosomes in the insect vectors have revealed details of how the

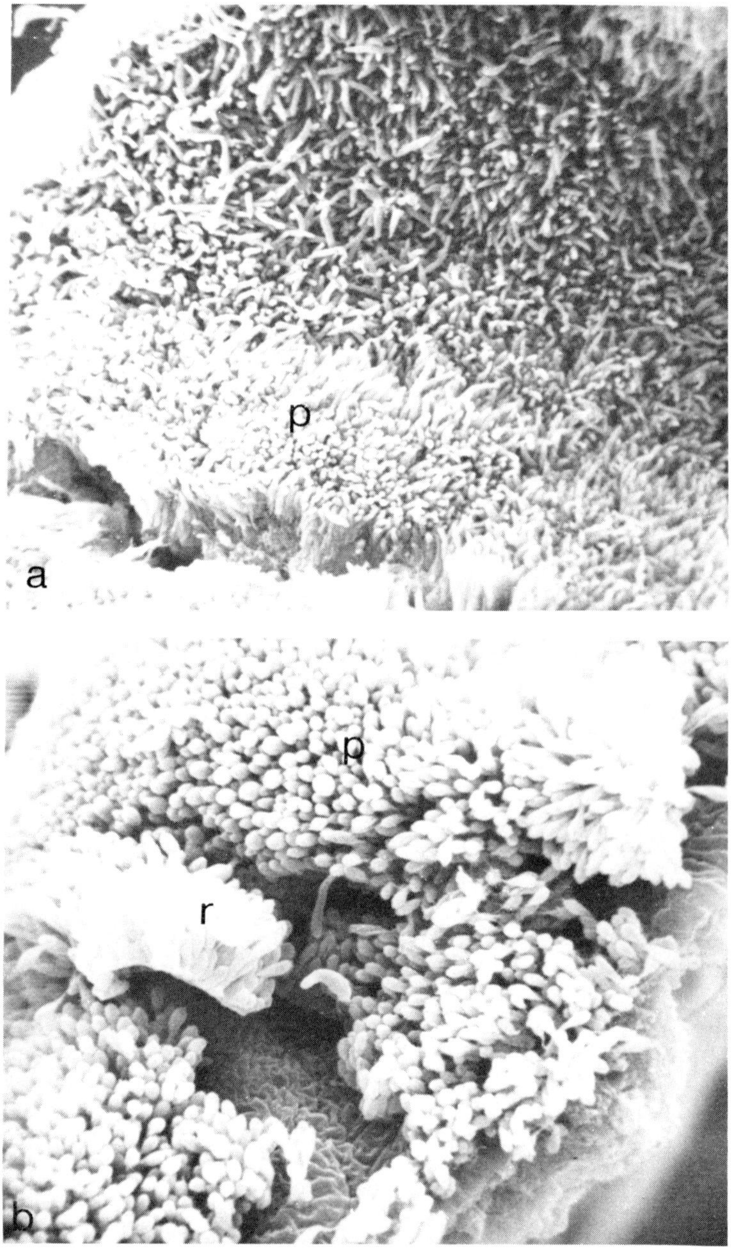

Figure 11. Electonmicrograph of parasites (*T. melophagium*) in a, the midgut (× 515) and b, the hindgut (× 1150) of a sheepked *Melophagus ovinus*, showing levels of infection observed in some insects where all of the surface is covered by parasites, p. Note the corrugated surface of the hindgut wall and the parasite rosettes, r.

Courtesy of *Acta Tropica*.

parasites become associated with or attached to surfaces, confirming transmission electron microscope observations and giving a three-dimensional view of the associations. This work is illustrated in figure 11 which shows parasites (*T. melophagium*) attached (*a*) to the sheepked's midgut with flagella inserted between microvilli and (*b*) the pylorus and hindgut where a mass of parasites associates with a cuticle lined epithelium.

Similar studies in the proboscis of *Glossina* have revealed an important association between mechanoreceptors and trypanosomes of the salivarian subgenera *Trypanozoon, Nannomonas* and *Duttonella* using the scanning electron microscope. It was only when this instrument was used that this association could be appreciated because of the problems of acquiring a thin section passing through the appropriate part of the receptor and parasite. It has been suggested that the interaction between these receptive sensilla and parasites changes the probing behaviour of the fly and increases the chances of parasite transmission. Studies of *Leishmania* parasites in the insect vector the sandfly have been undertaken and reveal the interaction between parasites and midgut wall as described by transmission EM.

Recent studies on *Leishmania* using the scanning electron microscope have aided elucidation of the mechanisms of entry of promastigotes into macrophages in culture. From these studies the penetration has been described as 'facilitated phagocytosis'. The flagellar tips become attached to macrophages and this seems to stimulate the production of lamellar sheaths, veils or pseudopodial whorls which progressively surround the parasite. In some experiments an inhibitor of phagocytosis, Cytochalasin B, prevented entry into macrophages. However, other workers found that even in the presence of this compound cells with low phagocytic ability could be penetrated, possibly indicating that there is an active contribution on the part of the parasite aiding its entry into cells.

LIFE CYCLES

Invertebrate parasites

The life cycles of monoxenous trypanosomatids have been briefly outlined in an earlier section. Transmission is via resistant cyst-like forms in *Blastocrithidia triatomae*, but the nature and structure of resistant stages in other genera is not clearly known. Some species such as *Crithidia fasciculata* must retain a free-living stage in their life cycle to ensure passage from mosquito to mosquito and must also tolerate the physiological changes associated with the host's metamorphosis from larva to adult. Contamination of mouthparts of either larvae or adults and subsequent entry to the gut seem to be essential for transmission to occur; this may happen by chance or may be enhanced by a behavioural trait such as the requirement of flea larvae for faeces deposited by the adults. There is a gap in our knowledge about the stages involved in transmission; few experimental studies have been undertaken. It is known, however, that the cysts of *B. triatomae* are highly infective and very resistant. They are structurally different from other kinetoplastid cells as they appear to lose structures such as kinetoplast, subpellicular microtubules, mitochondrion and nucleus. The cytoplasm is dense, and a labyrinthine structure appears. Normal structures only reappear during excystation. In *Leptomonas* changes in the plasma membrane occur in the rectum of the host, possibly associated with unattached stages in encystment.

Little is known of the free-living stages of *Herpetomonas muscarum* of muscids, but such stages have been observed in banana-mash media where *Drosophila* larvae are reared. This suggests that larvae are infected from contaminated food.

Insect stages of digenetic genera

The other genera of parasites in this group are digenetic, with two hosts in their life cycle. The sole exception to this is the equine trypanosome *T. equiperdum* which has secondarily lost the need for a vector, transmission from horse to horse occurring during coitus. The life cycles of the digenetic trypanosomatids other than the plant parasitic genus *Phytomonas*, namely *Endotrypanum, Leishmania* and *Trypanosoma*, involve vertebrate and invertebrate hosts alternately. The majority of invertebrate hosts are insects, but fish trypanosomes and some amphibian trypanosomes are transmitted by leeches. Further, some avian and possibly some mammalian trypanosomes develop in and are transmitted by the arachnids — mites and ticks. The digenetic life cycle involves cyclical development. This implies morphological and physiological changes in the parasite when they reach the appropriate host. These changes involve adaptation to different microhabitats in invertebrate hosts where conditions are clearly very different from those in the vertebrate blood or tissues. Adaptations and preadaptations are needed to survive and reproduce in the hostile environment of an insect gut. In the insect gut the parasite must be capable of resisting proteolytic digestive enzymes, become adapted to maintaining its position in a highly mobile peristaltic tube, change its enzyme systems to utilize not only different nutrient substrates but also adapt them to operate at different temperatures. Parasites must then reproduce sufficiently to provide a reservoir of infection. Forms infective to the vertebrate host may be produced either in the posterior station (hindgut/rectum) for transmission by contamination or in the anterior station (proboscis/salivary glands) if the vertebrate is infected by bite (figures 12 and 13).

The pattern of development in the insect has been used as a means of categorizing the parasites. The trypanosomes of mammals were divided into Stercoraria and Salivaria sections by Hoare. These categories refer to the location of the parasites within the host and hence to the method of transmission. The Stercoraria develop in the posterior station — the proctodaeal part of the insect gut, usually the hindgut and rectum — with some initial development in the midgut. Transmission may occur as a result of the vector depositing faeces con-

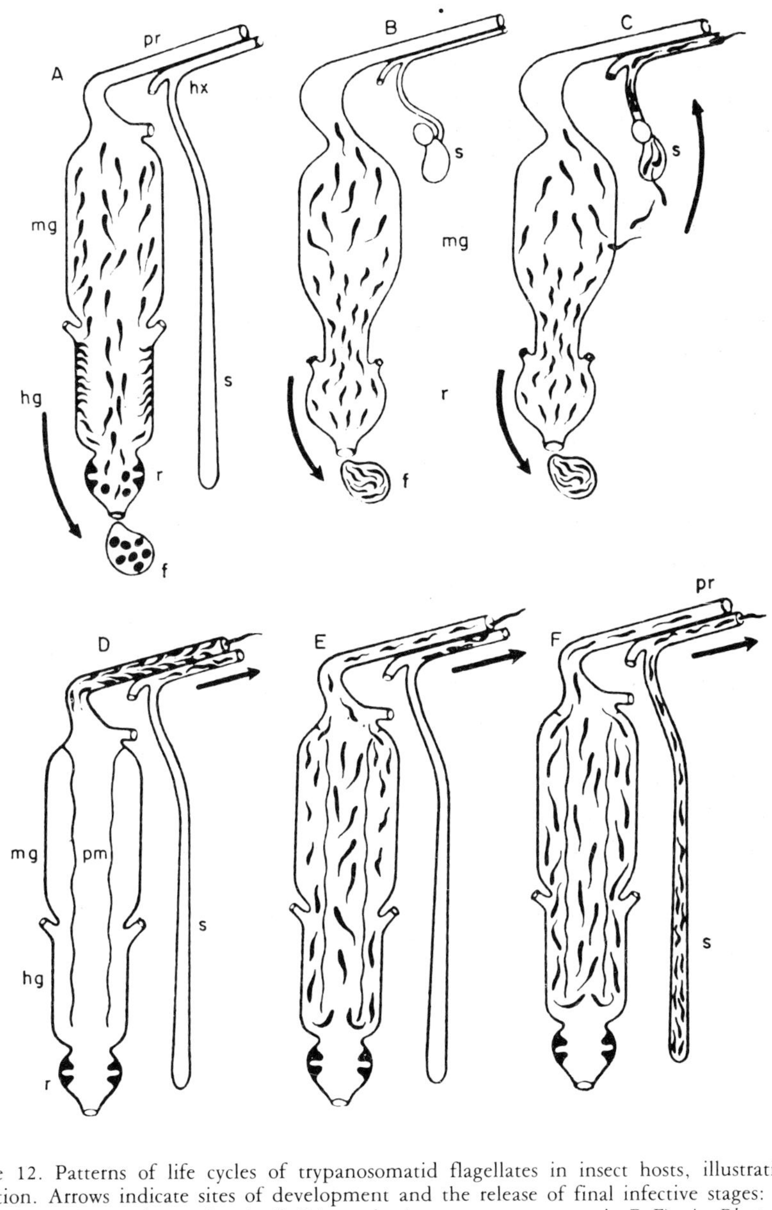

Figure 12. Patterns of life cycles of trypanosomatid flagellates in insect hosts, illustrating their evolution. Arrows indicate sites of development and the release of final infective stages: posterior station in A–C, anterior station in C–F (cysts in A, metatrypanosomes in B–F). A, *Blastocrithidia*, specific insect parasite. Stercoraria: B, *Trypanosoma cruzi*; C, *T. rangeli*. Salivaria: D, *T. vivax*; E, *T. congolense*, F, *T. brucei*.

Abbreviations: f = drop of faeces containing infective stages (cysts/metatrypanosomes); hg = hindgut; hx = hypopharynx; mg = midgut; pm = peritrophic membrane; pr = proboscis; r = rectum; s = salivary glands.

Courtesy of Academic Press, from Hoare, 1967, *Advances in Parasitology*, Volume 5.

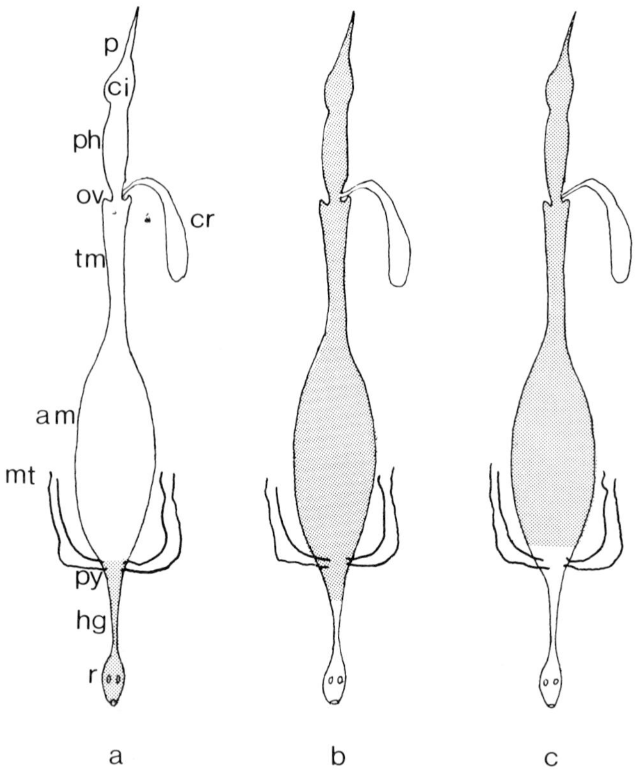

Figure 13. Diagrammatic representation of distribution of *Leishmania* infection in the gut of sandflies showing sites of parasite colonization: a, Hypopylaria; b, Peripylaria; c, Suprapylaria.

Hypopylaria infections are found in reptilian *Leishmania* and are restricted to the hindgut and rectum. Peripylaria infections are found in the pyloric region of the gut which is the initial site from where colonized infections move forward and colonize the midgut and foregut, e.g., *L. braziliensis*. Suprapylaria infections colonize the midgut and foregut and do not become established posterior to the midgut, e.g., *L. donovani* and *L. tropica*.

Abbreviations: p = proboscis; ci = cibarium; cr = crop; ph = pharynx; ov = oesophageal valve; tm = thoracic midgut; am = abdominal midgut; py = pylorus; mt = Malpighian tubules; hg = hindgut; r = rectum.

taining infective forms on the skin with subsequent irritation, provoking scratching which enables parasites to enter through lesions. Alternatively, the infected vector may be eaten or taken into the mouth during grooming and infection may occur by contamination of oral mucosal lesions.

The Salivaria occupy the salivary glands or mouthparts (*T. vivax* and *T. congolense*) of the tsetse fly (the invertebrate host) and are transmitted during feeding. Some organisms remain in the midgut, forming a reservoir of parasites throughout the duration of the infection in the insect (figure 14). Salivarian transmission would seem to be more efficient than stercorarian. It is mainly found in

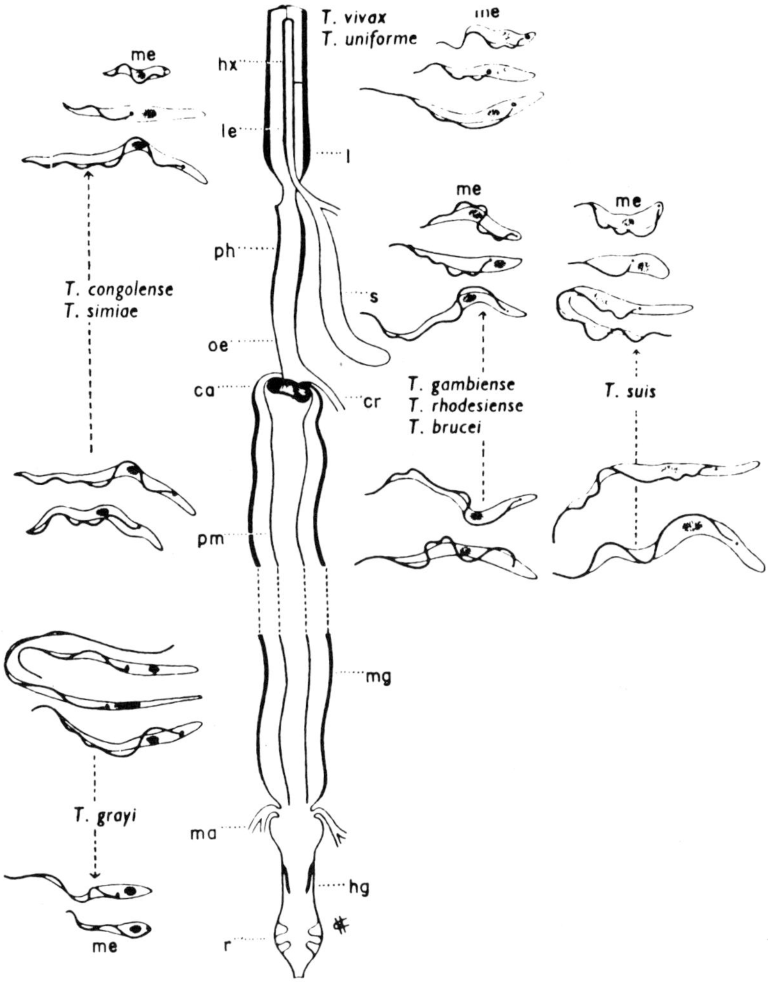

Figure 14. Developmental patterns of trypanosomes in tsetse fly. ca = cardia (= proventriculus); cr = crop duct; hg = hindgut; hx = hypopharynx; l = labium; le = labrum-epipharynx (hx + l + le = proboscis); ma = Malpighian tubules; me = metatrypanosomes; mg = midgut; oe = oesophagus; ph = pharynx; pm = peritrophic membrane; r = rectum; s = salivary glands (one cut off). *T. grayi* illustrates the stercorarian pattern; others are salivarian.

Courtesy of Academic Press, from Hoare, 1967, *Advances in Parasitology*, Volume 5.

the tsetse fly transmitted trypanosomes, but *T. rangeli* develops in the salivary glands of South American bugs, and fish trypanosomes develop in the anterior part of the gut of leeches. *Phytomonas* of plants also develops in the salivary glands of insects.

Although *Trypanozoon* infections are generally confined to the lumen of the gut, salivary glands and associated ducts, the haemocoele is involved in the life cycles of some trypanosomes (*T. brucei, T. rangeli* and some avian trypanosomes) and midgut cells are found infected. Monoxenous flagellates can also be naturally found in the haemocoele of insects.

The genus *Leishmania* has recently been divided, by Lainson and Shaw, into three sections, Hypopylaria, Peripylaria and Suprapylaria. The Hypopylaria develop in the midgut and hindgut (figure 13*a*), the Peripylaria have a phase of reproduction in the anterior part of the hindgut before migrating forward to invade the pharynx, cibarium and proboscis (figure 13*b*). The Suprapylaria do not enter the hindgut, but multiply in the midgut before migrating to the foregut (figure 13*c*).

The transmission of Peripylaria and Suprapylaria is by the bite of the sandfly but the exact mechanism is a matter of some debate: the presence of the parasites in the pharynx, cibarium and proboscis (figure 15) indicates that a sandfly would be capable of transmitting the infection. It is believed that only the reptilian *Leishmania*, which develop in the posterior station alone, are transmitted by contamination of the host oral mucosa. This requires confirmation in this little studied group. Recent studies indicate that '*Leishmania*' of reptiles may in fact be trypanosomes, e.g., *L. tarentolae* is in fact *T. platydactyli*.

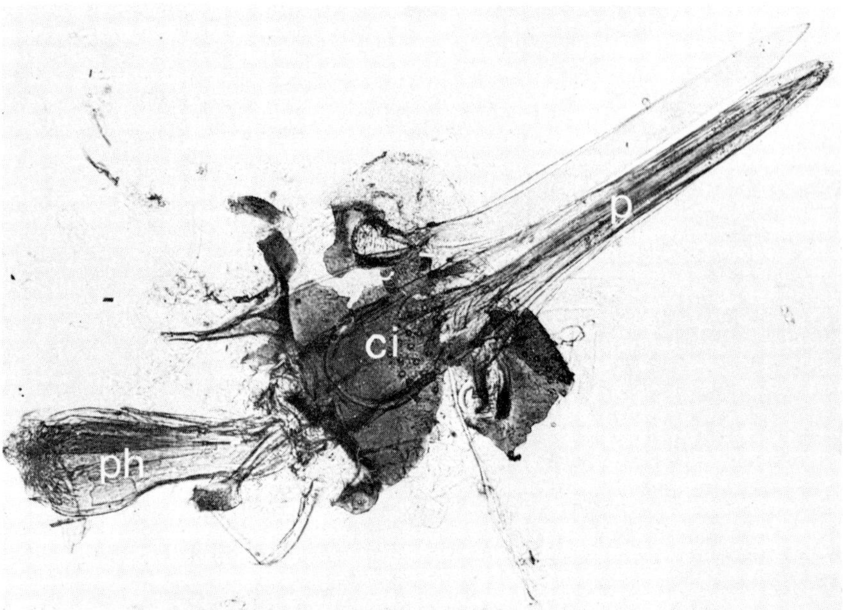

Figure 15. Dissection of the mouthparts of a sandfly, *Lutzomyia longipalpis*.
Abbreviations: p = proboscis; ph = pharynx; ci = cibarium.

Stages in the vertebrate host

The course of infection of *Leishmania, Endotrypanum* and *Trypanosoma* in vertebrate hosts is highly variable. The genus *Leishmania* has a predilection for cells of the mononuclear phagocytic series and division and multiplication occur in these cells, which are normally responsible for the body's defences. *Leishmania* are generally categorized as producing either cutaneous or visceral disease in man, depending on which populations of macrophages are predominantly infected — those of the skin, or those of the internal organs.

In animals naturally infected with *Leishmania* parasites, particularly wild reservoir hosts, infections are not usually apparent and lesions, if present, are difficult to detect.

The genus *Endotrypanum* is confined to the South American sloths and the forms in the blood are intraerythrocytic. The course of infection and involvement of other stages in the life cycle in the mammal is unknown, as is the mechanism of red-cell penetration. In the genus *Trypanosoma* there is a great variety of life cycles and patterns of infection in vertebrate hosts. Although usually regarded as parasites of the blood, many trypanosomes, in certain stages of their development, show a predilection for certain tissues and organs. The range of such tropisms is illustrated in table 5. Such tropisms may be transient or more durable; however the idea that trypanosomes are only blood parasites is not valid. Certainly they occur in the blood, but many species whose life cycles have been thoroughly studied reveal tissue preferences; these preferences are usually expressed in the reproductive phase of the infection. It is also possible that tissue sites, such as lymphoid organs, the vasa recta capillaries of the kidneys, testes and the choroid plexus, isolate the parasites from the host's immune response during a period of reproductive activity, thus providing privileged sites from which new variants may arise or appropriate disguise mechanisms may develop.

Non-cyclical methods of transmission

Although closely related to the *T. brucei* group of organisms and belonging to the subgenus *Trypanozoon, T. evansi* and "*T. equinum*" are found in Africa north of the known limits of *Glossina* distribution, and also in Asia and South America where *Glossina* does not occur. *T. vivax* is also found in South America and was found in Mauritius in the 1930s. Neither in Mauritius nor in South America can *T. vivax* be transmitted by *Glossina.* The trypanosomes which are so closely related to the pathogenic African species are, it is assumed, transmitted by biting flies — by contamination of the mouthparts with trypanosomes which are then inoculated at a subsequent probe or bite. Although many studies on this subject have been carried out, and Tabanidae and *Stomoxys* have been usually suspected as being responsible for most transmissions, fundamental problems remain to be solved, particularly in relation to *T. vivax* transmission in South America.

Also in South and Central America an unusual method of transmission of

Table 5. Trypanosomes of vertebrates showing hosts and sites of concentration of organisms at stage in life cycle when a tissue phase is present (see also Appendix 1).

Species	Host	Site
T. corvi	Corvids	Bone marrow in winter
Avian trypanosomes	Geese	Bone marrow
T. cruzi	Man, rodents, marsupials	Heart muscle, autonomic ganglia
T. brucei subspecies	Man, ungulates	Choroid plexus in late stage
T. lewisi *T. musculi*	*Rattus* *Mus*	Vasa recta capillaries in kidney in reproductive phase, placenta
T. microti *T. nabiasi* *T. evotomys*	*Microtus* (field voles), *Oryctolagus* (rabbit), *Clethriomonys* (bank voles)	Lymphoid tissues in reproduction phase
T. dionisii	Chiroptera	Heart muscle, intestinal epithelium
T. equiperdum	Equines	Genitals

equine and bovine trypanosomiasis takes place. This is a result of the mechanism of feeding of the vampire bat *Desmodus*, which also transmits rabies. During its blood meal a vampire bat ingests blood infected with trypanosomes from equines and bovines and becomes infected itself through the passage of parasites through the mucous membrane of the mouth or lesions in the gut. At subsequent feeds *Desmodus* can reinfect other animals, hence acting as a mammalian vector.

Oral infection has been demonstrated in pathogenic and non-pathogenic trypanosomes. This was initially suspected in East Africa where a high proportion of the large carnivores (lions and hyaenas) were infected with salivarian trypanosomes and yet were only rarely found to be blood sources for *Glossina*, which nevertheless had an opportunity to feed on them. It was therefore suggested that carnivores could become infected by feeding on prey. This was subsequently shown when dogs became infected after feeding on infected goats. Laboratory studies also indicate that oral infection can occur, as trypanosomes inoculated directly into the stomach survive despite the low pH. Hamsters have been experimentally infected with *Leishmania* by the oral route. *T. cruzi* is also suspected of being capable of transmission to man *per os* as a result of contamination of food or the oral area with infected faeces of bugs.

Transplacental congenital transmission is not known to occur frequently but cases of new-born children being infected with *T. b. gambiense* though they were born in areas where the disease is not transmitted have been described. It is also believed that *T. theileri* can be transmitted to the foetus in view of the frequent recovery of *T. theileri* in cultures of foetal bovine cells. *T. musculi* of the mouse, on the other hand, which concentrates on the maternal side of the placenta in very large numbers during the reproductive phase of the cycle, is not found in mouse foetuses.

Infection by transfusion is a considerable problem in the epidemiology of Chagas' disease. The risk of such infection in South America is high, as it is the lower social groups, the most frequently exposed to triatomids, who are frequently reduced to selling their blood; infection of recipients is prevented by the addition of gentian violet to blood in blood banks to kill the parasites. This route of infection has been recorded for *Leishmania donovani*, but is rare.

Transmission of *T. equiperdum* during coitus between mares and stallions has been referred to already. This is the only well documented case of transmission by this route amongst trypanosomatid parasites.

IDENTIFICATION OF THE PARASITES

Traditional morphological criteria have been developed for the identification of the Kinetoplastida and, combined with biological studies of the behaviour of parasites in the vector, these usually allow accurate identification at the generic or subgeneric levels. However, there is need for differentiation at the specific and subspecific levels, in particular for the identification of isolates causing human and animal disease as it is necessary to reliably distinguish pathogens from non-pathogens when they are isolated from reservoir hosts or vectors. The description and identification of *Trypanosoma* and *Leishmania* have been transformed over the past decade by the introduction of biochemical techniques which have amplified the hitherto imprecise morphological differentiations at the specific and subspecific levels.

Trypanosomes

The classical methods of identification and description of trypanosomes at the species level remained the same for some 60 years; these relied on the measurement of the parasites and the distances between the organelles carried out on stained preparations. The biometrical data so obtained were used until biochemical methods became available. The biometrical data were expressed by Dice–Leraas diagrams. Biometrical studies were used to determine similarity between species of trypanosomes of the subgenera *Herpetosoma, Nannomonas* and *Megatrypanum*. In the first of these subgenera cross-inoculation experiments with trypanosomes isolated from different but related mammal species were also used. The value of biometric data is very limited but microscopy still allows differentiation of parasites into subgenus purely on the basis of the relative positions of organelles, their size, the presence or absence of a free flagellum, the total length of the parasite and the shape of the posterior end. These criteria can only be properly seen on well prepared and stained thin blood films. Observations of living parasites with either phase contrast or, preferably, dark ground microscopy and the characteristics of their movement also enable differentiation of the subgenera, particularly in the Salivaria.

When measuring trypanosomes and the distances between their organelles, drawing equipment is required. This equipment is known as a camera lucida which produces a virtual image of the parasite in the same plane as a piece of drawing paper. The lengths or outline of the parasite are then drawn over the image and, knowing the magnification, the parameters used in the descriptions of the parasites are then measured.

The following measurements and conventional abbreviations are used: the total length of the parasite including free flagellum (L); the length of the free flagellum (F); the posterior end to the kinetoplast and nucleus (PK and PN); the distance from the kinetoplast to the nucleus (KN); and from the nucleus to anterior end (NA). These measurements can be expressed in tabular form if a series of parasite populations from different species of host are to be compared. This has been done for rodent and bird trypanosomes to emphasize similarities rather than differences.

Two indices are also used to express parasite mensural characteristics; these are the nuclear index (NI) and the kinetoplast index (KI). The nuclear index is the ratio PN:NA. The kinetoplast index is arrived at by dividing PN by KN; if the KI is less than 2 the kinetoplast is nearer the posterior end, if it is more than 2 it is nearer the nucleus, and if it is 2 the kinetoplast is equidistant between the posterior end and the nucleus.

These mensural techniques, however, can only be used as a guideline to subgeneric status; the more detailed characterization of an organism must now be undertaken, if this is experimentally feasible, by biochemical methods. This is not yet, however, possible with many species of non-pathogenic trypanosomes whose growth in culture is limited, and whose bloodstream forms may be scanty. Limited numbers of isolates are available for comparison, and the use of biochemical methods in non-pathogenic species is likely to be restricted for some time. However, biochemical methods have been used to considerable advantage in recent studies on trypanosomes of fish, bats and frogs. Experimental studies on host specificity, using blood passage, culture passage or cyclic transmission have been found useful in the identification of host specific species (or 'host restricted' species to use the term preferred by Hoare). Extensive cross-transmission experiments under laboratory conditions have aided elucidation of parasite identity in fish, bird and rodent trypanosomes.

Human volunteers were frequently used in East Africa in experiments to identify parasites of *T. brucei* from game animals. Trypanosomes isolated in laboratory animals were subsequently shown to be *T. b. rhodesiense*. The work was carried out in small but highly developed hospitals specifically maintained for treatment of sleeping sickness. In the absence of a suitable method of identification the only way to demonstrate the zoonotic nature of *T. b. rhodesiense* was by this method. Earlier studies on man were carried out in Zaire to demonstrate the possibility of *T. b. gambiense* retaining its infectivity to man after cyclical transmission by *Glossina* through up to 20 generations in domestic animals. The Tinde experiment in East Africa also demonstrated that *T. b. rhodesiense* retained its infectivity to man over 20 years while passaged cyclically in antelopes and sheep.

A breakthrough in the objective identification of *T. brucei*-like parasites came when Rickman and Robson, working for a WHO/UNDP team in Kenya in 1970, made use of the fact that human serum normally lyses *T. brucei brucei*, which is not infective to man, but has no such effect on *T. b. rhodesiense*. They developed the blood incubation infectivity test (BIIT) in which the organism whose identity it was required to know was incubated with human serum and then inoculated into susceptible rats. This bioassay of infectivity has, with much subsequent modification, been of considerable value in demonstrating potential infectivity of organisms to man: if an isolate which has been incubated in human serum retains its infectivity to rats, then it is potentially *T. b. rhodesiense*, whereas *T. b. brucei* is lysed during the incubation period and the inoculated rats do not become infected. Recent studies have demonstrated that the lytic factor in human serum is a high density lipoprotein and the equivocal results obtained during the early studies of the BIIT can apparently be explained by differences in infectivity to man of the different variant antigenic types (VATs) which arise during the course of *Trypanozoon* infections in animals. This has been shown by changes in BIIT results as VAT changes during the progress of a cloned infection. This demonstrates the importance of safety when handling organisms designated as *T. brucei brucei* as it is likely that at least at some time during the course of an infection variants which could infect man may appear. The lack of virulence of *T. b. gambiense* for adult rats prevented the original BIIT being used with that subspecies. However, the multimammate rate *Mastomys natalensis* has been found to be more susceptible to *T. b. gambiense* and a modified BIIT using *Mastomys* as the recipient has been successfully developed. The American montane vole *Microtus montanus* is also a suitable laboratory host for *T. b. gambiense* and has been used in the BIIT. Recent studies have also shown that *T. b. rhodesiense* isolates from man may, if cloned, lose the characteristic of BIIT positivity.

Further developments in the methods of biochemical and serological taxonomy were then found to aid understanding of the relationships between parasites. Analysis of antigenic structure by immunoelectrophoresis of soluble antigens has been used to distinguish *Trypanozoon* organisms and the indirect fluorescent antibody technique was also reported to be of use as there were significant differences in titre depending on whether homologous or heterologous antigens were used.

The most promising way of identifying trypanosomes is to examine the biochemical differences between parasites. The most appropriate starting point is the genome of the parasite. If the nucleotide sequence of the parasite or some aspect of that sequence could be examined, then the reason for the chemical uniqueness of the species would be clear. Differences in base pair composition can be shown by the percentage of guanine and cytosine (G & C) base pairs in a DNA molecule. This has been shown to be of value for studying relationships of bacteria as well as trypanosomatids.

The proportion of G & C in a DNA sample is determined by measuring its buoyant density in a caesium chloride (CsCl) density gradient; the buoyant density is related directly to G & C (and hence adenine and thymine, A & T) composition. As *Trypanosoma* and *Leishmania* have DNA in both the nucleus and kinetoplast two values of G & C can be obtained per organism. The technique is of value in identifying both *Trypanosoma* and *Leishmania* and considerably aids our understanding of parasite inter-relationships.

Around the same time as DNA analysis was developed, enzyme polymorphism was found in trypanosomatids. It was found that isoenzymes could be used to identify these parasites. An enzyme frequently occurs in a variety of different molecular forms (called isoenzymes). Such differences show up as charge differences which can be demonstrated by the different electrophoretic mobilities of the molecules (figure 16). The isoenzymes have been shown to be under genetic control and thus the differences observed between organisms reflect differences in the parasite genome. In view of the large number of enzymes within a cell the use of isoenzymes as indicative of relationships between these organisms is clear, as they are proteins coded for by the nuclear DNA. However, although these studies are valuable, caution is appropriate.

The same mobilities of enzymes on gels do not necessarily mean common molecular structure and, conversely, molecular differences are not necessarily reflected in a charge difference; further, small differences in charges of enzymes may not be revealed on gels.

Isoenzyme studies in trypanosomes have a wide application in enabling more precise identification. This is of great value in epidemiology as it is now possible, using isoenzyme markers, to distinguish between the members of the subgenus *Trypanozoon*, in particular *T. b. gambiense, T. b. brucei* and *T. b. rhodesiense*. The enzymes which exhibit seemingly consistent differences are alanine transferase (ALAT) and aspartate aminotransferase (ASAT). Isolates from pigs and dogs in Liberia and Ivory Coast had an ALAT pattern which had only previously been found in trypanosomes isolated from man. Studies have also revealed similar isoenzyme patterns in *Trypanozoon* isolates from kob and hartebeest in Upper Volta. This is to date the firmest evidence yet to support the existence of an animal reservoir of *gambiense* sleeping sickness (see Chapter 3).

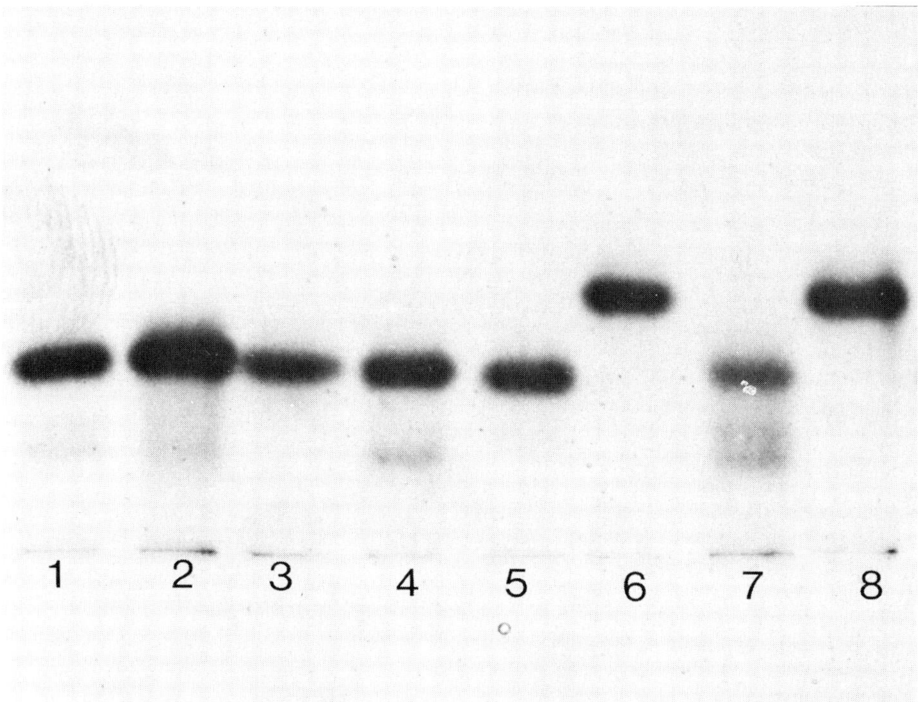

Figure 16. An enzyme electrophoresis plate showing the glucose phosphate isomerase pattern for six strains of *L. major* (1–5 and 7) and two of *L. aethiopica* (6 and 8). A single enzyme can reliably distinguish the two species in this case.

Isoenzyme studies on the subgenus *Nannomonas* have seemingly demonstrated that two types of *T. congolense* exist, one from the forest zone and one associated with the savannah. Subgenus *Duttonella* trypanosomes (*T. vivax*) of three distinct zymodemes (zymodemes are defined as 'populations of organisms that differ from similar, closely related, populations in the electrophoretic mobilities of one or more specified isoenzymes') were identified from cattle in Nigeria and on subsequent examination they were shown to be stable during experimental maintenance and in the field. The salivarian subgenera, being difficult to culture, are usually examined as bloodstream forms after passage through DEAE cellulose and centrifugation (see Chapter 4).

The application of isoenzyme analysis to *T. cruzi* has revealed most interesting features of the epidemiology of this important parasite. The parasites of the subgenus *Schizotrypanum* are morphologically identical and thus great difficulty is experienced in identifying the parasites responsible for the disease in man. The use of isoenzymes has demonstrated that in some areas man is only infected with parasites derived from peridomestic animals and bugs; and is not infected with the *T. cruzi* zymodeme circulating in a sylvatic cycle in the adjacent forest which is maintained by different bugs and forest mammals. The *Schizotrypanum* parasites of bats, morphologically identical with *T. cruzi*, have been shown to be isoenzymatically very different from *T. cruzi* of human origin (see Chapter 6).

The use of isoenzymes has shown that trypanosomes isolated from different species of fish, which were hitherto regarded as separate species, are in fact one species. The isoenzyme studies were supplemented in this case with morphological data as well as observations on the life cycle. Use of culture forms of stercorarian trypanosomes permits cleaner techniques and less animal manipulation than with salivarian parasites which are difficult to culture.

The use of isoenzymes for characterization of stocks of parasites from the wild, in particular for identification of reservoir hosts and vectors, will play an important role in elucidating the epidemiology of these diseases in future. Such techniques can also be expected to be useful for defining markers in genetic studies. This will be of great importance in *Trypanosoma, Leishmania* and other flagellates in view of the indication that trypanosomes are diploid organisms which undergo random mating, and that recombination between different stocks occurs. This work has been done by studies of isoenzyme variants of 19 different enzymes.

Genetic engineering techniques for the comparison of the variant specific antigen genes using complementary DNA (cDNA) have recently been employed to distinguish *T. b. brucei, T. b. gambiense* and *T. b. rhodesiense*. Such techniques may supplant other characterization techniques as they have potential for development into characterization and identification techniques which could be applied in the field.

Leishmania

Leishmania parasites in their mammalian hosts have frequently been regarded as being morphologically indistinguishable. This idea is not an acceptable one in view of the known size differences between amastigotes of *L. major* and *L. tropica*, *L. enriettii* and *L. donovani*, and *L. mexicana amazonensis* and *L. braziliensis*. Morphometric studies in the case of this last pair of parasites employed techniques similar to those described above for the biometry of trypanosomes. Electron microscope studies have also shown that size differences do indeed exist between *Leishmania* amastigotes, but differentiation by this method, as well as by counting microtubules around the periphery of the parasite and microtubule interval, is tedious. These methods are not, therefore, as rapid or as replicable for standard use as are biochemical methods. The only clear ultramorphological characteristic so far identified in the genus *Leishmania* is the presence of virus-like particles (VLPs) in the porcupine *Leishmania*, *L. hertigi*, in which all the isolates

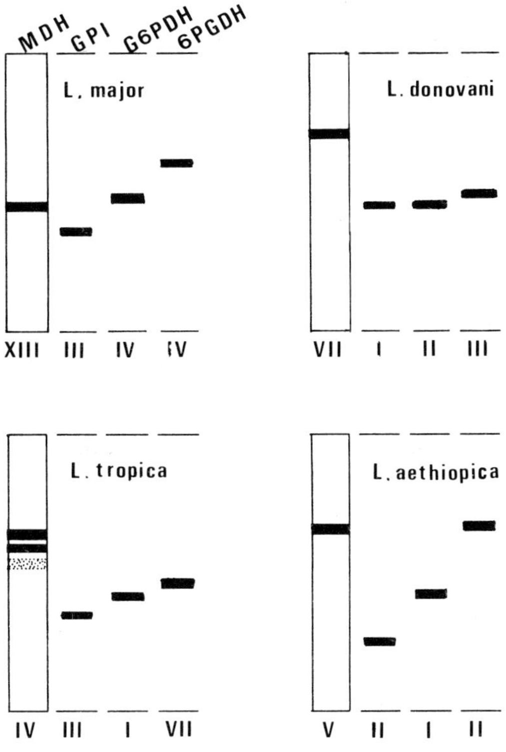

Figure 17. Biochemical profiles of typical strains of four Old World *Leishmania* species as shown by enzyme electrophoresis. MDH = Malate dehydrogenase; GPI = glucose phosphate isomerase; G6PDH = glucose-6-phosphate dehydrogenase; 6PGDH = 6-phosphogluconate dehydrogenase. No more than one enzyme type is shared by any two species.

Adapted from M. L. Chance with permission.

so far examined from Brazil and Panama have paracrystalline arrays of VLPs in the cytoplasm of promastigotes.

Since there are even fewer morphological characteristics in *Leishmania* than trypanosomes, isoenzyme and DNA buoyant techniques are of particular value in the identification of *Leishmania* isolates (figure 17); the results have, as with trypanosomes, made a major contribution to our knowledge of parasite epidemiology by the identification of vectors of human pathogens and reservoir animals (see Part III). Isoenzyme studies have clarified the relationship between simple cutaneous leishmaniasis and diffuse cutaneous leishmaniasis; they have aided characterization of a new species of *Leishmania, L. aethiopica*, have confirmed the identity of its reservoir (hyrax) and shown its ability to produce diffuse cutaneous leishmaniasis in anergic individuals. The relationships of the visceral leishmaniases and the neotropical cutaneous leishmaniases have also been elucidated; reservoirs and sandfly vectors have been identified with the aid of biochemical characterization techniques. In *Leishmania*, promastigotes are grown in culture and harvested by centrifugation and lysed for subsequent isoenzyme analysis. This avoids the difficulty of separation of host tissue from amastigotes in vertebrate hosts.

Adler developed a test in which parasites could be identified by culturing them in immune serum. In homologous immune rabbit serum, promastigotes in culture form enormous clusters or syncytia. In heterologous serum they grow normally. Soviet workers have extended this test, increasing its value by titrating the serum. The Adler test has not, however, proved to be adequately sensitive to differentiate certain clinico-epidemiologically different strains.

The Adler test was extended when it was demonstrated that promastigotes in culture excrete a factor (EF) which reacts with homologous rabbit antiserum in a precipitin test in agar gel. This has allowed the identification of two main EF types, each with two subtypes, which may occur singly or in combination and which are of value in identifying individual isolates.

Recent studies on *Leishmania* have analysed the extent of k-DNA nucleotide sequence homology by nucleic acid hybridization. The results have confirmed differences between *L. braziliensis* and *L. mexicana*, and are of potential value for all kinetoplastids as indicators of similarity. It is clear that the techniques referred to here are far more satisfactory than the earlier methods on which the classification of *Leishmania* parasites was initially based, which used clinical state, epidemiology and geographical distribution, none of which are valid taxonomic features; as in trypanosomes cDNA probes are being developed which are of considerable promise as additional characterization techniques with potential for field applicability.

Exciting new developments for characterization are radiorespirometry and monoclonal antibody techniques by which useful quantities of specific antibody are produced. These have already allowed identification of closely related New World strains and promises to allow rapid, accurate identification of many strains.

ANTIGENIC VARIATION

From the early days of the investigations on trypanosomiasis in man and his domestic animals in Africa workers have recognized that regular cyclical peaks and remissions of parasitaemia occur. In man these parasitaemic peaks are associated with the febrile periods. The first suggestion that parasites might change their antigenic properties came as early as 1905 when it was observed that *T. equiperdum* isolated from a horse was unaffected by antibodies in serum taken from the same animal earlier in the infection. The following year the observation that trypanosomes could survive antibodies during chronic infection provided an indication that some antigenic change was occurring in the parasites. The phenomenon of antigenic variation has attracted many scientists fascinated by the elegance and adaptability of the trypanosomes, and the scientific literature which has emanated since these observations is indeed vast. The ability of the pathogenic trypanosomes to change their surface antigen is clearly an important feature of their success, and the study of antigenic variation has an important role in the search for control methods. Drugs which block antigenic variation could clearly be of use in chemotherapy of trypanosome infections; the identification of circulating variable antigenic types (VATs) in man-derived isolates in the field has already been of value in producing more sensitive sero-diagnostic tests; the use of monoclonal antibody techniques as an aid to further development of diagnostic tests dependent on antigen detection will depend on a knowledge of antigenic variation, and an understanding of antigenic variation must contribute to any assessment of the feasibility of a vaccine for trypanosomiasis.

The initial observation of the periodically fluctuating parasitaemias and the association of the remission in parasitaemia with the production of antibody specific to the variant antigenic type which predominates at the peak of the parasitaemia is a fundamental starting point for the understanding of the biology of salivarian trypanosomes.

The variant antigen has been shown to be a glycoprotein and its location on the surface of bloodstream trypanosomes had led to its description as the variant surface glycoprotein (VSG) or variant specific surface antigen. VSG molecules are arranged on the surface of the trypanosome to form an electron dense coat 12–15 nm thick. This was demonstrated through the use of ferritin conjugated variant-specific antibody, which was shown by transmission electron microscopy to bind to the surface coat of the trypanosome to which the antibody had been raised. The variant antigens are lost during transformation to procyclics in the fly after 36–48 h and the surface coat is regained by the metacyclics in *T. brucei* and *T. congolense*.

It has been shown that there is a non-random sequence of expression of the variant antigenic types during the course of infection. The fact that the same variants recur in different infections in a semi-predictable fashion indicates that antigenic variation is not the result of mutations, but is a consequence of controlled expression from a family of antigen genes.

Antigenic variation is demonstrated and VATs are specifically recognized by a variety of immunological techniques: agglutination of trypanosomes in immune serum, neutralization, immune lysis and immunofluorescent tests.

This last has become more valuable in recent years in analysing the antigenic composition of trypanosome populations in the blood or in the salivary glands of tsetse flies. By initiating the infection with cloned populations, which contain a single VAT, it can be assumed that all the antigenic types detected in the course of an infection are lineal descendents of a single variant. Immunofluorescence tests can then be used to identify the different types present. Variant specific antibodies can be produced either by immunization with pure VSG or by infecting rodents with cloned trypanosome populations, followed by a curative dose of berenil, or hybridoma technology can be used to prepare monoclonal antibodies. These are particularly useful in identifying variant antigens on metacyclic trypanosomes since insufficient numbers can be obtained to purify VSG, and cloned populations of metatypes are antigenically unstable. Pure immunogens are not needed for the production of monoclonal antibodies since the cloning of antibody secreting cells governs the specificity.

Using immunofluorescence tests it has been shown that trypanosome populations which were hitherto believed to be of one antigenic type are in fact contaminated with a very small number (1:10 000) of parasites of a different VAT (these rare types are known as heterotypes; the predominant one a homotype).

The potential number of variant antigenic types which are expressed by an infection in a mammal is known as the repertoire of VATs. To date the limit of this repertoire has never been defined and it is as yet unknown if indeed there is a limit to the number of VATs capable of being expressed. Recent work has indicated that specific VATs can reappear during the course of a clone derived *T. brucei* infection.

It is also clear that VATs in the brain and lymph nodes of rodents may differ from those present in the blood at the same time. The suggestion has been made that slender trypanosomes invade the tissues and undergo antigenic variation.

Earlier studies indicated that the metacyclic trypanosomes in the tsetse fly carry the so-called 'basic strain antigen' and that a stock of *Trypanozoon* parasitic in a mammal, when it develops in *Glossina*, reverts to this basic antigenic type, known as the metatype, on production of the metacyclics; this basic antigenic type, on infecting the mammal, always produces the same sequence of antigenic types in the subsequent infections.

This idea has recently been challenged, and immunofluorescence tests on metacyclic trypanosomes using monoclonal antibodies have revealed that this population is antigenically heterogenous. Although it is possible that each stock of trypanosomes reverts to the same mixture of metatypes, the existence of such heterogeneity and the presence of many stocks expressing different metatype repertoires in the field cast severe doubts on the practicality of using metatype immunization as a basis for protection.

The biochemistry of the antigens themselves is becoming more clearly understood. The macromolecules which make up the surface coat in *Trypanozoon* parasites have been isolated and purified; they have been shown to be glycoproteins of around 60 000–65 000 daltons and consist of a single polypeptide chain of approximately 600 amino acid residues and 15–30 monosaccharide units (D-mannose, D-galactose, D-glucose and N-acetyl glucosamine). Recent evidence suggests that a galactose-rich oligosaccharide in the unexposed part of the VSG is a common factor. The sugar residues vary in number and location in the glycoproteins isolated from different clones of the parasites. The amino-acid composition of glycoprotein derived from different clones also varies. The immunological distinctiveness of each glycoprotein is reflected by the ability of a purified glycoprotein to induce an immune response which protects against homologous challenge but not against challenge with an organism displaying a different VSG.

The antigenic uniqueness of each VSG is derived from the uniqueness of its amino-acid sequence. Studies of the N-terminal amino-acid sequence demonstrated no homology between variants derived from the same clone. The only similarity in behaviour of the VSGs is the cleavage by trypsin which selectively attacks the molecules 150 amino-acid residues from the C-terminal ends. More extensive sequencing studies have recently shown that although the N-terminal two-thirds of the molecule are hyper-variable, the C-terminal domain contains both conserved amino-acid sequences and segments in which hydrophilic or hydrophobic qualities are conserved.

The structural orientation of the VSG in the cell membrane of *Trypanozoon* has been deduced from biochemical and cytochemical studies. The carbohydrate part of the molecule is closely adherent to the cell membrane near the C-terminal end. The N-terminal end covers the carbohydrate molecules; this is in accordance with the observation that carbohydrate is not apparently a major antigenic determinant. The association between the VSG and underlying plasmalemma requires further study to determine the molecular interactions.

There have been various theories to explain the method of control of antigenic variation; it has already been indicated that the theory that antigenic variation results from the random selection of mutants is not substantiated by the predictable sequence of types which arise. The alternative hypothesis that the variation is induced by antibody is not upheld by the rapid appearance of different antigenic types in immunosuppressed hosts infected by clones or by the similar rapid appearance of many heterotypes in unrelapsed clone infections at a time before antibody could be produced; indeed 19 separate VATs have been found during the first wave (patent) of a *T. brucei* parasitaemia. Nor is this view upheld by the reappearance of VAT in bovines infected with clones.

Recent molecular biological studies have clearly indicated that antigenic variation is controlled by genetic mechanisms. A change in VSG is associated with changes in the DNA sequence flanking VSG genes in the nucleus.

All the studies referred to above have been undertaken with *T. brucei* strains, most of which, for reasons of laboratory safety, have been believed to be non-infective to man; however it has been shown that different VATs derived from a clone vary in their resistance to human serum as determined by the BIIT (blood incubation infectivity test). This finding suggests that the characteristics of man-infectivity may be related to the nature of the VAT and thus the stocks of organisms may differ in this characteristic depending on the VAT expressed at a particular time.

Studies on *T. b. gambiense* have indicated that there are limited numbers of antigenic types in Nigeria and that even when isolates from Sudan, Uganda and Zaire are compared many antigens are common. *T. b. brucei*, however, seems to have a larger capacity for antigenic dissimilarity, perhaps because it is found in a wide range of animals and tends, even in cattle, to produce chronic infections. Field observation of *T. b. brucei* in cattle indicates that parasites do retain antigenic characters in the field over periods of years.

Work on antigenic variation in *T. congolense* and *T. vivax* has not been as extensive as on the *T. brucei* group. However, neutralization and immunolysis tests have shown that antigenic variation occurs in both *T. congolense* and *T. vivax*. *T. congolense* displays autoagglutinating properties which prevent the use of agglutination tests and *T. vivax* causes practical difficulties for study in view of its general lack of infectivity for laboratory rodents. Biochemical and molecular characterization of VSGs of these subgenera are in the process of being determined.

Recent studies on *T. vivax* using recently isolated strains infective to mice suggest that different sequences of variable antigens are expressed in different hosts. Further, a tsetse transmissible stock of *T. vivax* gave rise to an antigenic type at the first parasitaemia peaks in goats which was different from that injected by the fly.

Studies on *T. congolense* indicate that antigenic variation is similar to that observed in *T. brucei* and the effects of cyclical transmission on the process of variation are also similar.

Recent studies on *T. cruzi* have revealed that the same cell surface antigens are present in epimastigotes from culture as well as trypomatigotes and amastigotes isolated from the host. The major cell surface glycoprotein (90 000 daltons) from a number of geographically distinct isolates did not vary and any differences that did exist were not associated with the major surface glycoprotein. The results of peptide mapping show no differences in the *T. cruzi* glycoprotein. Small changes in amino-acid sequence or carbohydrate structure could themselves change the antigenic properties, but the overall evidence is against antigenic variation in *T. cruzi*. Host serum components are incorporated into the surface membrane (particularly bloodstream trypomastigotes) by binding in *T. cruzi*, a phenomenon also associated with salivarian trypanosomes. The glycoprotein of *T. cruzi* has been shown to protect mice against virulent challenge.

In *Herpetosoma* (*T. lewisi*) it has been demonstrated that changes in antigenicity occur during the course of infection but it is not clear if these antigenic changes are related to the surface. Surface agglutinins of *T. lewisi* are specific to reproducing and adult forms but reproducing variant agglutinogen is not apparently immunogenic. It is interesting, however, that there is a marked difference in surface antigen between *T. musculi* and *T. lewisi* as judged by agglutinating activity of mouse serum from mice infected with or immune to *T. musculi*.

Detailed cytochemical studies of the surface coats of *T. lewisi* and *T. musculi* have demonstrated its fuzzy appearance and it is known from studies using lectins that polyanionic carbohydrates are present; host serum protein is also known to be absorbed onto the parasite surface.

TECHNIQUES FOR THE ROUTINE STUDY OF TRYPANOSOMATIDS

Detection of infections in vertebrate hosts

Trypanosoma

Trypanosomes found in thick, thin or wet blood films and stained with Giemsa's or Leishman's stain may be identified to subgenus level. However, these methods have limited sensitivity in detecting very low parasitaemias. Recently devised techniques enable the detection of parasitaemias as low as 100 organisms per millilitre of blood. The most effective techniques for detecting parasites so far developed for bovine and human trypanosomiasis are based on centrifugation and filtration micro methods.

The microhaematocrit centrifuge with 70 μl capillary tubes was originally used to detect low-grade trypanosome parasitaemias in birds; this has been extended for use in human and animal trypanosomiasis. Parasites are found in the buffy-coat region of the centrifuge tube when examined unopened, using immersion oil to reduce diffraction. Zernicke condensers and objective lenses with a long working distance increase the available working distance and improve parasite detection. The sensitivity of this technique for detection of *T. congolense* and *T. vivax* has been improved by breaking the tube and examining the buffy coat and its contents under a coverslip with dark ground illumination. In parallel with these developments the use of DEAE cellulose columns to separate trypanosomes from red blood cells on the basis of the charge differences when blood was diluted by different buffer solutions (the pH depending on the host animal erythrocyte charge) provided a further technique for separation of trypanosomes from red blood cells. The red cells are retained in the cellulose and the parasites pass through into the eluted buffer (the eluate). The eluate is then centrifuged and parasites, if present, are found in the sediment after the supernatant has been removed. Extensive development of this technique has been carried out recently to produce a field-test technique based on miniaturization of a DEAE column with incorporation of the appropriate buffer for dilution of human blood. This technique, known as the miniature anion exchange centrifugation technique, has been found to be much more sensitive for detecting parasites in human sleeping sickness than thick blood film examination and lymph-gland juice examination. Moreover the test is rapid and has been developed for field use (see the section on human trypanosomiasis diagnosis in Chapter 3).

Subinoculation of blood for the detection of pathogenic mammalian trypanosomes of Africa has been widely recognized as a technique of great sensitivity. Mice are frequently used as hosts and it is appropriate to use six mice per animal to increase the sensitivity of the technique. However, *T. vivax* is not usually detected by this method as only some isolates are infective to rodents. Nursling rats or the multimammate rat *Mastomys natalensis* are more sensitive for detecting *T. b. gambiense* from man or stocks of *T. b. brucei* of low virulence originating from animals.

Trypanosomes can be detected in the lymph-gland juice of man infected with West African sleeping sickness and animals infected with trypanosomes. However, the value of lymph-node biopsy as a technique for the detection of parasites in cattle and small ruminants on a large scale is probably limited.

For the clinician it is important to know whether the central nervous system has been invaded in sleeping sickness. Parasites may be detected in cerebro-spinal fluid from a lumbar puncture, in a wet preparation in a Neuebauer haemocytometer, or they may be concentrated by centrifugation and then examined.

The stercorarian trypanosomes, frequently difficult to find in thick blood films, can be detected by techniques of blood centrifugation. Subgenus *Megatrypanum* species which have very low parasitaemias, for example *T. theileri* of cattle, *T. melophagium* of sheep and *T. theodori*, a goat trypanosome the bloodstream forms of which have never been seen, can be detected by the inoculation of blood from the host into cultures. Blood agar slopes have been used in the past for this but more defined and efficient systems now exist: see the section on cultivation pp. 54–61. Six cultures per animal per day have been used to detect fluctuations in parasitaemia of *T. theileri* in the expectation that not every culture will become positive.

Cultures are particularly valuable in detecting the very low-grade parasitaemias in chronic infections with *T. cruzi*, the causative organism of Chagas' disease. In some cases parasites would not otherwise be found. The use of culture for diagnosis of *T. cruzi* is, however, not as valuable a tool as xenodiagnosis. Xenodiagnosis involves the use of clean vector bugs reared in a laboratory. A batch (usually 6–12) of a susceptible species (*Rhodnius prolixus, Panstrongylus megistus* or species of *Triatoma*) is fed on a suspect and after a period of 2–3 weeks the bugs are dissected to determine if *T. cruzi* has developed. The presence of the parasite indicates the suspect was infected. Comparisons have been made recently between haemoculture and xenodiagnosis which have shown that xenodiagnosis is a more sensitive technique for the detection of *T. cruzi* infections. A serious disadvantage in the techniques of culture and xenodiagnosis is the time required for a definitive result to be available.

The trypanosomes of the subgenus *Herpetosoma* parasitic in rodents do not grow particularly well when inoculated from the low parasitaemias which are found in most naturally infected wild rodents. The non-reproducing so-called 'adult' forms in these infections seem difficult to grow in blood agar media. Only *T. lewisi* and *T. musculi*, which produce higher parasitaemias, are readily cultivated and then subpassage may be difficult.

In non-mammalian trypanosomes parasitaemias are frequently low and detection of infection is recommended by microhaematocrit centrifugation, possibly followed by dark ground examination of the buffy coat. However, cultivation has also been used for the detection of trypanosomes, particularly in birds where it was found that inoculation of the bone marrow rather than blood into cultures demonstrated a higher prevalence of infections than would be found in blood examination; it was found also that in winter *T. corvi*, a parasite of British corvids, is present in the bone marrow but not in the circulating blood.

The ability of trypanosomes from most non-mammalian hosts to grow in simple culture media such as NNN has been demonstrated; fish (both teleosts and elasmobranchs), amphibians and reptiles all have trypanosomes which may be grown in this way.

Leishmania

Compared with trypanosomes, which are motile organisms, *Leishmania* parasites pose a more difficult problem for the diagnostic parasitologist. *Leishmania* are rarely found in blood films and biopsies of skin lesions, internal organs and normal skin are necessary. These are best prepared as impression smears, followed by Leishman's or Giemsa's staining to detect the organisms. The material obtained at biopsy is used to cultivate the promastigote forms. Cultivation and animal inoculation techniques are of value in isolating organisms for further study but, as with trypanosomes, the delay in obtaining a result limits their diagnostic value.

Biopsy procedures for the detection of the cutaneous leishmaniases involve the aspiration of material from the edge of the lesion followed by staining to detect amastigotes and inoculation into cultures and/or animals (usually hamsters). For the diagnosis of visceral leishmaniasis biopsy of bone marrow, liver and spleen are undertaken to determine if parasites are present. This material may also be cultured if the microscopic examination is negative; recently it has been found that the insect tissue culture medium of Schneider, used for *Drosophila* cell cultivation with the addition of 30 per cent foetal calf serum, is more sensitive than blood agar (NNN) media for the detection of visceral leishmaniasis due to *Leishmania donovani*. Hamsters and cotton rats (*Sigmodon hispidus*) are susceptible to *L. donovani* but, as in cutaneous leishmaniasis, the use of animal inoculation as a clinical diagnostic procedure is often precluded due to the time required for the parasites to develop. Animal inoculation is of particular value for the isolation of parasites for experimental study.

The widespread occurrence of reservoir hosts requires the isolation of parasites, particularly from wild animal (rodents, carnivores, edentates) reservoirs. Standard techniques used are the cultivation (usually in blood agar with antibiotics added to reduce contamination) of blood and organs (particularly liver, bone marrow, spleen, heart and lungs) but also the removal of skin and the search for small lesions (particularly the pinna of the ear, nose and base of the tail in rodents) and the subsequent inoculation of such material into culture media and animals, respectively. Hamsters are usually the animals of choice. Inoculation of apparently normal skin from South American mammals has yielded positive cultures and/or infected hamsters on many occasions.

Impression smears or dabs of internal organs of suspected reservoirs are also prepared in association with the above techniques to determine which organs are parasitized. However, their value may be limited in view of the possibility that amastigotes found in organs, particularly in Central and South America, may not necessarily be *Leishmania*, but other trypanosomatids which can produce amastigotes in tissues (e.g., *T. cruzi*, *Endotrypanum*, *Herpetosoma*). Mixed *Leishmania* infections may also occur; thus isolation of parasite material for later study and possibly cloning of cultures obtained is necessary.

Detection of infections in vectors

The most commonly used technique for the identification and detection of infections in insects is the dissection of the gut, mouthparts and/or salivary glands (or removal of haemocoelic fluid) and the examination of the various constituent parts in a drop of isotonic saline. The parasites may be either in the lumen of the tubes themselves or in the fluid surrounding the dissected gut, as dissection frequently results in the parasites breaking out of the gut. Phase contrast microscopy increases the chance of detecting parasites. Permanent preparations may be made if the coverslip is removed, the saline rapidly dried and the material fixed and stained with Giemsa's or Leishman's stains.

Although dissection is clearly the key to the detection of infections in insects, inoculation of material into susceptible animals is of value in some circumstances where, for example, infection rates may be low. In this situation pools of insects may be macerated and inoculated into susceptible animals. The detection of *T. brucei* infections in *Glossina* is infrequent in view of the low infection rates, and the ideal situation would in this case be to allow each *Glossina* to bite a susceptible animal to test the true infection rate. However, this is clearly not a viable approach, particularly in the field. Differentiation of *T. vivax* and *T. congolense* in *Glossina* is difficult as both develop in the mouthparts; the presence of a midgut infection of *T. congolense* will permit differentiation as *T. vivax* does not develop in this site; examination of haemocoelic fluid of *Glossina* for trypanosomes is suggested as *T. brucei* has been found in the haemocoele.

Sandfly dissections for *Leishmania* parasites are more difficult due to the smaller size of the insect. Inoculation of parasites found during dissection of sandflies into hamsters and cultures is important for later identification of the parasites. However, the group to which the *Leishmania* belong can be identified from their position in the gut of the sandfly, but the precise identity will require confirmation by laboratory studies. Sentinel animals in cages have been used to detect the presence and types of *Leishmania* parasite circulating in parts of Central American forests, although the technique does not enable identification of the vector species.

Some field workers have used liquid nitrogen to cryopreserve insects (*Glossina* and sandflies) caught in the field for transport to the laboratory; experiments can then be carried out on any parasites detected in the vectors. One limitation of this technique is the time the liquid nitrogen supply can last in possibly extreme conditions.

Rodent trypanosomes (*T. lewisi*) can be isolated by the the inoculation of pools of macerated fleas into susceptible rats. This technique avoids the need to dissect numbers of fleas and if the rat becomes infected the isolate so obtained is of value as it has been clearly recently isolated; recently isolated stocks of known provenance are of great value in laboratory studies.

Cryopreservation

Cryopreservation can be defined as the storage of organisms or other biological materials (e.g., semen) at low temperatures. Prior to the advent of storage of micro-organisms at low temperatures it was necessary to maintain parasites by sub-passages through susceptible animals for laboratory studies; large numbers of laboratory animals (mice, rats and rabbits) are required for the maintenance of virulent organisms, which is expensive in terms of laboratory space, animal food and the time of technicians. The characteristics of organisms maintained by continual animal passage are liable to change. Organisms thus lose many of their original characteristics. Maintenance of organisms in culture presents similar problems (time, expense and organism stability), in addition to the need to continue to provide sterile media and expensive chemicals for sera for cultures. Cryopreservation of organisms thus saves time and money but also maintains the original biological properties of organisms. The term 'stabilate' has been introduced to define the preparation of *Trypanosoma* and *Leishmania* parasites for storage of living organisms on a 'unique occasion'. The process of preparing a 'stabilate' is described as stabilation.

Protozoa have been known to display 'cryoresistance' since the time of Van Leeuwenhoek in the seventeenth century, and as long ago as 1904 it was demonstrated that trypanosomes could survive for several minutes in liquid air (− 191 °C). Attempts in the 1930s to maintain viruses and spirochaetes led to attempts by protozoologists to preserve parasitic protozoa in dry ice (solid CO_2) and it was demonstrated that trypanosomes and malarial parasites maintained their infectivity after storage at − 70 to − 80 °C for periods of up to 5 months using no cryoprotectant but only reducing the temperature gradually to the final storage temperature. Storage of micro-organisms and spermatozoa was found to be more successful and the recovery of infective forms after freezing more likely if compounds such as glycerol and dimethyl sulphoxide (DMSO) were used as 'cryoprotectants' (substances which protect organisms from the results of freezing and subsequent thawing).

Trypanosoma and *Leishmania* from both the vertebrate and insect stages are now maintained as a matter of routine in a cryopreserved state. They are usually maintained as blood cultures or occasionally in insect tissues with the addition of serum or isotonic saline containing glucose and glycerol or DMSO at concentrations of 5–10 per cent. Dry ice cabinets, mechanical freezers or liquid-nitrogen fridges are used to store the materials, the last being the most commonly used. Trypanosomes, related flagellates and *Leishmania* have been found to survive cryopreservation best if the rate of freezing between 0 and −40°C is slow and it is recommended that this is around one degree per minute until −40°C is reached; at this point the material can be placed directly into the temperature of the storage vessel. Slow freezing is usually achieved by incubating the tube containing the parasites in a dry ice/absolute alcohol mixture until the required temperature is reached or by slowly introducing the vial, ampoule or tube into the flask of the liquid-nitrogen fridge using a specially designed apparatus which fits into the neck of the container and is slowly lowered. Provided the parasites have been frozen slowly and kept at the low temperature their viability and infectivity will be retained for at least several years; there is no reason why viable preservation of organisms in this state should not last for decades. Good labelling and record keeping of frozen materials is essential. Plastic ampoules or tubes rather than glass ones are recommended as they are safer.

Cultivation

The need to cultivate *in vitro* trypanosomes and *Leishmania* has been recognized ever since the organisms were discovered. The reasons for their cultivation are varied: purely for maintenance to avoid using an animal host, for diagnosis (e.g., in visceral leishmaniasis and *T. cruzi*), for experimental studies related to biochemistry, for the production of antigen, for the production of *Leishmania major* promastigotes for vaccination, and for the production of large numbers of forms which resemble the parasites found in the vector (e.g., stercorarian trypanosomes and *Leishmania* species).

The first medium produced for the growth of trypanosomatids still remains widely used. This is the so-called NNN medium which is a blood agar medium with a liquid overlay. The diphasic medium was developed by Novy, Nicholle and McNeal in 1903. The medium has a solid phase of agar or nutrient agar ('4N media') and defibrinated mammalian blood (usually rabbit or outdated human blood from blood banks); to the sterile melted agar the defibrinated blood is added and prior to solidification the tube into which the agar and blood is poured is 'sloped' in such a way as to allow the surface of the solid phase to be at an angle when the culture tube is kept upright. The slopes are then incubated for 24–48 hours to ensure that they are sterile prior to the addition of the liquid overlay which is usually a Lockes balanced salt solution to which the antibiotics penicillin and streptomycin are added at a concentration of 200 iu and 200 μg/ml respectively. This medium has been used extensively for the growth of stercorarian trypanosomes, *Leishmania* species (except *L. b. braziliensis*) and many species of monogenetic flagellates. However, more defined or semi-defined media are now available for various trypanosomatid parasites and the last few years have seen the introduction of tissue culture techniques for the growth of *Leishmania* species and salivarian trypanosomes.

The trend over the past decades has been the production of defined media for monogenetic flagellates resulting from and enabling a contribution to our knowledge of the nutritional requirements of the group. It would not be appropriate here to discuss details of media, but many are available which differ in subtle ways. However, defined media have been developed for monogenetic flagellates such as *Crithidia fasciculata* whose basic constituents are salts, trace elements, magnesium sulphate, potassium as citrate, low molecular weight organic acids (malic, succinic), 12 amino acids, vitamins and co-factors, carbohydrates as sorbitol, and haemins. However, *C. fasciculata* can also be grown in a carbohydrate-free medium. If the flagellates contain endosymbionts it is possible to markedly reduce the number of amino acids present; for example *C. oncopelti* requires only methionine and *C. deanei* methionine and tyrosine, although growth is more rapid if tryptophan and phenylalanine are also present. A supply of purines may be necessary in flagellates which contain endosymbionts; for example *C. oncopelti* requires adenine whereas *C. deanei* does not.

The use of chemically defined media is clearly essential for many biochemical and nutritional studies, but for routine cultivation of many trypanosomatids media have been devised which are cheap and easy to prepare for situations when chemical definition is not essential. Media containing proteose peptone, liver digest, glycerol, triethanoline, haemin and folic acid are suitable for growth of *C. fasciculata* at pH of 8·0–8·2.

Leishmania parasites have been grown as promastigotes for experimental and diagnostic studies (Montenegro skin test)in NNN or 4N media; however, defined media are now available which support the growth of the more fastidious species of *Leishmania* such as *L. braziliensis* subspecies; as with monoxenous flagellates such defined media contain basic salts, glucose, 17 amino acids, purines and vitamins together with other constituents such as haemin and defatted bovine albumin. Semi-defined media for *Leishmania* differ in that the only undefined constituent is a serum component. This is usually foetal calf serum and is used at concentrations of 5–30 per cent. The commercial availability of tissue culture media has led to the development of highly effective culture media for the growth of *Leishmania* promastigotes based on these. One such medium, known as HO-MEM, is based on the Eagle's minimal essential medium (MEM) with commercially available salt solutions, MEM amino acids and non-essential amino acids, pyruvate, sodium bicarbonate, glucose, biotin and para-aminobenzoic acid; to the filtered sterilized medium 5–10 per cent foetal calf serum is added. Further development of media for the growth of *Leishmania* has been achieved by the use of commercially available insect tissue cultue media such as Schneider's, Grace's and Mitsuhashi–Maramorosch's. Amastigotes transform to promastigotes rapidly in these media and yields of promastigotes are up to five times greater than from blood agar based media; the optimal concentration of foetal calf serum is 15 per cent. Comparative trials with Schneider's *Drosophila* medium supplemented with 30 per cent foetal calf serum for diagnostic cultures in cutaneous leishmaniasis have shown it to give positive results faster and to be more sensitive than blood agar based medium (37/55 positives compared with 8/55 on NNN).

It is recommended that if a stock of *Leishmania* parasites is proving difficult to culture then a diphasic 4N-type blood agar medium solid phase with a tissue culture medium (e.g., Medium 199) and 10 per cent foetal calf serum as an overlay may succeed when other media have failed.

The ability to grow in culture and the speed of that growth have been used to indicate the species complex to which members of neotropical *Leishmania* belong. Lainson and Shaw demonstrated that *L. braziliensis* complex parasites are 'slow growers', not only in blood agar media but also in hamsters when compared with the fast growing *L. mexicana* complex stocks. These problems have now largely been overcome through the use of the HO-MEM medium or an enriched overlay in 4N; even so, true *L. b. braziliensis* grow less well than parasites which cause the simple cutaneous lesions (*L. mexicana* complex).

Cultivation of *Leishmania* amastigotes in media which do not contain cells has not been very successful probably due to the nature of the metabolic and nutritional requirements of amastigotes which are likely to be related to the intra-cellular habitat. However, cultivation of amastigotes in tissue culture cell lines has been achieved and the use of such infected tissue culture cell lines has been a valuable tool in experimental chemotherapy, but only certain cell lines have been shown to be capable of acting as host cells of *Leishmania* amastigotes. The two most successful are a Sticker Dog Sarcoma and a Hamster Peritoneal cell line; similarly, not all species of *Leishmania* grow well, with *L. mexicana* and *L. donovani* being perhaps the most easily grown. *L. mexicana* and other cutaneous species of *Leishmania* are usually maintained at 32 °C whereas the visceral stocks of parasites should be maintained at 35–37 °C in tissue culture cells (figure 18).

Dog Sarcoma and Hamster Peritoneal cell monolayers can be infected initially with promastigotes which invade these cells despite their low phagocytic ability and transform to amastigotes and multiply profusely; infected cells are not usually passaged continously but uninfected cells are easily infected.

For experimental studies on the cell biology and host–parasite relationships extensive work on the relationship between *Leishmania* and macrophages has been carried out using macrophages derived from mouse peritoneal exudates; the utilization of macrophages with limited life closely mimics the *in vivo* situation as the parasites are rapidly phagocytosed and transform to amastigotes, but the

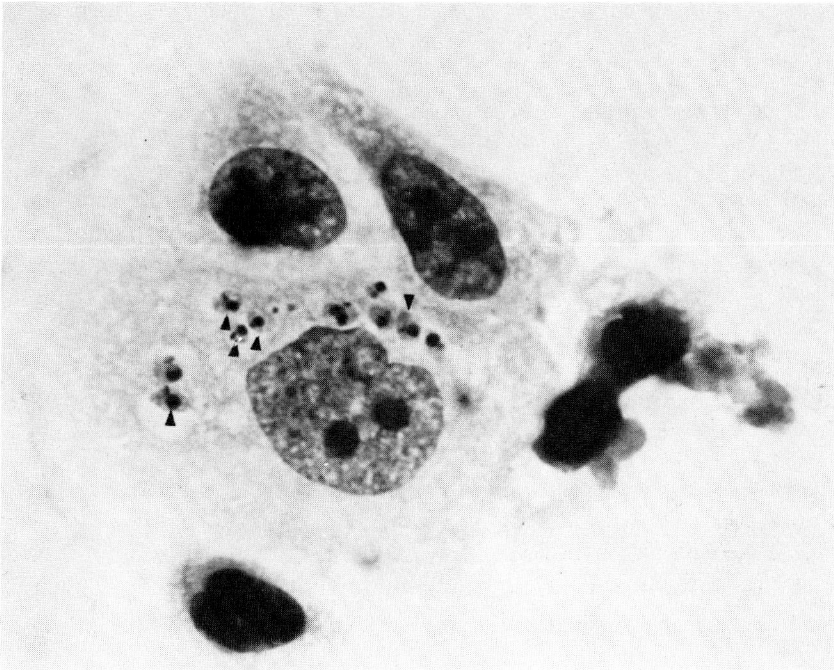

Figure 18. Amastigotes (arrowed) in a Giemsa stained slide of a preparation of tissue culture of Dog Sarcoma cells infected with *Leishmania m. mexicana* (× 1600).

medium and cells have a restricted use as a means of cultivation. A macrophage-like cell line (P-388), however, is now available. P-388 is of tumour origin and allows continuous cultivation of host cells.

Trypanosoma cruzi

In common with many stercorarian trypanosomes *T. cruzi* is cultivated easily as the insect stages on NNN or 4N-type media. The multiplicative forms in culture are epimastigotes and metacyclic trypomastigotes are produced which are infective to mammalian hosts. However, defined and semi-defined media have been developed which support *T. cruzi* growth; in the same way such media have been used for the growth of other trypanosomatids at around 25 °C. Cultivation of the amastigote stages of *T. cruzi* in tissue culture cells, for example, Girardi human heart cells as monolayers, and in macrophage cultures has been shown to be possible; such *in vitro* cultures of *T. cruzi* in tissue culture cells also enable experimental chemotherapy studies as in *Leishmania*. Haemoculture on NNN or 4N media can be used as an alternative to xenodiagnosis using triatomid bugs. Trypanosomes of the subgenus *Schizotrypanum* (e.g., *T. dionisii*) which are parasitic in Chiroptera (bats) and are non-infective to man have been shown to be capable of growing in blood agar culture media as well as in tissue culture cell lines and in peritoneal macrophages as amastigotes.

Other stercorarian species

Both *Herpetosoma* and *Megatrypanum* subgenera can be grown in NNN- and 4N-type media and the use of these media has been widespread, in particular for the detection of *Megatrypanum* species (e.g., *T. theileri* in cattle, *T. melophagium* in sheep and *T. theodori* in goats). The parasitaemia of these species is so low that cultivation is the only effective technique for detecting them. Up to six tubes may be used on a single occasion in attempts to isolate the parasites. *T. theodori* has never been observed in the blood of its host the goat.

T. theileri is frequently grown inadvertently at 37°C when cultivation of bovine cells in tissue cultures is being carried out; some authors have detected trypanosomes in foetuses of bovines when primary foetal bovine kidney monolayers have been initiated.

T. lewisi and *T. musculi* are capable of growing in blood agar medium at 25–27°C and in various tissue culture systems at 35–37°C. Little work has, however, been carried out on these species in relation to their behaviour in defined or semi-defined media. However, many members of this subgenus which have been found difficult to culture could probably be grown in more sophisticated systems. Studies on a trypanosome of voles, *T. evotomys*, have been carried out in cell culture which have demonstrated attachment mechanisms *in vitro* at 25–27°C using a cell line to which the parasite had to be adapted over several weeks by media changes.

Chicken embryos

Chicken embryos have also been used for the cultivation of *Leishmania* parasites and trypanosomes. *Leishmania* promastigotes cause a high mortality when inoculated into chick embryos, but passage can be achieved if the embryonic membranes remain intact although the embryo may be moribund. Growth is optimal at 23–28°C for *L. donovani*, *L. tropica* and *L. braziliensis* and promastigotes are found in the allantoic fluid if inoculated into the allantoic cavity. Inoculation of *Leishmania* into the chorioallantois results in parasites being found in that site and in the heart. Intracellular stages have been observed near the region of inoculation. Inoculation of *T. cruzi* results in the dispersion of parasites throughout the embryonic organs. When the inoculations are made into the chorioallantoic cavity the chorioallantoic membrane becomes infected and the amastigotes cause lesions in the chorioallantois. Various trypanosomes have been passaged through chick embryos but *Trypanozoon* parasites may be fatal to the embryo. Embryos should be inoculated at six days old.

Salivarian trypanosomes

For many years the cultivation of this group of parasites proved extremely difficult and success was elusive. If successful cultivation is to be achieved, recently isolated stocks or those cryopreserved after a minimum number of passages prior to cryopreservation offer the best chance of success. Semi-defined media are available for the routine growth of the procyclic forms of *Trypanozoon* from *Glossina*. The liquid media are modified and improved from standard tissue culture media such as TCM 199 or Eagle's minimal essential medium.

Recently, procyclic parasites of *T. brucei* from cultures containing explants of alimentary canal of *Glossina morsitans* have been inoculated into culture media containing heads and salivary glands of *Glossina* which were freshly dissected from sterilized puparia from which they had been about to emerge; when maintained at 28°C with the medium replaced every two days a 25-fold increase in parasites was observed over a period of 48 hours and 10 per cent of the salivary glands became invaded by parasites within 12–17 days; a proportion of forms were epimastigote and infective metacyclic trypanosomes.

The cultivation of the form which infects mammalian hosts at 37°C was a goal achieved recently. The implications of this achievement in terms of antigen preparation, studies of antigenic variation, chemotherapy and biochemistry are profound. Haematozoic trypomastigotes of *T. brucei* were grown at 37°C on bovine fibroblast-like cell lines with an overlay of RPMI 1640 medium with HEPES buffer and 20 per cent foetal calf serum; the parasites were maintained for long periods in this system as typical bloodstream trypomastigotes which were infective for mammals and retained the surface coat typical of bloodstream forms. Similar tissue culture systems for the growth of different stocks of the *Trypanozoon* subgenus have been subsequently developed using cells from different hosts such as hamster and buffalo lung tissue culture cells which were fibroblast-like as well as rabbit fibroblast-like cells. The latter system allows the propagation of pleo-morphic stocks of *T. brucei*, and even single (cloned) metacyclic forms from *Glossina* could initiate this culture system. Clusters of parasites were grouped among the feeder layer of rabbit fibroblast-like cells 48 hours after inoculation; once these intercellular parasite clusters were formed the medium could be changed daily; the cultures when inoculated into mice produced a pleomorphic infection typical of normal *T. brucei* infections (figure 19).

Progress towards methods of cultivation of *T. congolense* and *T. vivax* has also recently been made. Early success was achieved by Trager who grew *T. vivax* in a tsetse salivary gland tissue culture system which produced forms infective to sheep. More recently limited success has been achieved with *T. vivax* in a TCM 199 medium with HEPES buffer and supplemented with foetal calf serum and plasma from animals of the same variety as those which were used as the source of the parasites. A three-fold increase over a 24-hour period has been observed in this system. Recently the long term cultivation of haematozoic forms which retain infectivity to cattle has been achieved in a tissue culture system.

Cultures of epimastigotes and trypomastigotes of *T. congolense* have been established after infected proboscides of *G. morsitans* were placed in a bovine dermal-collagen explant. Parasites emerged from the mouthparts and established

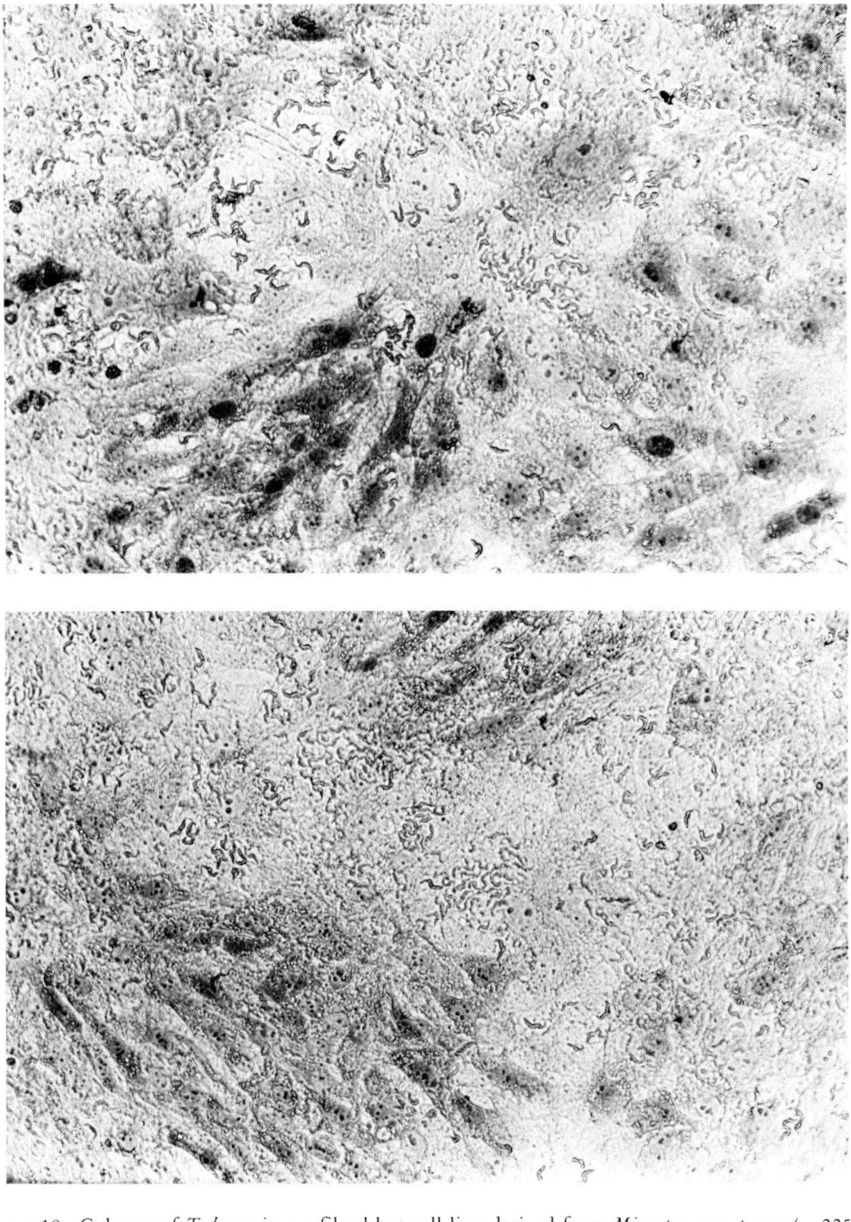

Figure 19. Cultures of *T. brucei* on a fibroblast cell line derived from *Microtus montanus* (× 225). Courtesy of Dr L. Jenni.

clusters adherent to the plastic surface of the culture vessel. Subcultures have been successful and parasites maintained for 200 days.

Rearing of vectors

A major handicap for many years in laboratory studies of these parasites was the difficulty of maintaining laboratory colonies of suitable insect vectors. The vectors of African trypanosomes and *Leishmania* were particularly difficult to maintain, which meant that these infections could not be transmitted cyclically. The absence of a regular supply of insect material also prevented many studies of the insects themselves, such as physiological and genetic studies or tests on their susceptibility to insecticides. The founding of a colony, initially of *G. austeni* and then *G. morsitans morsitans*, at Langford near Bristol, England by Nash and his colleagues was and remains the basis of extensive research; pupal material is disseminated from this colony to workers throughout the world including, ironically, Africa. The colony was initially reared on goats, and flies were fed six days a week. More recently an *in vitro* feeding system has been developed where flies are fed five days a week through artificial silicone rubber, agar or parafilm membranes on defibrinated pig's blood. Constant relative humidity (RH) of 70 per cent and 25°C temperature are maintained. The membranes overlie pools of blood in grooved glass plates which themselves rest on horizontal rectangular glass radiators through which warm water passes to maintain the blood at 35–37°C. The reproductive performance of tsetse flies thus maintained *in vitro* is comparable over a long period of time with that of flies maintained on living hosts. It has been found, however, that cow's blood is not a satisfactory food for the maintenance of tsetse *in vitro*. Larvae deposited by female *Glossina* are collected and the pupae either disseminated for research or returned to the colony. Eclosion (emergence) of adult flies usually occurs approximately one month after larviposition.

The methods originally developed at Langford have been used in laboratories in Europe and Africa where *Glossina* of other species (*palpalis* group in particular) are being reared either for laboratory studies or Sterile Male Release campaigns. Hosts used in Africa for *Glossina* breeding are goats and rabbits, but *in vitro* systems are being developed.

The success in rearing *Glossina* in the laboratory with the production of surplus material for dissemination for research has been followed by the successful rearing of sandflies; self-supporting colonies of *Lutzomyia longipalpis* and *Phlebotomus papatasi* have now been reared for many generations allowing experimental studies on transmission and life cycles of *Leishmania* as well as physiological studies. The sandflies fed on hamsters are maintained at 95 per cent RH and 25°C prior to oviposition. Eggs of sandflies are reared on wet filter paper in plastic pots roughened with acetone and lined with plaster of Paris; the open end is closed with fine gauze; humidity is maintained by keeping the pots in sealed polythene food containers. Larvae are fed on desiccated liver powder and the containers are kept in the dark.

After emergence from pupae the flies are released into a larger cage containing 120 flies; a 30 per cent sucrose solution is available; high humidity is provided by keeping each cage in a clear plastic bag with a swab of wet cotton wool; mating takes place easily in these cages.

Female flies are offered an anaesthetized hamster or a new-born rat on which to feed 3–5 days after emergence: engorged flies are held individually in 4 × 2 cm glass tubes with a 30 per cent sucrose solution on swabs of cotton wool always available; they are kept on a 12 h dark–light regime and the relative humidity is maintained at 85 per cent by standing the tubes over dilute sulphuric acid of approximately 0·1 M (specific gravity, 1·1). Three days after engorgement the filter paper in the tubes is wetted with a syringe and hypodermic needle. This stimulates oviposition, which is usually complete six days after engorgement. Engorged females can alternatively be kept in plastic pots. These techniques have enabled extensive studies to be carried out on sandfly biology in relation to leishmaniasis.

Triatomine bugs, vectors of Chagas' disease, have been maintained in the laboratory for many years. *Rhodnius prolixus* has been used extensively in insect physiology research because it is so easily bred; nymphal stages and adults feed on blood and are fed every 2–4 weeks. Bugs are maintained in glass jars with folded filter paper; eggs are collected and placed in a separate jar for first-instar nymphs to hatch. Colonies of such bugs are maintained for xenodiagnosis in South American hospitals and laboratories.

The other vectors of trypanosomes which are easily bred in the laboratory are the flea vectors of the subgenus *Herpetosoma*, and *Aedes* mosquitoes which transmit some avian trypanosomes. Other vector groups are less easily bred or cannot be bred in captivity, for example, tabanids, leeches and *Melophagus ovinus*.

Chapter 2. The Vectors

GLOSSINA: VECTORS OF SALIVARIAN TRYPANOSOMES

The insects

Glossina species are the insect vectors of the pathogenic salivarian trypanosomes of Africa and are thus among the most economically important vectors. They are commonly known as tsetse flies. Although fossil species of *Glossina* have been found in Colorado, living *Glossina* are restricted to sub-Saharan Africa north of the Kalahari. An unconfirmed record of *Glossina* was made in southern Arabia in the first years of this century. there are 22 described species of *Glossina*. Various subspecies have been described. *Glossina* belong to the family Glossinidae, order Diptera but were formerly included in the Muscidae, along with the houseflies. Tsetse flies are of similar size to this more common group of Diptera, varying in size from the smaller species around 7 mm in length to larger species which can be twice that. *Glossina* are nondescript in colour, being of brownish-grey hue occasionally with darker bands on the abdomen. They rest with their wings overlapping horizontally in a characteristic scissor-like manner above the six-segmented abdomen. The proboscis or haustellum, with piercing mouthparts, arises from a bulb-like structure at the base of the head; at rest it projects anteriorly (figure 20).

There are two absolutely distinctive features of the genus *Glossina* which separate them from other Diptera. The first is the presence of a so-called 'hatchet cell' in the wing venation. This 'cell' lies between the longitudinal veins IV and V and gives the appearance of a cleaver used by butchers (figure 21). The second characteristic is the secondary branching found on the hairs of the arista, arising from the third segment of the antenna.

Glossina species are all haematophagous, totally dependent on the blood sucking habit. Different species of *Glossina* have host preferences for sources of food. These host preferences are important in the epidemiology of the diseases

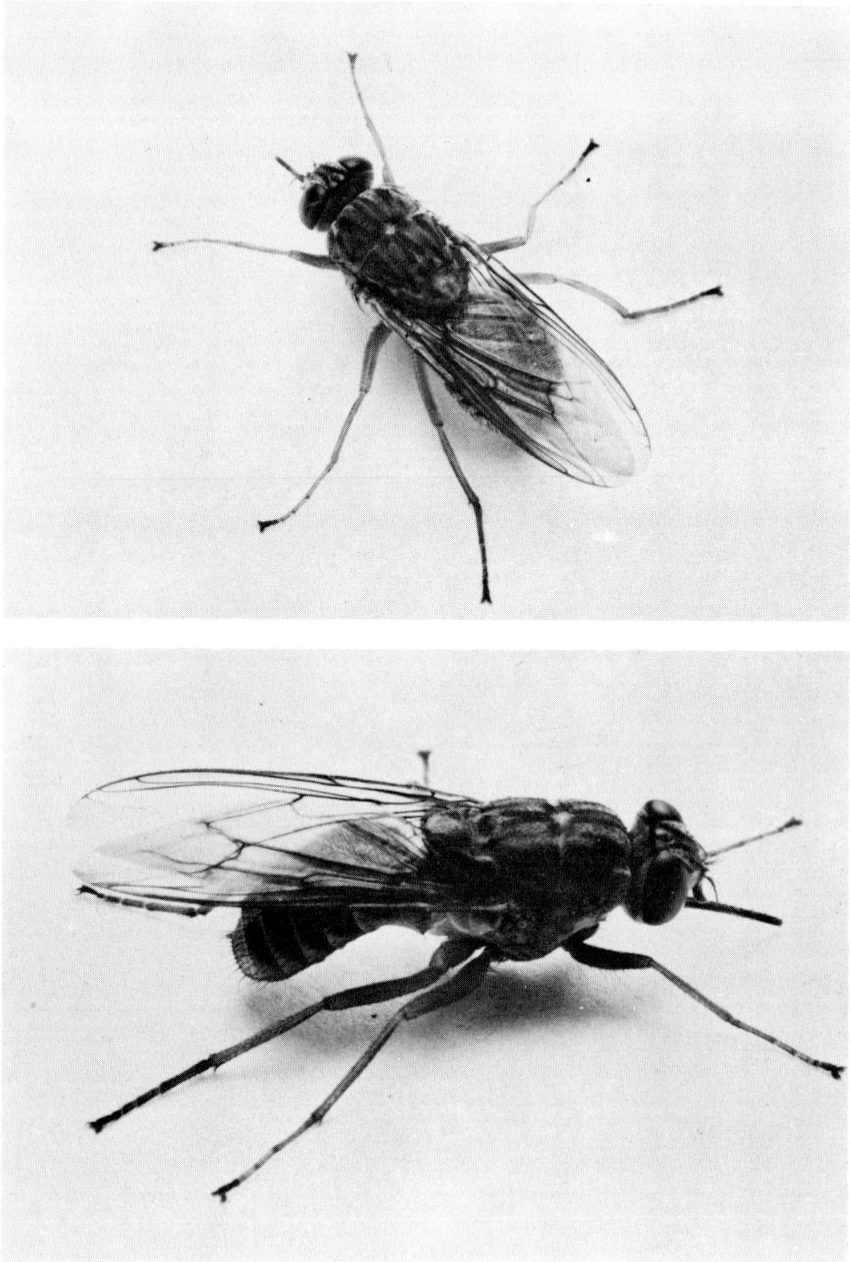

Figure 20. *Glossina morsitans* viewed from above (× 5) and the side (× 8).

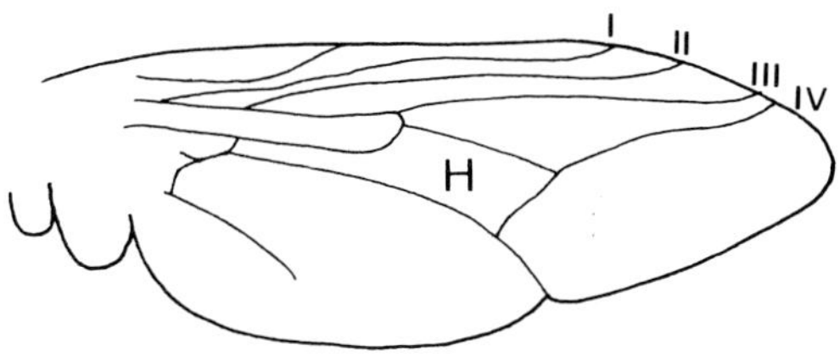

Figure 21. Diagram of wing venation of *Glossina* showing the 'hatchet cell' H, which is characteristic of the genus.

transmitted by *Glossina*. As both males and females take blood, both are vectors of trypanosomes.

Glossina are surprisingly successful insects when their method of reproduction is considered. They are larviparous. A single female *Glossina*, which usually mates only once, at the time of its first blood meal, a few days after emergence, will produce approximately 8–12 larvae during its life-span of 3–5 months. During mating sperm is transferred from male to female by a spermatophore. Mating itself is believed to control ovulation, probably as a result of the mechanical stimulus. However, endocrines from median neurosecretory cells are also involved. Mating is aided by a contact pheromone which has been isolated from the cuticle of females, and has been analysed and synthesized. It is a long chain paraffin wax of low volatility.

The incubation period of the developing larva, between ovulation and the deposition of the third-stage larva in a suitable place — the larviposition site — is approximately 9–12 days, depending on temperature. The egg is fertilized by sperm which are stored in the spermathecae. The egg hatches within the uterus, where the developing larva remains until it is mature. The developing larva is fed from milk glands which enter the uterus anteriorly; the larva takes the fatty nutrient fluid through its mouth and is totally dependent on this food source. There are three larval instars within the uterus.

The females require regular blood meals for the development of the larvae, and any reduction in the frequency of blood meals will adversely effect larval development by inducing abortion or a larva which has a reduced weight at larviposition. The deposited larva, which possesses posteriorly two characteristic polypneustic lobes which are black at the time of larviposition, immediately burrows into the moist soil or sand, usually under fallen logs, bushes, large stones and tree buttresses, through peristaltic movement and pupates. The black puparium (more frequently mis-termed the pupa) remains in the ground for a period of 30 days (longer if temperatures are lower) until the adult fly emerges as a teneral fly. The puparium is shaped like a barrel and is 6–8 mm in length. There are transverse rings around the puparium. Teneral flies are soft, more lightly coloured and have an everted ptilinum — a sac on the anterior of the head between the eyes which has aided the emergence from the puparium. After emergence the fly must pump up its wings and allow its cuticle to harden before flight. The eyes are widely separated on the head of the fly and are usually large and dark brown in colour. The males are distinguished from females by the presence of a structure known as the hypopygium which is a paler knob-like structure found underneath the last abdominal segment; the female fly does not possess such a structure. The hypopygium when folded away from the abdomen reveals the male terminalia which are important in distinguishing *Glossina* species and subspecies.

Glossina require to feed approximately every two days; female flies live longer than males. The blood is obtained from vertebrate hosts as a result of the piercing of the skin by the mouthparts, which are equipped with specialized teeth (on the labellum) for penetrating the skin and creating a 'pool' of blood from which the fly feeds. Engorgement usually takes around 60 seconds, depending on the size of the fly and the ease with which blood can be obtained from the pool. The size of each blood meal is around 20–60 mg, depending on the physiological state of the fly and its size.

The blood is sucked through a food canal which is a complex structure made up of the labrum which forms a median gutter along which lies the hypopharynx; the hypopharynx is an extension of the common salivary duct of the long salivary glands and the saliva which passes down the hypopharynx has an anticoagulant effect. The paired salivary glands, the site of development of trypanosomes of the subgenus *Trypanozoon*, stretch posteriorly into the abdomen. The hypopharynx and labrum are also sites of development of trypanosomes and the narrow hypo-

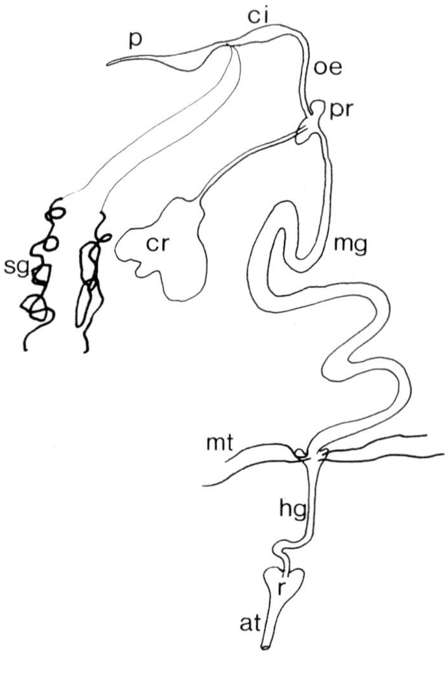

Figure22. Diagrammatic representation of the gut of the tsetse fly *Glossina*.

Abbreviations:
p = proboscis;
ci = cibarium;
oe = oesophagous;
pr = proventriculus;
sg = salivary glands;
cr = crop;
mg = midgut;
mt = Malpighian tubules;
hg = hindgut;
r = rectum;
at = anal tube.

pharynx is the site from which infective forms of trypanosomes reach the mammalian host.

The food canal leads into the cibarium, pharynx and oesophagus which form the foregut of the fly. The proventriculus forms the junction between foregut and midgut and the crop. A diverticulum in which blood is initially stored, prior to its passage to the midgut, leads off the proventriculus. The proventriculus is an important region, from which the peritrophic membrane is formed, which passes back into the midgut where *T. brucei* and *T. congolense* develop. The peritrophic membrane extends throughout the midgut and plays an important role in the life cycle of the trypanosomes. There are four Malpighian tubules at the midgut–hindgut junction and the hindgut leads to a bulb-like rectum before the anus is reached (figure 22).

Ecology and trapping methods

A vast amount of information has accumulated over the past 70–80 years on the ecology of *Glossina* species. These data have been of direct value in epidemiology and in the planning of control campaigns. Sound ecological data are a prerequisite for a determination of appropriate methods of control.

Ecological information is dependent on the accuracy of methods of sampling populations. The methods available for sampling tsetse flies have been improved markedy over recent years with the introduction of more efficient trapping methods. Early studies depended on 'fly-rounds' which were carried out by two catchers over a predetermined track of 10 000 yards; the catchers stopped every 500 yards to collect the flies attracted to them; bait cattle replaced human bait in some areas, or a black screen or animal skin supported on poles was used. Tsetse can also be caught by vehicle capture as hungry flies are attracted to moving objects. The proportion of females, particularly of *G. morsitans,* which came to flyrounds was much less than the 50:50 ratio which would be expected if males and females were equally attracted. Studies on traps demonstrated that flies could be caught by objects which simulated hosts and that a higher proportion of females were then caught. Important recent studies have demonstrated that man is repellent to *G. morsitans* and indeed many flyrounds carried out in *G. morsitans* habitats could have been influenced by this. Flyround data can also be influenced by circadian activity cycles of *Glossina*.

Interest in the development of traps has been accelerated recently; it has been found that there is an active ingredient in ox breath which is capable of increasing the catch of *G. m. morsitans.* Attempts to identify the active component indicate that ketones may be important. When carbon dioxide and acetone are incorporated in a trap the catch is increased by eight times. A biconical trap developed in West Africa without any chemical attractant has proved of value in many areas for collecting tsetse flies, particularly riverine *G. palpalis* group species and *G. pallidipes* in East Africa (figure 23).

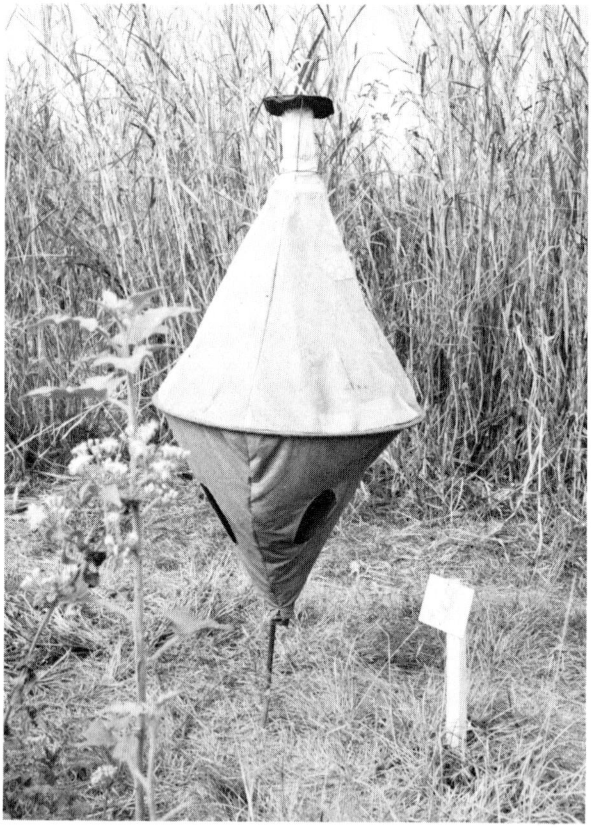

Figure 23. Biconical tsetse trap developed for the capture of riverine *Glossina*, with a blue lower cone. Traps are placed adjacent to rivers in fringing riverine vegetation, or around villages or in plantations, to catch *G. palpalis* and *G. tachinoides*. Traps are approximately 1·5 m in height.

Electric grids through which high voltages (3–6 kV) are passed have been used to assess the effectiveness of different types of trap and bait (figure 24). Mark–release–recapture methods have been developed to estimate the absolute density of *Glossina*. A method based on 'trapping-out' of fly populations using biconical traps can also be used for absolute population estimates.

Populations of *Glossina* fluctuate greatly depending on the time of the year. These changes are primarily related to meteorological changes or availability of host animals. Such changes have usually been monitored over long periods by flyrounds or traps. Fly populations are highest at the end of the rainy season and decline as the dry season advances due to an increase in the temperature, a decrease in humidity and a reduction in the availability of suitable habitats. As the dry season advances, *G. morsitans* populations, which usually live in open savannah, become restricted to densely vegetated areas near water courses;

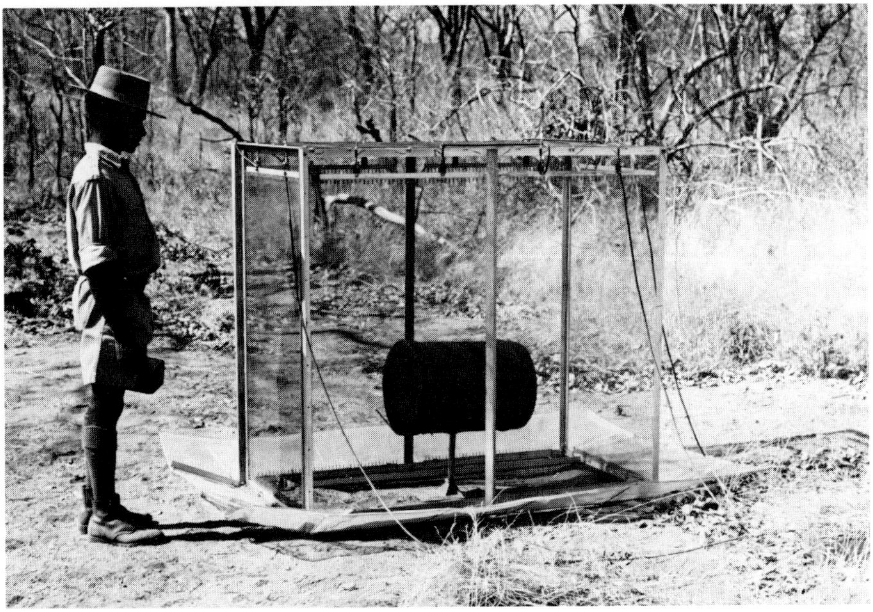

Figure 24. A cylindrical visual bait surrounded by a cage of electrified netting. Flies attracted to the target are killed or stunned as they collide with the netting and fall, to be retained in a sticky hopper at ground level.

Courtesy of Dr. G. Vale.

conversely, *G. palpalis* group flies which are normally restricted to more humid habitats, especially at the end of the dry season, are more widely distributed in savannah during the rainy season. In Nigeria the times of maximum and minimum fly populations (*G. morsitans*) are dependent on the vegetation zone in which the flies are found. The minimum population of *G. morsitans* is found earlier in the dry season (March) in the more northerly Sudan savannah zone where the dry season is more intense; the maximum population reaches a peak earlier due to the shorter rainy season. In the northern Guinea savannah, however, the minimum population is in May and the maximum in December. Detailed studies of *G. morsitans* distribution throughout Africa have revealed that its distribution is largely controlled by climatic conditions, especially mean temperature and mean saturation deficit.

Glossina species have invaded many types of habitat within the area of the distribution of the genus (see figures 25 and 26). The genus is usually regarded as being divided into three groups based on the morphology of the genitalia, but which correspond generally with the habitat: the riverine species of the *palpalis* group; the woodland/savannah *morsitans* group; and the *fusca* group of flies associated with the more humid forested areas. However, this categorization into species groups infesting particular habitats is not absolute. As has already been pointed out above, *G. morsitans* group flies are found in riverine vegetation at the extremes of their range; *G. palpalis* group flies, in more humid forested areas of forest/savannah transition zones, can be found well away from standing or running water. The latter group has also become associated with peridomestic habitats in some parts of West Africa, living and breeding in close proximity to man and his domestic animals (particularly pigs). Invasion of peridomestic habitats in East Africa by *G. fuscipes*, which is normally confined to lakeshore and riverine vegetation, was aided by the invasion of the villages by *Euphorbia* and *Lantana camara* which produces thicket-type vegetation, and provides an ideal habitat for flies. Dense continuous thickets are also a favoured habitat of *G. pallidipes* in Eastern Africa (see figure 51, p. 125).

G. morsitans subspecies each have characteristic habitats in the different parts of Africa in which they occur. *G. m. submorsitans* is usually associated with doka (*Isoberlinia doka*) woodland of the northern Guinea savannah; *G. m. morsitans* with the mopane (*Colophospermum mopane*) and miombo woodlands of Central and Southern Africa. The miombo woodland where *G. m. centralis* is found in East and Central Africa is similar to doka of West Africa with *Isoberlinia*, *Brachystegia* and *Julbernardia* being the dominant trees. There has, however, been a recent appreciation that although *Glossina* species have characteristically

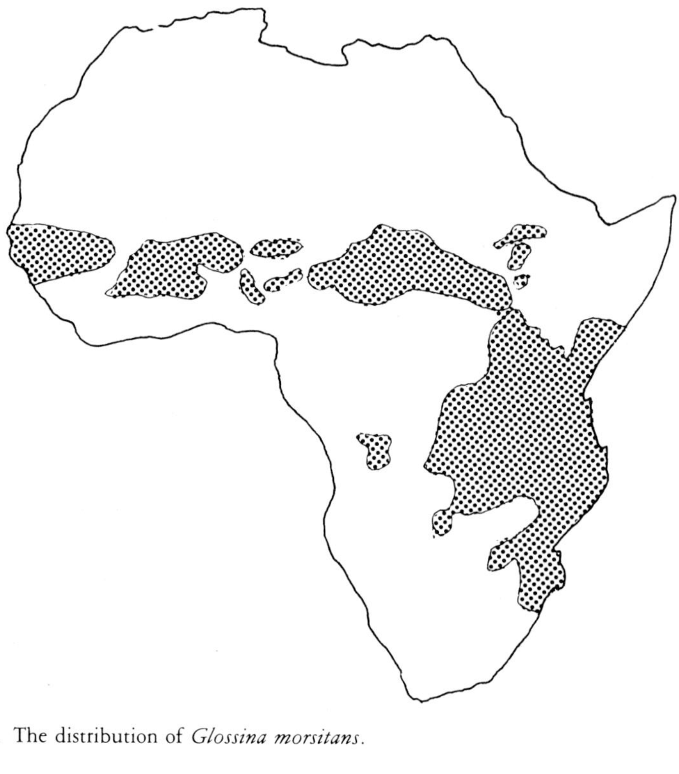

Figure 25. The distribution of *Glossina morsitans*.

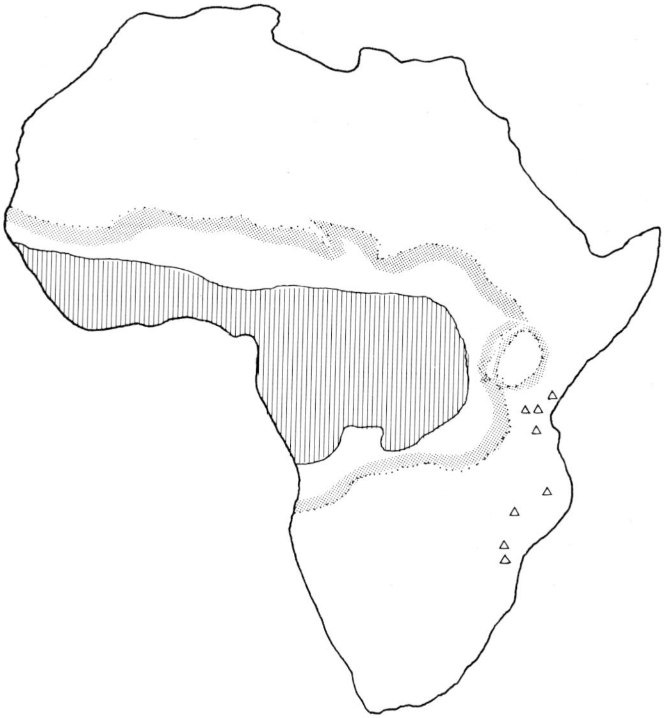

Figure 26. The distribution of *G. fusca group* ||||||||||||||||, *G. palpalis* group and *G. brevipalpis* △△△ .

occupied these classical habitats they are also capable of invading vegetation planted by man. In West Africa *G. palpalis* group species can be found in mango, oil palm, banana, cocoa and sugar cane plantations and can form peridomestic populations. *G. pallidipes* has recently been found to invade coniferous plantations in Kenya.

Activity

The behaviour and activity of *Glossina* are important aspects of their biology in relation to control and disease transmission. In the laboratory *G. morsitans* has a circadian rhythm of activity known as a U-shaped activity pattern. Peak spontaneous activity is recorded during early morning and evening with reduced spontaneous activity during the middle of the day when temperature in nature would be at its highest and hosts inactive. In nature there are marked seasonal differences in activity, which is largely limited to an ambient temperature above 13–17 °C; for example in the cool season, in the northern parts of *Glossina* distribution, peak activity occurs at midday as it is too cool during the early morning and evening. During the wet season, however, in the Zambesi Valley activity is uniform throughout the day as the temperature changes are small. Thus, although an intrinsic circadian rhythm has been demonstrated in the laboratory, the activity of flies in the field is also governed by temperature, humidity, light intensity and season.

Glossina have been shown to respond to various stimuli both in the laboratory and the field. The hungrier the flies become the more responsive they are to visual and olfactory stimuli. In the laboratory flies respond to stripes moving with an angular velocity of 3–7 degrees per second, which is equivalent to a man walking at 5 km/h at a distance of 10–30 m from the fly. Flight capacity of *Glossina* is limited to several minutes in every 24 h period due to the extensive metabolic requirement of flight activity.

Glossina respond to olfactory stimuli in addition to visual ones. Ox breath odour (see above) has been found to be a powerful attractant. Acetone and CO_2 have been found to be attractive but not as attractive as ox breath. An attempt to identify the active component in ox breath is currently underway and would be of great significance for control if it could be isolated. Studies so far indicate that odour stimulates fly activity but that visual stimuli orientate the fly to the target. Sounds are also emitted by *Glossina* which may play a role in host finding or orientating flies to a certain part of a host. The significance of sound in *Glossina* biology remains to be elucidated.

Feeding habits

The feeding behaviour of the more important species of *Glossina* is summarized in Table 6. It has become clear that although well defined feeding patterns exist, these may be modified depending on host availability; there are several examples of unusual *Glossina* feeding patterns associated with invasion of peridomestic habitats or habitat modification in some way. The development of accurate serological methods for the analysis of the sources of *Glossina* blood meals has made a most important contribution to our knowledge of fly ecology and disease epidemiology. The most important test, which enables the host to be identified to species, is the haemagglutination inhibition test; a highly sensitive complement fixation test has also been developed. A wide range of mammals, some birds and reptiles have been identified as hosts of *Glossina*, but some species of mammal are common but not frequently fed on. These include carnivores, zebra and impala. Impala have a vigorous muscular skin twitch which seems to render them difficult for *Glossina* to feed upon. Even though *Glossina* do not normally feed on impala they can digest the blood meal as efficiently as that of other hosts if able to acquire a meal. Some hosts may also be either visually unattractive or emit unattractive odours. However, even though a host may be unattractive under normal circumstances and not form a part of the normal diet, a really hungry fly will take a blood meal from more rarely used hosts. Species of *Glossina* can be grouped into those species which take their meals predominantly from Suidae, such as *G. swynnertoni* and *G. austeni*; from Bovidae, *G. pallidipes*, *G. longipalpis* and *G.*

Table 6. Blood meal sources of various *Glossina* species (in per cent).

Species of *Glossina*	Primates	Suidae	Bovidae	Other mammals	Birds	Reptiles
palpalis	39	6	22	4	2	27
fuscipes	18	3	38	5	1	34
tachinoides	43	2	30	16	–	9
pallidipes	3	13	80	4	–	–
longipalpis	2	4	90	2	–	–
fusca	–	14	74	13	–	–
morsitans subspecies	7–18	36–46	22–45	7–15	1–5	–
swynnertoni	4	65	23	7	1	–
austeni	5	58	36	2	–	–

fusca; and the *G. morsitans* subspecies which take meals equally from Suidae and Bovidae. The *G. palpalis* group species feed on man and any available animals, the percentage of blood meals depending on the local availability of hosts which may be pig, bushbuck or reptiles (crocodile or *Varanus* lizards). The *palpalis* group are said to be catholic feeders. Some species of *Glossina* are more highly specialized and depend consistently on certain species of host for their food, for example, *G. brevipalpis* feeds predominantly on hippopotamus and *G. longipennis* on rhinoceros.

Resting sites

The resting behaviour of *Glossina* is of considerable importance in view of the need for information as to where residual insecticides can be most effectively applied. Flies can be marked with fluorescent powders, paints, small patches of reflecting paper or radioisotopes (^{55}Fe). Some studies have been carried out in large cages, but results from this type of experiment are not as satisfactory as in uncaged conditions. Resting sites vary with sex, species and season, and between day and night. During the day *G. morsitans* rests mainly on trunks and lower branches, particularly the underside of horizontal branches of trees, and at night flies rest in the upper foliage of trees. *G. swynnertoni* rests on the underside of branches 2·5–10 cm in diameter 1·3–3 m above the ground. Selective application of insecticides to these sites would be an appropriate method of control.

Riverine flies of the *G. palpalis* group rest closer to the ground. When in the proximity of water they are usually found within 1–2 m of the water edge and resting, by day, on twigs and small woody parts. At night they move to the lower surfaces of leaves where the stomata provide a more humid microclimate. Peridomestic populations of *G. tachinoides* have been observed resting very close to the ground level on the dried fronds of palms used as fencing material. There are considerable variations in the resting behaviour of a given species in different areas and vegetation types and this topic must be studied in relation to each part of Africa.

Age determination

Glossina populations can be aged using two techniques. The most accurate method is applicable to females only. Males and females can be aged approximately by the degree of fray on the trailing edge of the wings. This fray is induced by activity which results in the appearance of a series of scar or scar-like indentations in the wing edge. A scale of one to six is used where one is a perfect, undamaged wing and six is where there is damage along the whole edge of both wings. The mean wing fray of a population is calculated and from this figure an estimate of the mean age of the population is derived.

The physiological age of females can be determined accurately by dissection of the reproductive system. The number of ovulations which have taken place can be assessed, up to a maximum of seven, from the size of the ovarioles and their relative positions. Ovulation always takes place in a regular sequence and is repeated in that sequence: there are two ovarioles on each side of the mid-line and the sequence of ovulations, as viewed from the dorsal side, is right inner, left inner, right outer and left outer. After four ovulations the sequence is repeated but the remnants of the follicles remain visible. This information, the state of the uterus and the age of any larva in the uterus, can give very precisely the age of female *Glossina*. These data, together with that on mean temperature in the area of origin of the fly (which determines the rate at which the various reproductive processes occur), will have important bearings on control operations.

Age estimations are important during non-residual insecticide applications and in assessing, after residual insecticide applications, the effectiveness of the application and level of reinvasion. Dissection of females can also give values of natural or induced abortion (e.g., after insecticide application) rates in the population.

Control

The most effective method of controlling trypanosomiasis is to avoid being bitten by tsetse. This may be achieved by concentrating populations in areas free from tsetse or by controlling the fly. Control of *Glossina* has been and continues to be undertaken by a variety of methods. These can be categorized as: alteration of habitat; pesticide application; genetic control; traps; biological control; and physiological interference.

Alteration of the habitat

(*a*) by removal of vegetation either by hand or by mechanical means such as bulldozers or tractors dragging chains;

(*b*) by removing, usually by shooting, preferred wildlife hosts or keeping game away from areas where livestock will be kept by parallel game and stock fences, reinforced by 'tsetse pickets', with the area between the fences cleared of trees and scrub.

These latter techniques have largely been abandoned but occasionally cleared barrier areas are used to prevent reinvasion of areas cleared by other means or to protect areas where experimental sterile male release programmes are undertaken.

Perhaps the most effective habitat changes are achieved almost incidentally when populations exceed about 40 people per square kilometre, destroying much woodland and driving out game animals. It is unusual for tsetse to be able to maintain populations with only man or cattle to feed on.

Pesticide application

Insecticides can be applied from the ground or from the air. Groundspray application uses either knapsack sprayers or vehicle sprayers for residual application to specific resting sites (selective application) or motorized mist-blowers for non-residual aerosol applications (figure 50, p. 125). Aerial application can be made either using fixed-wing aircraft (see figures 51 and 52) or helicopters. Fixed-wing aircraft are usually only used for non-residual application. This type of application of insecticide, particularly with endosulfan, has been made in Botswana, Kenya and Zambia. Five to six sequential applications of 10–20 g/ha of endosulfan are applied. Helicopters (Bell 47G) are used to apply both non-residual and residual insecticide formulations. Helicopters, though more expensive to operate than fixed-wing aircraft, produce a downdraft from the main rotor blades which aids the penetration of droplets through the vegetation, particularly in riverine forest galleries. More discriminative applications are possible using helicopters whereby only certain vegetation types are sprayed.

Effective aerial insecticide applications depend on the correct equipment, formulations of insecticide and meteorological conditions to allow the droplets to reach the *Glossina* resting sites.

Insecticides in common use for *Glossina* control are DDT, dieldrin and endosulfan. The synthetic pyrethroids, permethrin, cypermethrin and deltamethrin, can also be used. Unlike many insects of medical importance there is as yet no evidence of resistance to these insecticides, although biochemical studies and computer simulations predict that it could occur. However, as may be expected, side effects of pesticides on non-target organisms have been recorded. DDT and dieldrin cause mortality in some exposed vertebrates, particularly insectivorous birds; endosulfan is particularly toxic to fish whilst the synthetic pyrethroids are toxic to freshwater Crustacea. All insecticides kill non-target insects but the more rapid reproductive rate of insects other than *Glossina* and the discriminative and selective application of the insecticide reduces long-term effects on non-target insects and permits a recovery of the populations. *Glossina* eradication or control, if successful, will result, in the long term, in far more extensive habitat change and loss of species following changes in land use, than due to any insecticide application. Insecticides (deltamethrin) can be incorporated into traps in order to reduce *Glossina* populations and impregnated traps, screens and car tyres are in use for purposes of control.

Genetic control

Sterile-male techniques have been advocated for the control of *Glossina* following the success of attacks on other Diptera such as screw worm and Mediterranean fruit fly using mass-release techniques. These techniques have been tested in the field, but rearing *Glossina* is labour intensive due to the low reproductive rate and haematophagy. It is suggested that sterile-male release cannot alone be a method for large-scale control. However, sterile-male release could possibly contribute to integrated control programmes, where initially the population is reduced by the application of non-residual insecticides. In pilot schemes to date non-residual insecticides were used to reduce the population by around 90 per cent prior to the release of irradiated males. Male *Glossina* puparia or adults are exposed to a gamma irradiation source of 11 kilorads in a nitrogen atmosphere. Male flies thus irradiated must compete for wild females for mating as effectively as wild males. Release can be as puparia or adults. Adults are released after a blood meal has been taken in the laboratory in areas where sleeping sickness is endemic. Pilot projects in Tanzania and Upper Volta indicate that the technique is theoretically possible, but a great effort is required in capital outlay and to date it is only effective in very small areas compared with the vast total area infected. An earlier project in Zimbabwe used chemosterilants for sterilization.

Sterile-male techniques dependent on mass release methods depend on efficient fly rearing facilities, and clearly if several species are vectors in an area all species need to be bred for control to be effective. Genetic control using hybrid sterility has been experimentally tested by the introduction into a population of flies which, when mated with wild flies, produce sterile offspring. These methods have not as yet been shown to be practical in a large-scale programme. Sterile male flies when released are also capable of becoming infected with and transmitting salivarian trypanosomes.

Traps

Traps of various types have been developed to reduce *Glossina* populations; these initially incorporated sticky materials to retain flies or, more recently, have used a non-return system. The biconical trap has been shown to be capable of reducing *Glossina* populations and to be of value in itself in reducing disease transmission. Perhaps more promising are odour baited traps. These can attract vast numbers of flies which can be automatically chemosterilized and then released back into their habitat. This could be an important and viable future technique of *Glossina* control. Hand catching has also been used as a method of *Glossina* control.

Biological control

Biological control using pathogens or parasitoids has been advocated, but as a large scale practical solution this seems unlikely to be of use. A parasitoid of *Glossina* puparia, the tiny hymenopteran wasp *Nesolynx* (= *Syntomosphyrum*) has been used on a small scale, as it can be reared in large numbers in puparia of house flies. However, when released in areas where *Glossina* was found it was not found to be effective in reducing the *Glossina* population. Other potential parasitoids include dipterans of the genus *Exhyalanthrax* (Bombyliidae) and the hymenopteran genus *Chrestomutilla* (= *Mutilla*). Adult *Glossina* are subject to predation by Asilidae (robber flies). Flies may be trapped in spider webs, for example of the genus *Nephilia*, or be caught by the jumping spiders *Plexippus* or *Hersilia*. Predation requires to be more extensively evaluated as a potential tool in *Glossina* control. Although various micro-organisms have been found in *Glossina* (bacteria, viruses, *Rickettsia*, mermithid nematodes), no use of them can as yet be suggested in biological control.

Physiological interference

Physiological methods have been suggested for *Glossina* control. Although pheromones have been identified, the short distance (2–3 cm) over which they act probably prevents their use; however, some insect growth regulators (IGRs) such as dimilin (diflubenzuron), have been found to inhibit chitin synthesis, thus preventing the development of viable larvae. A topical application of an appropriate dose to a fly will induce a female to produce, throughout her life, larvae which cannot pupariate and are thus non-viable. IGRs are in use in agricultural entomology for the contol of pests and a suitable formulation of one for *Glossina* control is now awaited for field trials.

Although tsetse control has been pursued using many techniques, it should be remembered that the objective throughout must be the control of trypanosomiasis. The present approach is one of evaluating the land-use potential of particular areas prior to embarking on any strategy; such an approach requires detailed surveys of distribution of the fly and the problem of the disease — human or animal. This is followed by the planning of an appropriate strategy for the region in question.

TRIATOMINAE: VECTORS OF *TRYPANOSOMA CRUZI*

The insects

Blood sucking bugs belonging to the family Reduviidae (sub-order Heteroptera, order Hemiptera) are the vectors of *Trypanosoma cruzi*, the causative agent of Chagas' disease (figures 27 and 74). These bugs are widespread throughout Central and South America as well as in the southern states of the USA (figure 28); there are 14 genera and about 111 species recognized as valid in the subfamily Triatominae, and most of these are recorded as being infected with *T. cruzi* or closely related organisms. Although many of these species are restricted to specialized sylvatic habitats, some species, particularly *Triatoma infestans*, *Panstrongylus megistus* and *Rhodnius prolixus*, have become associated with domestic and peridomestic habitats and have therefore become important vectors of Chagas' disease to man. The major vectors and the ecology of the bugs in relation to disease transmission and epidemiology are discussed in Chapter 6. In addition to the American species there are six species of *Triatoma* found in South-east Asia and one genus (*Linsheosteus*) in India. The cosmopolitan *T. rubrofasciata* has been associated with the transmission of the rat trypanosome *T. (Megatrypanum) conorhini* in Japan.

The family Reduviidae are known as cone-nosed, assassin or kissing bugs. In Spanish they are known as 'chipos' or 'vinchucas' and in Portuguese 'barbeiros'. Both males and females and all 5 nymphal stages are haematophagous. They are

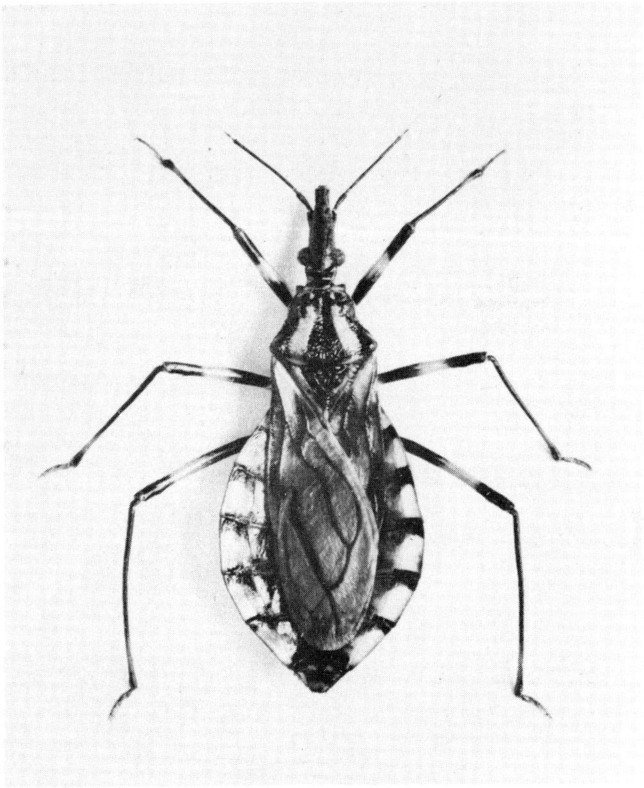

Figure 27. A female triatomine bug, *Triatoma braziliensis* (× 3).

characterized by the possession of piercing and sucking mouthparts and a transverse sulcus which divides the head into two lobes. The rostrum is reflexed below the head and has three distinct segments with the terminal segment coming into contact with a stridulatory furrow. There are two pairs of scent glands on the metathorax.

Adult triatomines vary in size from as small as 1 cm to the largest species such as *Dipetalogaster maxima* which can be 4 cm in length. The head is elongated and has a pair of laterally positioned compound eyes. A pair of ocelli are also present in the adults of most species. A pair of four-jointed antennae are located on the head. There are two pairs of wings. The forewings are known as hemielytra, as the basal part of the wing is hard and thickened whereas the distal area is membranous. There is great variation between species in the use of wings for flight. Bugs are sometimes attracted to light at night and can be caught at considerable heights. Adult bugs fly in response to inadequate food supply and are capable of flying considerable distances, which is important in the colonization of new habitats as well as in spreading Chagas' disease. The wingless nymphal stages

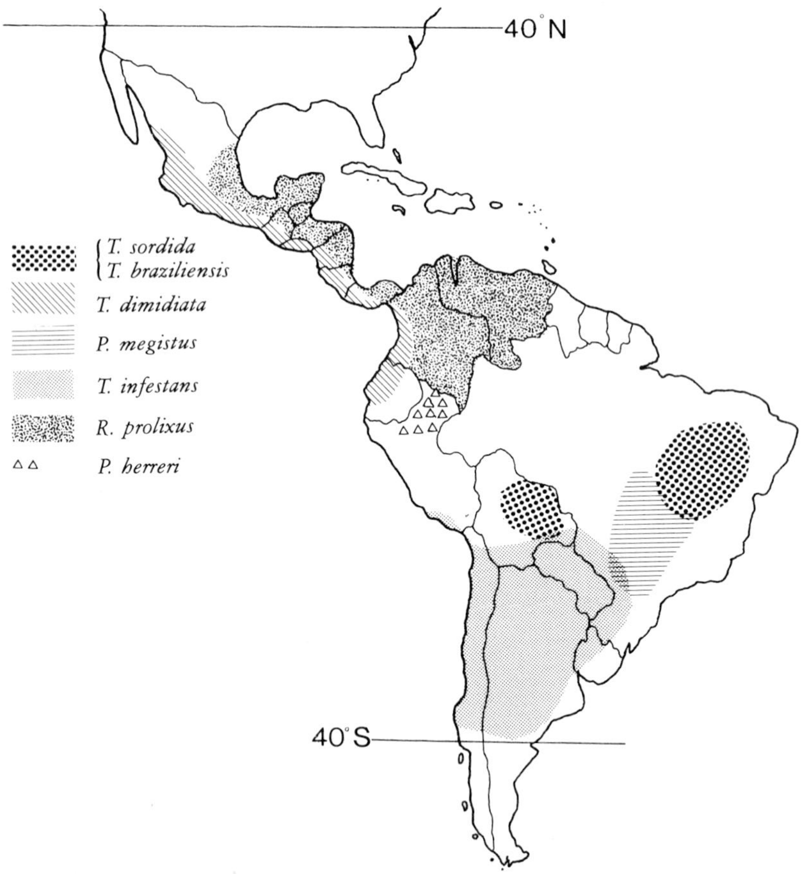

Figure 28. The distribution of important vectors of Chagas' disease in Central and South America.

do not fly and remain within the area in which the eggs are deposited. Eggs are laid in the microhabitat of the adults such as cracks or crevices in homes, burrows or nests of the mammalian or avian hosts of the bugs. Eggs of some species are laid loose, others glued in clumps to the substrate.

The eggs are usually faintly coloured white, pink or yellow and 1·5–2·5 mm in length with a characteristic constriction in the egg just in front of an operculum. The adult female can commence depositing eggs within a week or so of the final moult from the fifth instar nymph; the number of eggs that can be laid during any period is highly variable (200–2000) and depends on many factors but particularly the availability of blood meals; bugs can remain without food for long periods and such starvation will not effect the persistence or viability of trypanosomes in the gut. The eggs hatch in 1–2 weeks but this period may be extended under low tempertures. There are five nymphal instars which may require between 4 and 48 months between hatching and the final moult of the fifth instar to adult bugs. The rapidity of the life cycle is dependent on the temperature and on the frequency and volume of blood meals. There are optimum conditions at which the highest percentage of eggs or nymphs will develop for each species, but these conditions may not be those at which development occurs most rapidly. Nymphs can imbibe between 6 and 12 times their own weight in blood. Adults generally only take in three times their own weight. Blood-meal weights increase through each nymphal stage, adult bugs usually ingesting 100–300 mg. Some fifth instar nymphs can take considerably more blood than this. Adult females take more than males. Most triatomines can be easily reared in the laboratory: indeed *Rhodnius prolixus* has been used extensively in research on insect physiology. Females copulate within 1–3 days after emergence and males can inseminate females 5–9 days after emergence. A period of 10–20 days elapses between copulation and oviposition. Unfed females may lay fertile eggs if they had maintained a high nutritional status as nymphs. Triatomines can copulate on more than one occasion though multiple mating seems of no importance in maximizing fertility ot fecundity. Blood meals are necessary for viable egg production. In the laboratory adult males tend to live longer than females. Laboratory studies indicate that some species of bug show 100 per cent survival until 11–13 months after emergence but this high rate of survival is not to be expected in the field.

Ecology and sampling methods

Sampling

Sampling triatomines involves simple collection techniques. In homes which harbour bugs, timed manual collection by experienced collectors, following a 0·3 per cent pyrethrum spray to induce bugs to emerge from inaccesible crevices, provides relative population estimates. Homes in infested areas may be purchased, the whole structure systematically demolished, the bugs collected, and their positions recorded. An artificial refuge can be used, the Gomez–Nunez box, which is filled with folded paper and then nailed to the wall. The box is left for 2–4 weeks and then examined for bugs, eggs, exuviae and faeces — it is particularly useful for low density infestations or in post-control monitoring. This technique is more effective for *R. prolixus* than *T. infestans* and *P. megistus*. Light trapping by black, ultraviolet or normal light can be used, but generally catches are only adult males.

An interesting method has recently been described for finding bugs in the nests of sylvatic mammals. The mammals are captured, then released carrying a long reel of thread which plays out as the animal returns home. The line can then be followed and the nest discovered.

Absolute population size can be estimated by mark–release–recapture methods. Bugs are colour-marked with acrylic paints on the legs, pronotum or sternum of the abdomen. The generous application of paint on legs enables exuviae to be recognized after moulting. The Zippins withdrawal sampling method has also been used for calculating the total population. The graph of successive captures is extrapolated to zero, and the original population thus calculated.

Host location and feeding

Triatomines locate their hosts over short ranges by orientation to temperature gradients detected by the antennae; carbon dioxide produces increased activity of the bugs. Pheromones have been identified in the faeces of nymphs of *Rhodnius* and *Triatoma*; with the habit of defecation soon after feeding — important in transmission of *T. cruzi* — the pheromone in bug faeces might attract unfed bugs to a source of food. The 'faecal aggregation pheromone' may also be important in the maintenance of the correct gut fauna by coprophagy. As with other exclusively haematophagous insects, bacterial and fungal symbionts are essential for the development of *R. prolixus* and *Triatoma infestans* as well as other species. Bugs will, however, only seek a blood meal if other physiological parameters, particularly food remaining in the gut from a previous meal are fulfilled. This is probably determined by the degree of abdominal stretch which exists. The structure of the gut is shown in figure 29. If hungry, bugs will probe on any warm surface and sample underlying fluid; provided the appropriate engorgement factors such as adenosine triphosphate (ATP) are present, as detected by sensilla in the proboscis, then engorgement will occur until the amount of blood imbibed is sufficient, as determined by abdominal stretch receptors. The distension of the abdomen also triggers the moulting cycle in nymphs. Bugs are capable of withstanding long periods without food, the later instars being able to tolerate longer periods of starvation. Fourth and fifth instars can survive between five and seven months without a blood meal. Many species of bugs are ecologically restricted (see Table 7), for example, to the burrows or nests of particular mammals such as armadillos (*Dasypus*) or wood rats (*Neotoma*), and have host preferences associated with this ecological restriction. However, from collated information it is clear that the most important vector bug species are quire opportunistic in their host selection and a wide variety of hosts are fed upon. Occasional reptile and amphibian meals have been recorded. The host preferences are indicated by blood-meal identification, but host proximity is perhaps the most important factor in host selection. This is underlined by the ease with which triatomines can be fed on unusual hosts in the laboratory. The apparent feeding preference will therefore vary depending on the habitat, ecology and presence of suitable hosts. Thus *T. sordida* feeds largely on birds (chickens) and is found in chicken houses in Brazil, but on oppossums and rodents when found in natural sylvatic habitats in a farming area.

Palm trees of over 20 species throughout South America are habitats of *Rhodnius*, *Triatoma* and *Panstrongylus* species. Other biotopes of triatomines include bromeliads, bark of trees, hollow trees and fence posts.

Although it is evident that some triatomines are habitat-specific and are unable

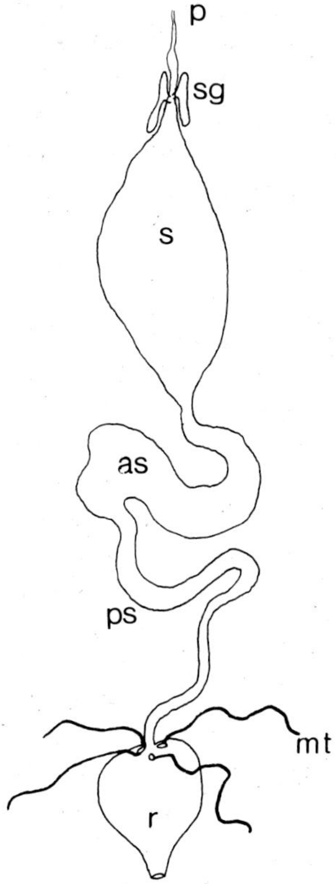

Figure 29. Diagram of the gut of a triatomine bug such as *Rhodnius prolixus*.

Abbreviations:
p = proboscis;
sg = salivary glands;
s = stomach;
as = anterior segment of midgut;
ps = posterior segment of midgut;
mt = Malpighian tubules;
r = rectum.

Table 7. Summary of habitats and behaviour of triatomine species.

Bug species	*Habitat*	*Food host*
Panstrongylus geniculatus	Armadillo burrows	Armadillos
Triatoma dimidiata	Hollow trees, stockpiles of domestic fuelwood, inside houses	Oppossums, man, domestic animals
T. infestans	Inside houses	Man, dogs, cats, chickens
T. maculata	Inside houses	Birds (chickens)
T. protracta	Wood rat nests	Wood rats
Psammolestes tertius	Birds nests	Birds esp. thornbirds *Phacellodomus*
Rhodnius prolixus	Palm trees (*Scheelea lumboltiana*), inside houses	Mammals, birds and man
Dipetalogaster maxima	Under rocks, stones	Mammals, lizards
Cavernicola pilosa	Bat roosts	Bats

to occupy other habitats, the important vector species have been able to colonize peridomestic habitats. The means by which dispersal and new colonization occur is not well documented. Some adults have considerable flight range. Transfer of bugs by transportation of infested articles, such as luggage and blankets, in trains and buses, as well as in firewood have been described; *T. dimidiata*, which inhabits hollow trees where it feeds on oppossums, is brought into homes with fuelwood.

R. prolixus, which is an arboreal species and lives in palm trees, is transferred by the passive transport of eggs to human dwellings. The eggs are cemented to the substrate of palm fronds used as roofing material. Nymphal stages are transported on birds and migratory birds may play an important role in dispersal. Attraction of adult bugs to the lights of new homes may also enable colonization. However, colonization of restricted sylvatic habitats is less easy to explain.

Bugs are active at night and exhibit well defined circadian rhythms. Activity commences at 1800–1900 h in the major vector species, *R. prolixus*, *P. megistus* and *T. infestans*. The cycle can be reversed within 3–5 days by reversal of the photoperiod regime. However, sylvatic species (e.g., *D. maxima*) are aggressive in daylight; they are also swift runners, enabling them to escape rapidly under rocks and stones.

Vector control techniques

The most effective method of reducing the problems of Chagas' disease is undoubtedly the provision of housing in which bugs cannot breed.

Mud or adobe wall structures provide cracks and crevices for triatomine populations. The use of concrete bricks or other suitable materials for walls of homes would appreciably reduce the frequency with which man is bitten. Roofing materials such as zinc or aluminium to replace dead vegetation such as straw, palm fronds or leaves would have a similar effect.

Metal roofs, however, are not always acceptable as they become very hot in the South American climate. Even well constructed houses may provide bug habitats in furniture, behind wall decorations or in building materials. These measures are, however, expensive and unlikely to be realized soon, and although this is recognized as the most effective long-term solution more practical steps have been taken, mainly the use of persistent insecticides such as dieldrin and BHC. However, bugs are highly tolerant of organochlorines, and DDT is usually ineffective. The aim of insecticide application has been to interrupt disease transmission. Applications of BHC at a dosage of one gram per square metre at intervals of 50 days have given highly effective control for a period of three years. Resistance to organochlorine compounds has been reported from limited areas of Venezuela (*R. protracta* and *T. maculata*) where they have had to be replaced by malathion and propoxur.

Spraying homes in antimalarial campaigns has had some impact on bug populations, but although it does reduce transmission, it will not kill the sylvatic bugs. Similarly, when the persistence is lost there can be reinvasion from other areas of infestation, either domestic or sylvatic.

Alternative methods of control using juvenile hormones (JH) and their analogues have been tested in laboratory and in field trials. The juvenile hormones and analogues block development, preventing acquisition of adult features; JH mimics are persistent in the field but also affect other insects. They are not regarded as a commercially viable product for bug control. In the field topical application is clearly inappropriate but formulation for tarsal pick-up in a paint or as a dust has been shown to work well, some bugs camouflage themselves with dust and thus cover themselves with dust or wettable powder formulations.

Although various parasitoids of eggs, for example, the microhymenopteran *Telenomus*, predators such as the bug *Cosmoclopius*, and pathogens, for example, the fungus *Metarhyzium*, have been described from triatomine bugs, no suitable biological control technique is presently available. However, a nematode of the family Steinernematidae, *Neoaplectana*, does show some promise. It is, however, unfortunately limited by its poor tolerance of low humidity as Chagas' disease transmission is usually in fairly arid areas. It may have some application in coastal areas of Brazil and Venezuela.

SANDFLIES: VECTORS OF *LEISHMANIA*

The insects

As far as is known, the natural vectors of all *Leishmania* species belong to the subfamily Phlebotominae of the family Psychodidae. The Phlebotominae are minute pale-brown to black hairy midges, which are readily identified by the way they hold their wings above their backs (figures 30 and 31), and by their jerky gait as they half fly, half run on a surface.

Some 600 species are distributed in all zoogeographical regions. They extend north to Central Europe, California and northern China and south to Australia, South Africa and northern Argentina.

The greatest concentrations of species are in the forests of South America where the genus *Lutzomyia* predominates. The main genus in the Old World is *Sergentomyia,* which is particularly well represented in the savannah belts of Africa but extends throughout the Aethiopian and Palaearctic Regions with a few representatives in the Oriental Region. *Phlebotomus* is distributed largely in the arid and semi-arid zones of the Palaearctic, with representatives in the Oriental and Aethiopian Regions. The Far Eastern and Australasian forms mostly belong to distinctive genera and subgenera.

The New World genera are conventionally separated from those of the Old World, but this has recently been questioned, and the generic classification of the group is the subject of active investigation and controversy.

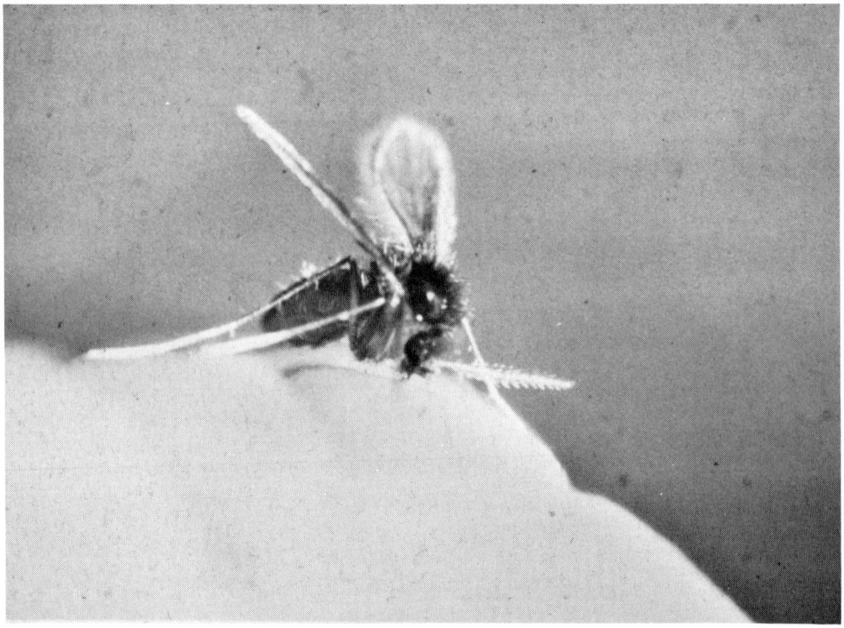

Figure 30. *Lutzomyia longipalpis* ♀, the main vector of *L. donovani* in South America. A laboratory bred specimen feeding (× 20).

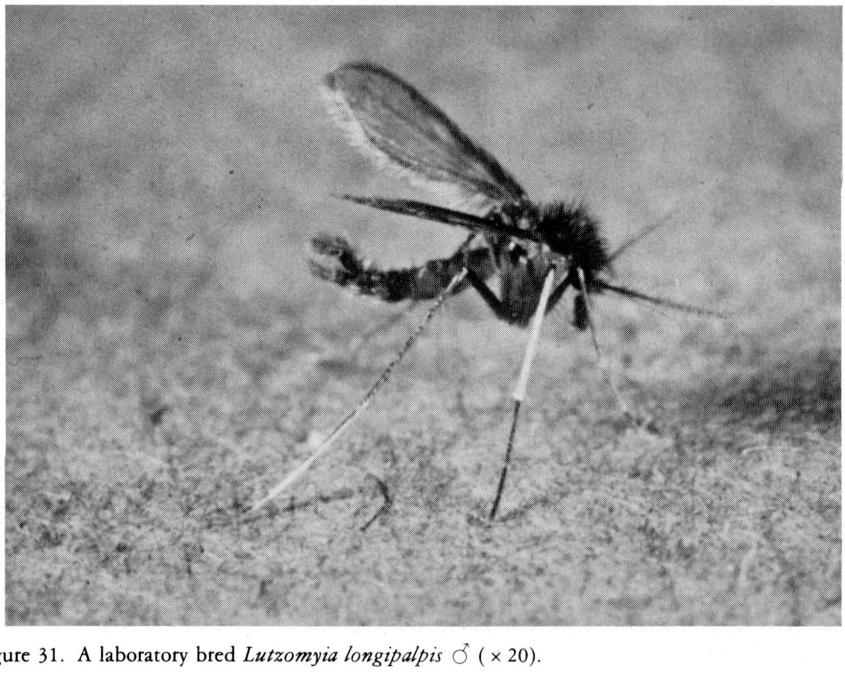

Figure 31. A laboratory bred *Lutzomyia longipalpis* ♂ (× 20).

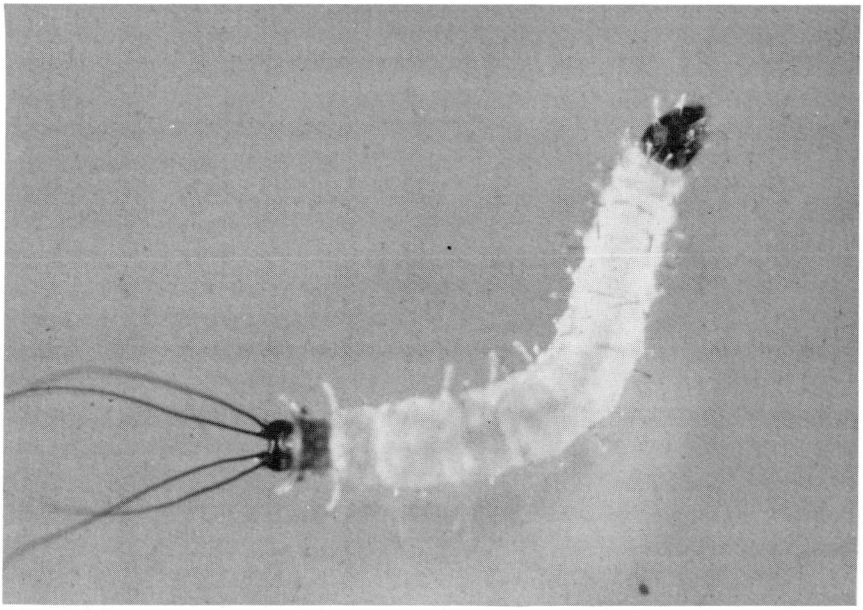

Figure 32. A fourth instar larva of *Lutzomyia longipalpis* from a laboratory colony showing four terminal bristles and 'matchstick' hairs (× 40).

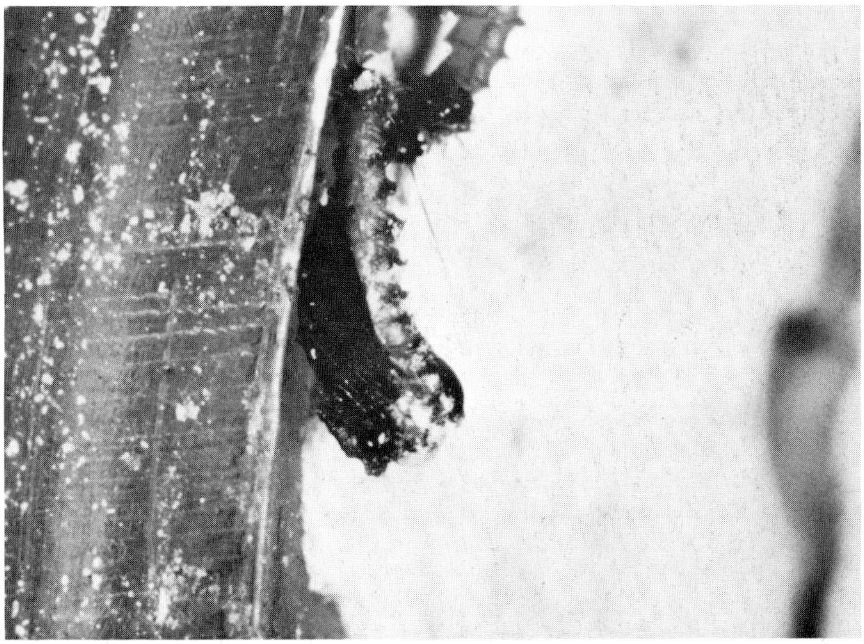

Figure 33. A pupa of *Lutzomyia longipalpis* from a laboratory colony showing the characteristic larval exuvium attached (× 40).

Most of what is known of the breeding biology of sandflies has been learned in the laboratory. Very few studies have been carried out in the field because of the great difficulty in finding sandfly larvae. Trapping newly emerged adults is less informative than finding larvae, but has given useful indications on larval habitats in the USSR, and, recently, in Panama. The aberrant cavernicolous forms from Central Africa are perhaps the only sandflies whose life history can be said to be well worked out.

Eggs are readily obtained from most species by allowing gravid females access to damp filter paper, plaster or soil. The normal batch of eggs is around 70. The eggs are spindle shaped, not operculate, about 0·3–0·4 mm in length and are either scattered or loosely stuck together. The surface of the egg is sculptured in a way which corresponds broadly with the classification of the group, and presumably also corresponds with as yet unknown ecological requirements. As the female in the laboratory usually dies during or shortly after laying, conditions are clearly not optimal, and the pattern of egg laying thus may not resemble that which occurs in nature. Larvae hatch in a few days depending on temperature, and feed by browsing on decaying organic matter and fungal growth.

Larvae are cylindrical, usually white, with a distinct, dark head. Like many dipteran larvae they move by ventral pseudo-legs. On each segment are characteristic 'matchstick' hairs with serrated stems and swollen heads (figure 32). At the posterior end four (two in the first instar) very long bristles extend like a fan at right angles to the body. The function of these bristles is not clear: they may be hygroscopic, tactile, defensive or may form a float when the habitat is flooded.

As mentioned above, larvae have rarely been found in nature. Heroic efforts in Sudan produced a single larva of *Sergentomyia africana*.

Many other authors have spent long hours in frustrated searches for sandfly larvae. Soviet workers over a period of many years searching have found numerous larvae on very rare occasions in rodent burrows. In Iran researchers have separated larvae from debris extracted from rodent burrows using a Berlese funnel. In India flotation techniques have been used to extract *P. argentipes* larvae from peri-domestic debris, particularly the accumulations beneath the drinking and feeding troughs used by village cows. Flotation was also used in Panama where the commonest larvae extracted from forest litter belonged to species which were rare or unknown as adults, but larvae of the commonest adults were not found. A few larvae of *P. longipes* were found in Ethiopia in cavities excavated in sandy banks.

Emergence traps placed over the ground or over rodent holes catch adult flies and indicate that rodent burrows are favoured breeding sites in the USSR for a variety of species. Adults of *P. dubosqi* have recently been bred from material collected from rodent holes in West Africa.

From this scattered information it can be seen that some sandfly larvae grow in humid micro-environments without free water and with considerable organic debris. Further information on their exact requirements and the factors which determine the fauna in a given area is largely wanting.

The larval development is relatively slow, as far as it is possible to ascertain, usually lasting 20–30 days. In areas with seasonal climates the final, fourth instar larvae undergo a diapause in the cold or dry season.

The larval skin remains attached to the pupa which can thus be identified by the four caudal bristles and matchstick hairs (figure 33). In laboratory colonies the pupae are usually attached to a firm substrate in a slightly drier part than where the feeding larvae congregate. The pupa is usually pale brown initially, becoming blackish when the adult is ready to emerge, usually in 1–2 weeks.

Adults emerge from the pupae in an immature state. Both sexes have a considerable volume of meconial fluid which is retained for the first day or two. The external genitalia of males rotate through 180° within a few hours of emergence; males with unrotated genitalia are occasionally found in the wild. Adults of most species measure 2–5 mm in length; they are yellow-brown to black in colour, usually with little pattern. The entire abdomen, much of the thorax and the wings are covered in scales. At rest they stand high on their long legs, holding their wings in a characteristic 'V' shape above the thorax. The females have mandibulate sucking mouthparts whose detailed structure varies according to the preferred blood source. Males have lapping mouthparts. The main structural features used in identification are the spermathecae of the females and the external genitalia of the males. The pharynx and the toothed structure in the cibarium are also important in certain groups (see figure 15).

The adults seek a dry surface, usually a vertical one, in a humid atmosphere, and are thus found in cracks or hollows in rocks or trees, as well as rodent holes. Under some conditions they rest openly on plastered walls, but in most habitats they soon disappear from view in the day-time as the atmosphere becomes too dry.

No elaborate social activities are known, but some species will congregate in large clusters on a warm rock surface at the entrance to their resting site at dusk. Males of *P. orientalis* have been observed 'dancing' — they flutter their wings, making short runs — possibly dispersing a pheromone, as females flock to the site and are rapidly engaged in copulation. There is no audible sound from the halteres of males or females so the attraction between sexes is probably olfactory and visual. Sometimes males are attracted to a blood source and meet females there. Mating takes place between males and females of all ages.

Ecology and sampling methods

Feeding

It is characteristic of haematophagous insects without symbiotic micro-organisms that they require extra nutrients in addition to the blood meal. Both males and females usually contain clear sugary liquid in their crops. The source of this sugar meal is in doubt, but they have been seen apparently feeding from the surface of green leaves. Whether honeydew or extrafloral nectaries, secretions or simple condensation is being consumed is not clear. The gut structure is illustrated diagrammatically in figure 34.

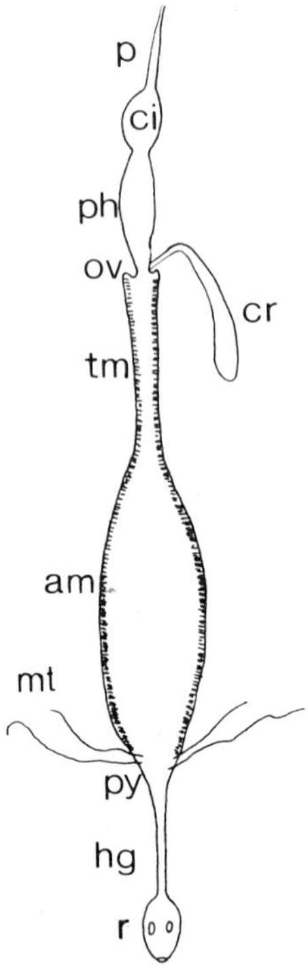

Figure 34. Diagram of a sandfly gut.

Abbreviations:
p = proboscis;
ci = cibarium;
ph = pharynx;
cr = crop;
ov = oesophageal valve;
tm = thoracic midgut;
am = abdominal midgut;
mt = Malpighian tubules;
py = pylorus;
hg = hindgut;
r = rectum.

Only females take blood and a blood meal is usually required before the eggs can develop. Some *P. papatasi* are autogenous, laying viable eggs without a blood meal. Reptiles, amphibia, birds and mammals are potential hosts; host selection depends partly on availability and partly on preference. Most species of *Sergentomyia* are reptile feeders but some will take, or even specialize in mammalian blood. *Phlebotomus* feed mainly on mammals, but some species take reptile blood and many will readily take bird blood. Host preference among *Phlebotomus* may have considerable epidemiological significance. For example, it has been suggested that the decline in kala-azar in India was due to the reduction of the anthropophilic section of the *P. argentipes* population by the malaria eradication programme, while the flies feeding on cattle remained relatively unaffected. In the genus *Lutzomyia* there are species which prefer mammals and others which specialize in reptiles. Having approached a host, the female fly usually probes two or three times before engorging. It is postulated that the probe rate of flies infected with *Leishmania* may be very much greater than that of uninfected flies. This could account for the large number of *Leishmania* lesions which sometimes appear simultaneously on a single person.

Breeding

Although breeding sites are poorly known, it is generally thought that feeding and breeding occur close together. Many *Sergentomyia* cluster in cracks used by resting lizards and probably never travel more than a few metres. Forest species feeding in the canopy may breed on the forest floor. Considerable movements have, however, been demonstrated for some *Phlebotomus* species, which may travel up to 2 km in search of food or between feeding and breeding sites.

Many species show gonotrophic concordance, with the females producing a batch of eggs after each complete blood meal. The oocytes in the ovaries of hungry females are immature; following a blood meal the oocytes begin to develop and within three of four days the digestion of the blood meal is complete and the eggs are fully developed. Frequently a double meal is taken, and occasionally one or two eggs remain unlaid. A few species show less concordance in the blood meal, and generally sugar meals may be taken at any time. Parasitic infections of bat trypanosomes in sandflies have been shown to disturb gonotrophic concordance.

Longevity

Since female flies in captivity usually die following egg laying, longevity studies in the laboratory have little bearing on what happens in nature.

Parous flies can be distinguished with difficulty from nullipars. A gross difference between young and old flies is in the volume of fat bodies, which is reflected in the specific gravity. Thus young flies float in saline solution in which older flies sink. Glands in the female genitalia become packed with granules during egg development, and many of these granules usually remain after laying. Examination of these accessory glands is easy, but is not very reliable in distinguishing flies which have laid from those which have not. The most reliable estimates depend on meticulous examination of the ovarioles, which is very tedious and skilled work.

The few relevant studies indicate that two or three cycles of feeding and egg laying are normal and that more than five cycles would be exceptional. Each cycle is usually completed in about seven days. As an infected fly may not become infective until its next-but-one-feed, survival and transmission of *Leishmania* parasites are dependent on the longevity of the vector.

Populations

Sandfly populations rarely become sufficiently dense to cause a nuisance. In the New World forests man biting rates may greatly exceed 100 per hour, but this is under conditions where people would not normally be exposed. In the Old World a biting rate of ten per hour during the peak hour around dusk is quite normal. Occasionally much higher rates occur, as with *P. perfiliewi* in northern Italy where 100 bites per hour have been recorded from man and where cows are bitten at such a rate that 20–30 specimens at a time can be collected from a single cow.

Sampling adults

Adult sandflies can be collected by a variety of methods. Catching using human bait gives valuable direct information on biting rates, but is unfortunately unethical where infection rates are high.

Animals such as dogs, cows or rodents may also be used as bait, and may be enclosed in a tent-like net in which the sandflies are trapped. Alternatively, the bait animals may be caged in the centre of a tray of oil (Disney trap) in which sandflies become trapped. This system can be used to determine host preferences.

The most extensively used sandfly trapping method in the Old World is to insert papers or cards soaked in castor oil into likely habitats — crevices, drainage holes in walls and rodent burrows.

These papers can be collected after 24 h or even longer, and the sandflies are

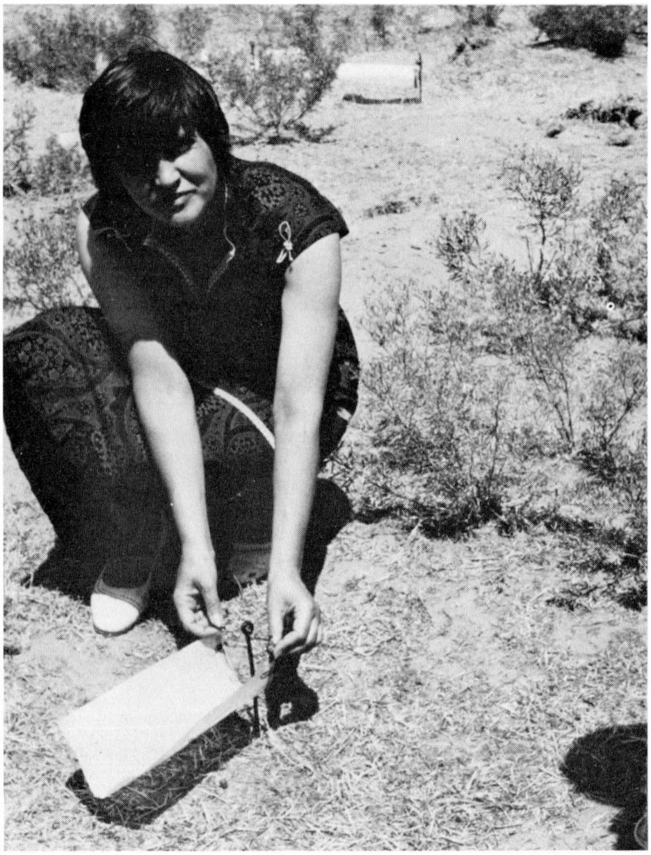

Figure 35. Sandfly sampling in a *Rhombomys opimus* colony in Uzbekistan, USSR using oiled paper flags.

picked off either in alcohol or in a drop of castor oil. Oiled papers usually provide damaged specimens unsuitable for taxonomic study but the collections can give relative population estimates, and the flies can still be dissected.

Oiled papers are only suitable in dry climates (figure 35). In more humid conditions, searching with a flash-light and aspirator is fruitful, and gives direct information on resting sites. Funnel traps may be placed over rodent burrows and may indicate probable breeding sites.

Light traps can be used but are very selective. In fact, no method is known which can be used to sample a sandfly fauna randomly, or to sample all adult stages of both sexes of a given species indiscriminately. Quantitative assessment of results should therefore be made with great discretion.

PART II

TRYPANOSOMA OF ECONOMIC IMPORTANCE

Chapter 3. African Human Trypanosomiases

> "The long history of West African civilisation is . . . the history of the evolution of human societies along paths that have enabled them to avoid frequent periodical decimation by trypanosomiasis."
>
> John Ford 1971

INTRODUCTION

Although only 10 000 cases of human trypanosomiasis are recorded annually in Africa the fear engendered by the disease resulting from its virtually inevitable fatal outcome if untreated, its dramatic clinical effects, the difficulties of its treatment, and the threat of devastating epidemics mean that it is accorded a relatively high priority by governments in the endemic area despite their limited financial resources. In West Africa, for example, the cost of surveillance for the disease is approximately US $ 0·5 per capita per annum which, in some countries, is as much as 25 per cent of the total health budget. Recent estimates indicate that some 45 million people live in the endemic areas of whom only about five million are under regular surveillance.

Although the disease has been recognized since the 18th century, it is believed that epidemics only occurred at the time of, or after European colonization. Previously the difficulties of communication and the isolation of communities may have prevented the spread of infection. The possibilities for expansion increased greatly with the opening up of Africa and the development of roads, river communications and railways which allowed rapid movement of people between infected and uninfected areas.

Recent political events in Africa have underlined the great importance of continued awareness and of financial commitment to surveillance and control to maintain low levels of endemicity and to prevent the tragic resurgences of disease such as have occurred over the past two decades in Zaire, southern Sudan and more recently Uganda. The history of epidemics at the beginning of this century alone indicates the potential threat which the disease poses today. During the years shortly before and for some time after 1900, devastating epidemics of sleeping sickness occurred in the Congo Basin and around Lake Victoria. It has been estimated that during this time half a million people died of sleeping sickness in Zaire and more than a quarter of a million died in Uganda. These epidemics stimulated great interest in the disease and resulted in several expeditions which, in the space of ten years, determined the aetiological agent, the vector and the life cycle in the vector and devised methods for control based on avoidance of the tsetse fly.

The epidemic of sleeping sickness in Zaire (Congo Free State, at that time) in the early part of the century gradually spread northwards and westwards and during the following decade provided enormous problems for medical services throughout Central and West Africa. It was the activities of these services which laid down principles of control of *T. b. gambiense* sleeping sickness which remain in existence today.

To begin with the health services relied on the control of population movements and treatment with the arsenical Atoxyl to stop the spread of the disease. The relative success of Atoxyl despite its serious toxic side effects paved the way for research on arsenicals as chemotherapeutic agents in human trypanosomiasis. Tryparsamide became the drug of choice in advanced cases and then was followed by Suramin for acute cases and later by Mel B which remains the best available drug for any stage of sleeping sickness. However, the drug itself causes a mortality of up to ten per cent due to fatal side effects.

While epidemics of chronic *T. b. gambiense* sleeping sickness held the attention of the medical services in West Africa and Uganda, a more acute form of trypanosomiasis was recognized in Central and East Africa. Owing to its far greater virulence in man, its different vectors and distinct differences in infectivity in experimental animals together with susceptibility to arsenicals, the organism was given separate specific status and called *T. b. rhodesiense*.

The authors subscribe to the view that the less virulent *T. b. gambiense* and the more virulent *T. b. rhodesiense* represent extremes of behaviour in man of a spectrum of similar parasites. In this chapter, nevertheless, we shall discuss the organisms separately where appropriate, referring to them as *T. b. gambiense* and *T. b. rhodesiense*, and draw attention to differences and/or similarities. In the coming years, it is probable that stocks of *Trypanozoon* will be referred to according to biochemical characteristics (e.g., zymodemes) rather than the classical terminology, but time is not yet ripe for this.

The virulence of *T. b. rhodesiense* and its known origin from animal reservoir hosts means that man usually becomes infected sporadically and only rarely does man-fly-man transmission take place. In this respect *T. b. rhodesiense* sleeping sickness represents a different problem compared with the chronic *T. b. gambiense* type disease where man himself, being able to continue working over long periods despite the infection, can be an effective reservoir. However, epidemics of *T. b. rhodesiense* have occurred, notably in Uganda and Kenya where the parasite has escaped from its zoonotic cycle and interhuman transmission has occurred through *G. fuscipes*.

The disruption caused by World War I created a situation which was of great benefit to the parasite and a disaster for the population. Epidemics of *T. b. gambiense* occurred in West, Central and East Africa. Recent civil disturbances in Zaire, Sudan and Uganda seem to be a repetition of history. After World War I, the foci of sleeping sickness were identified by surveillance, and cases were treated by Atoxyl and population movement was strictly controlled. These measures were successfully adopted in Uganda and in what is now Zaire and in the Congo and Cameroon. Outbreaks affecting the then French Equatorial Africa, now OCEAC countries (Cameroon, Central African Republic, Chad, Congo, Gabon) were identified in the mid–1920s. Here, and in Nigeria, surveillance and curative drugs as well as bush clearing were employed. In Cameroon, by the time the epidemic had subsided in 1935, 18 000 cases had been identified and treated in the Lake Chad basin. The actual numbers who died in Nigeria and other parts of West and Central Africa at this time can only be guessed at, but the disease clearly had a major depopulating effect and also caused wholesale movement of settlements away from rivers. The pattern observed in Nigeria was repeated in Upper Volta where the authorities were caught unawares. Investigations in Ghana, Togo and Benin in the early 1930s similarly revealed the presence of the disease on an extensive scale. By the beginning of World War II the work of the field teams had brought the disease under some semblance of control but success was limited by the insensitivity of the diagnostic methods available, the problem of treatment and the administrative costs of constantly deployed field teams. The discovery in 1940 of the effectiveness of Pentamidine as a prophylactic gave those responsible in West Africa some fresh hope for the future.

Despite occasional epidemics the disease in West Africa settled into a state of smouldering endemicity, being confined to so-called residual foci from which epidemics repeatedly arise. Melarsoprol (= Mel B and Arsobal) was developed by Friedheim in 1946 and, although highly toxic, the drug was effective in late stages of sleeping sickness at a time when Tryparsamide resistance was becoming apparent. Later, control was aided by the introduction of the chlorinated hydrocarbon insecticide, DDT, to combat tsetse. A focus of *T. b. gambiense* was eliminated from western Kenya by spraying riverine vegetation with DDT in the early 1950s. DDT was also used on a large scale by the Veterinary Department in Nigeria. Anti-tsetse campaigns in areas of sleeping sickness reduced the prevalence of the disease markedly in the northern Guinea savannah. Tsetse control in West Africa, either by removal of vegetation or insecticide application, has played an important role in reduction of riverine *Glossina* populations and insecticides remain a vital weapon. As yet no insecticide resistance has been reported in this vector.

During the 1960s, despite the lack of progress in the search for new and effective trypanocides, the introduction of serological techniques of diagnosis greatly improved the possibility of detecting early cases and those with low parasitaemia. Immunofluorescent techniques, however, necessitate a second visit to the field to retrieve suspects for detailed examination and treatment. This results in a high percentage loss of those examined on the first occasion. Serological tests giving an immediate, on-the-spot, result are being developed and this gives reason for renewed hope for future control of the disease by surveillance and treatment.

GEOGRAPHICAL DISTRIBUTION

Trypanosoma brucei rhodesiense sleeping sickness

The disease is found in East and East Central Africa (figure 36). Its southernmost limit is in the Okavango region of Botswana, and it occurs as far north as Ethiopia. Between these two extremes all countries in eastern Africa have recorded *T. b. rhodesiense* sleeping sickness. These are Burundi, Ethiopia, Kenya, Malawi, Mozambique, Rwanda, Sudan, Tanzania, Uganda, Zambia and Zimbabwe.

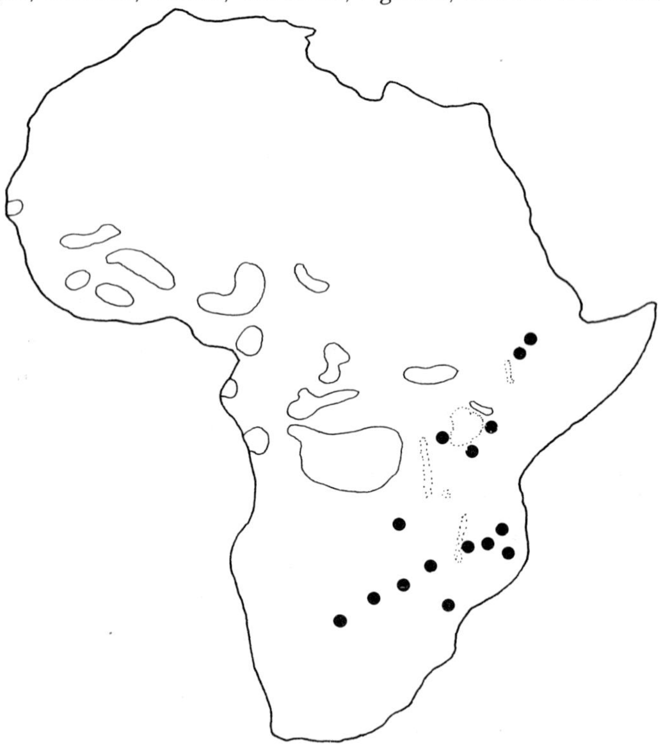

Figure 36. Sleeping sickness distribution in Africa. The solid dots indicate areas of *T. b. rhodesiense* endemicity and the open areas *T. b. gambiense* foci. These areas of *T. b. gambiense* sleeping sickness are areas where there is a higher level of endemicity and from such foci epidemics arise.

Trypanosoma brucei gambiense sleeping sickness

T. b. gambiense overlaps with the distribution of *T. b. rhodesiense* in the region of the East African complex of great lakes, particularly the northern shores of Lake Victoria in Uganda (figure 36). Countries west of those infected with *T. b. rhodesiense* sleeping sickness and south of the southern limit of the Sahara have all reported cases of this disease. Currently the most active foci of *T. b. gambiense* are in Cameroon, Congo, Ivory Coast, southern Sudan, Uganda and Zaire, but other countries of West and Central Africa continue to report sporadic cases of the disease which reflects the low levels of endemicity in the well defined residual foci of the disease. In Nigeria extensive vector control activities directed against the animal disease have made an impact on the number of human cases reported, and a vector control programme combined with treatment has practically eradicated *T. b. gambiense* sleeping sickness in Kenya and Tanzania.

THE ORGANISMS

Life cycle of *Trypanosoma brucei* in the mammalian host†

The cyclically transmitted trypomastigotes which occur in the bloodstream and tissues of animals and man vary widely in size and shape (12–42μm) (figures 37 and 38). This variation was known formerly as polymorphism, but the term pleomorphism is preferable as it has been recognized that the forms in the blood grade from one to another rather than being distinct morphological types. These changes in morphology are closely correlated with physiological changes in infectivity to mammal and fly. Pleomorphism was initially thought to be associated with sexual processes and the possibility of male and female forms of trypanosomes. However, although there is now stronger evidence for sexual processes in the life cycle of trypanosomes the likelihood is that it takes place in the vector, not in the mammalian host. There has also been considerable controversy over many years about the significance of tissue phases in the life cycle of *T. brucei*. Initial infection of *T. brucei* as a result of the bite of an infected *Glossina* produces a local lesion at the site of the bite which is known as the chancre. Although this is not commonly observed, recent studies have shown that parasites divide and proliferate in the skin at the site of the bite before dispersing throughout the body via the lymphatic system. During this initial stage of proliferation and dissemination throughout the body the parasites are trypomastigotes capable of undergoing antigenic variation before a parasitaemia can be easily detected. The duration of the prepatent period in *T. brucei* in mammals is dependent on the virulence of the stock as well as the numbers of metacyclic parasites inoculated.

---

† We use *T. brucei* to refer to the species as a whole or to stocks whose subspecific status has not been determined. *T. b. brucei* refers to stocks which do not infect man, while *T. b. gambiense* and *T. b. rhodesiense* are the subspecies which can infect man.

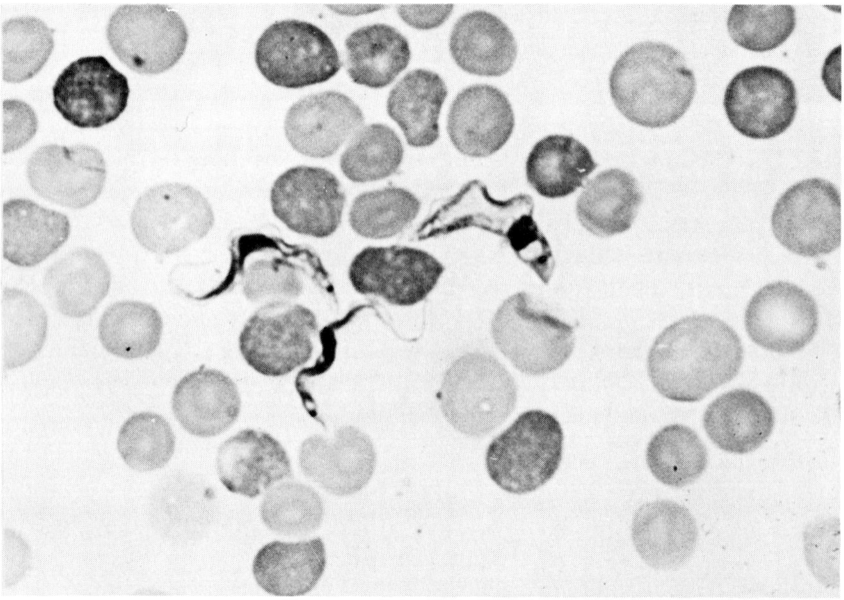

Figure 37. *T. brucei* in mouse blood; short stumpy and long slender forms (× 1600).

Waves of parasitaemia associated with multiplication of long slender forms during the rising parasitaemia are observed; during remission the short stumpy forms form an increasing percentage of parasites in the blood. The parasitaemia is controlled by changes in antibody levels and a specific antibody is produced to a specific antigen (see section on antigenic variation, p. 45) which causes the parasitaemia to fall; slender organisms appear more susceptible to antibody. However, the new surface coat is carried in small numbrs of heterotypes, which have survived the antibody directed against the antigens expressed in the previous parasitaemic waves, thus permitting survival of the parasite for a further cycle (figure 39). The ability of slender forms to continue to multiply prior to their differentiation to intermediate and stumpy forms, which are short lived and more immunogenic (probably because they are dying), may be an important determinant of virulence. There appears to be a correlation between the rapid capacity to differentiate to intermediate and stumpy forms and the levels of parasitaemia and resistance.

In *T. b. gambiense* infections and in chronic animal infections of *T. brucei*, trypanosomes are frequently very sparse in the blood. The concentration of *T. b. gambiense* in lymphatic tissues has been exploited for diagnosis of early stages of the disease. Experimental studies on *T. brucei* in laboratory animals have shown that trypomastigotes live extravascularly in the tissues as well as in the blood stream; in the extravascular sites they are responsible for tissue damage and destruction. Thus, although *T. brucei* is frequently referred to as a blood parasite, many if not all organs are infected. The major site of reproduction is usually recognized to be

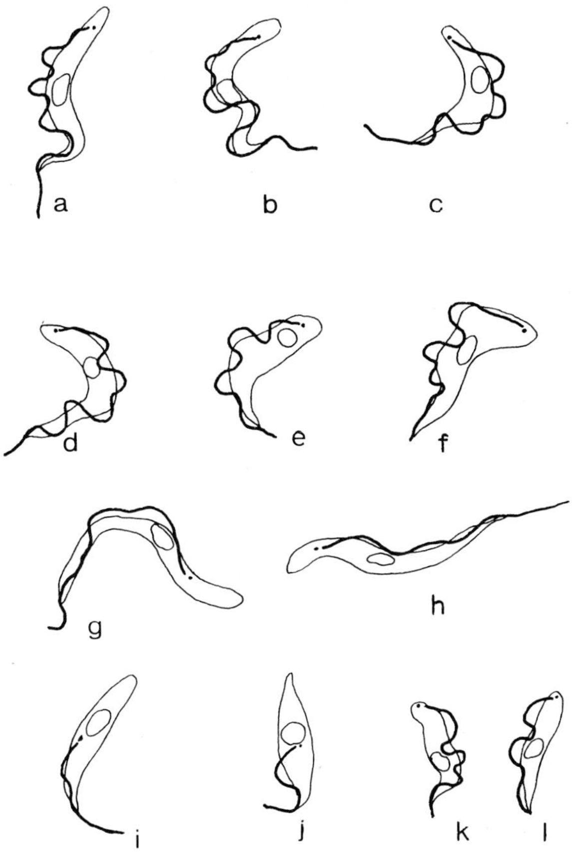

Figure 38. *T. brucei* and other *Trypanozoon* species (× 1300).

a–c = Long slender forms of subgenus *Trypanozoon*, e.g., *T. b. brucei*, *T. b. gambiense* and *T. b. rhodesiense*.

d–e = Intermediate forms of *T. brucei*.

f = Stumpy form of *T. brucei*.

g–h = Trypomastigote procyclic forms from the midgut of *Glossina*.

i–j = Epimastigotes from the salivary gland.

k–l = Infective metacyclic trypanosomes from the salivary gland.

the bloodstream where slender trypomastigotes divide by longitudinal binary fission. However, division of trypanosomes also occurs in lymphatics and this may result in a constant flow of trypanosomes into blood. It has long been thought that other types of parasite are present in tissues, and such occult or tissue stages have recently been demonstrated conclusively. Some early workers believed the amastigote and sphaeromastigote forms seen in tissues were distorted moribund organisms. Extravascular trypomastigotes are found, particularly in the interstitial matrix of the choroid plexus, where they cause oedema and destruction of collagen, and where immune complex deposits are found. Parasites in cerebral

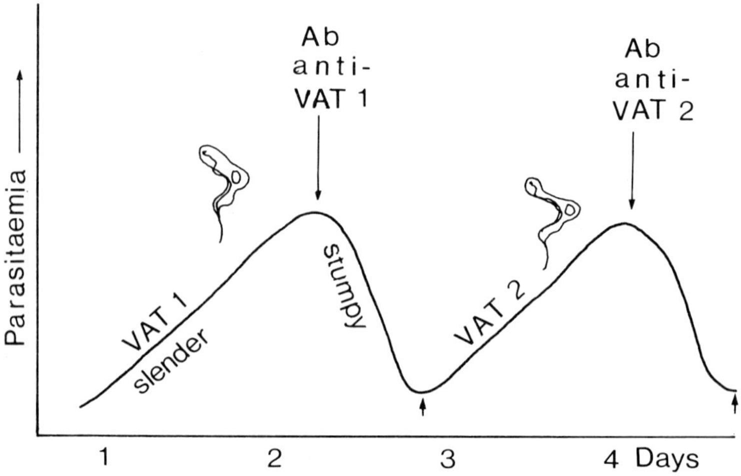

Figure 39. Diagram of events in a parasitaemic wave in a *Trypanosoma brucei* infection. Multiplication of the antigenic variant VAT 1 on slender forms leads to a peak of parasitaemia. Specific anti-VAT 1 antibody (Ab) is produced which rapidly kills the slender forms, but the stumpy forms are more resistant to antibody. Slender forms are less infective to the fly. A reduction in the proportion of slender forms leads to an increase in stumpy forms as the parasitaemia recedes. The emergence of small numbers of heterotypes of VAT 2 or other VAT at the arrows initiates a new wave of parasitaemia.

parenchyma, however, appear to be degenerate compared to organisms in the choroid plexus. The existence and significance of amastigotes and sphaeromastigotes is still controversial.

Evidence for a cryptic phase of *T. brucei* in the brain has also been obtained from experimental chemotherapy. In one study, *T. brucei*-infected mice treated with a substantial Berenil dose in the first week of infection were all cured, whereas older infections invariably relapsed. Subsequent subinoculation of tissue homogenates and blood into untreated mice identified the brain as the sole source of trypanosomes surviving the Berenil treatment. The fact that these recipient mice were then cured by the same large Berenil dose, if treated within the first week of infection, demonstrated that the trypanosomes were not intrinsically drug-resistant, but had merely been protected by their location. This may explain many clinical relapses hitherto ascribed to inadequacy of treatment or to intrinsic trypanosome drug-resistance.

Occasionally in infections of *T. brucei* in mammals multinucleate forms are observed in various sites; the significance of these forms remains to be elucidated, but it is not believed that they play a major role in the life cycle in the mammal.

Life cycle in the vector

As far as can be ascertained, all members of the subgenus *Trypanozoon* which are transmitted cyclically by flies of the genus *Glossina* (tsetse flies) have similar if not identical life cycles. The first description of this cycle was by Muriel Robertson in 1913 who described *Trypanosoma brucei gambiense* in *Glossina fuscipes*. *Glossina fuscipes* was fed on a monkey; development initially occurred in the midgut and proventriculus and, following this, the parasites migrated to the hypopharynx and salivary glands. This early work showed the separation of the *Trypanozoon* life cycle into a midgut phase and a phase in the salivary glands. It was also found that the life cycle was completed in about three weeks.

The first part of the midgut phase involves the transformation of the bloodstream parasites into slender so-called procyclic or midgut forms, which retain the trypomastigote configuration. These forms develop in the space between the peritrophic membrane and the midgut epithelium, the ectoperitrophic space. The role of the peritrophic membrane in the life cycle of *T. brucei* in *Glossina* was first recognized by Hoare who described the migration of parasites to the posterior 'open' end of the peritrophic membrane in the hindgut and their subsequent migration forward within the ectoperitrophic space to the proventriculus region of the midgut. Within the ectoperitrophic space intense multiplication of procyclic parasites takes place. Recent electron microscope studies have shown that trypanosomes penetrate the middle sections of the peritrophic membrane 9–11 days after the experimental feed. Prior to this it was believed that access to the ectoperitrophic space was by penetration of the soft part of the peritrophic membrane near its point of secretion at the proventricular valve (the 'press') or at the posterior end, as stated by Hoare. The view that entry was anterior was supported by the observation that flies fed on infected animals for their first blood meal (tenerals) had a greater chance of becoming infected than non-teneral flies. However, this observation has now been shown to be associated with the increased crop emptying time of teneral flies which allows trypanosomes more time to adapt to life in the endoperitrophic space after they are passed from the crop. There is much controversy still as to whether stumpy or slender forms initiate infections in the midgut of *Glossina*. On theoretical grounds it seems most likely that stumpy forms are physiologically more suited to transform to midgut forms as they have mitochondrial cristae. However, blood supposedly containing only slender forms whose mitochondria are acristate and which hence lack a functional Krebs-cycle pathway has been shown to be infective to *Glossina*.

Around days 12–20 after the infective feed the parasites leave the ectoperitrophic space to infect the proventricular region, having penetrated the softer part of the peritrophic membrane. The rate of development is dependent on temperature, and at higher temperatures the development and maturation of parasites is more rapid.

Electron microscope studies have also demonstrated a further midgut phase of *Trypanozoon*: intracellular parasites have been found in epithelial cells of the midgut as well as between the epithelial cells and the basal lamina bordering the haemocoele. Multinucleate cyst-like forms with daughter cells have been described. The significance of these forms is unclear, but in view of the finding of haemocoelic infections in experimentally as well as naturally infected *Glossina* it is possible that such intracellular stages are en route to the haemocoele. However, the extent of haemocoelic infection in nature is uncertain, as is its overall significance in the life cycle.

The possibility that parasites can invade the salivary gland from the haemocoele remains to be conclusively demonstrated. The classical life cycle is that procyclic (midgut) forms pass anteriorly through the food canal and then invade the salivary glands via the salivary duct or hypopharynx. The parasites transform to epimastigotes in the salivary glands and massive multiplication occurs in this site. The parasites attach themselves to the microvilli which border the epithelial cells of the gland by means of a junctional complex (hemidesmosome) between the flagellum and microvilli. Around 15–35 days after infection the fly becomes infective to a vertebrate host; metacyclic trypomastigotes possessing a surface coat develop. Transformation commences while epimastigotes are attached; the metacyclic forms are free in the lumen of the gland.

Anterior migration from the proventriculus to the hypopharynx before invasion of the salivary gland is suggested by the recent finding of procyclic parasites attached to mechanoreceptors in the proximal part of the labrum. These sensilla monitor flow-rate and the attachment of parasites to them impairs their function, interfering with probing behaviour. Infected flies probe more frequently than uninfected ones and also feed more frequently and more voraciously. These findings illustrate an adaptation of the parasite to increase its chances of successful transmission.

The complexity of the life cycle of *T. brucei* in *Glossina* is probably in part responsible for the low infection rates observed in the field. The efficiency of transmission and interference with normal behaviour may account for the survival of the parasite despite the low infection rates.

Some of the many factors which affect the chances of an individual fly becoming infected and transmitting the infection are listed below. The factors may be divided into intrinsic factors, ecological factors and parasite and host factors.

Intrinsic fly factors include the age of the feeding fly, its sex, genetic differences between fly species and possible intraspecific differences in susceptibility, various behavioural factors, the physiological or biochemical state, and intercurrent infections of the fly.

Ecological factors include meteorological conditions, the availability of infected hosts and hosts available for subsequent feeds.

Parasite–host factors include the number of parasites ingested by the fly, the proportions of the different pleomorphic types of parasite available and the strain of parasite, intercurrent infection in the host, behaviour and other factors affecting attractiveness of the host to the fly. These factors are described and brought together in Table 8.

Table 8. Web of interaction of epidemiology of trypanosomiasis.

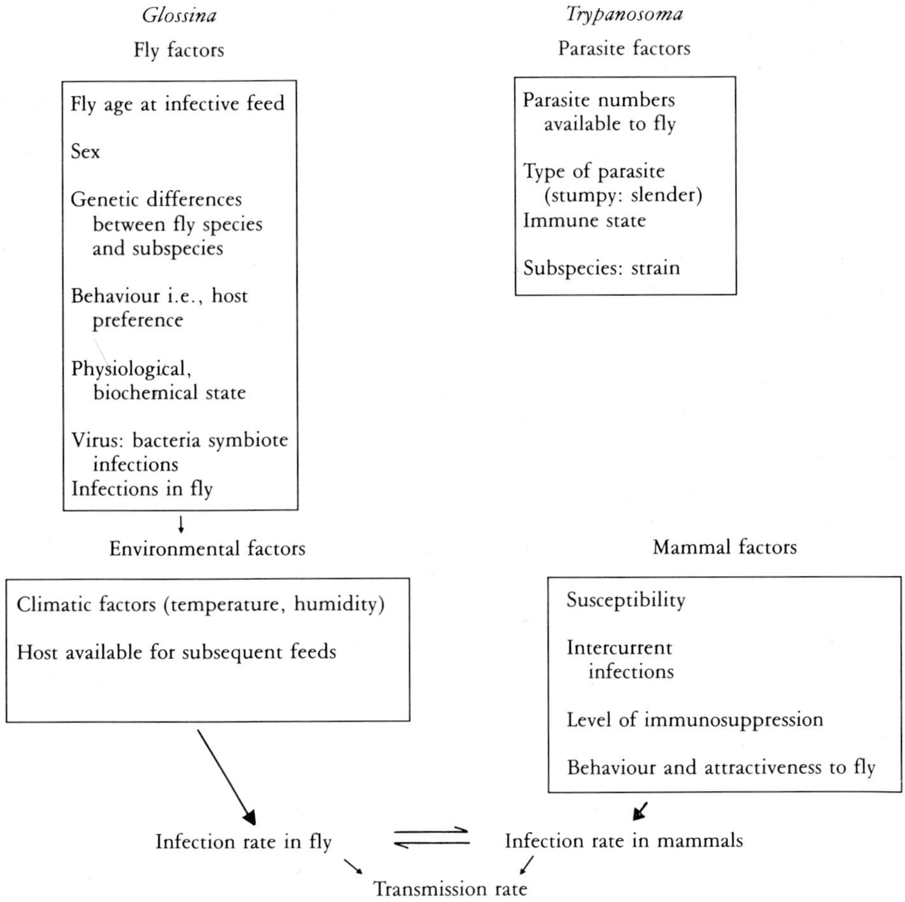

THE DISEASE

Diagnosis

Parasitological diagnosis: Trypanosoma brucei rhodesiense

The virulence of this organism means that parasitological diagnosis poses fewer problems than for *T. b. gambiense* because of the higher parasitaemias found in man during the febrile period. However, the parasitaemia fluctuates in *T. b. rhodesiense* infection, so that the organisms are not always detectable in the peripheral blood in the early stage and several daily examinations may need to be made. It is frequently found that patients reporting to fixed medical units for diagnosis have lost their parasitaemia as the fever has subsided by the time they reach medical help.

Centrifugation, using microhaematocrit centrifuge followed by buffy-coat examination under dark ground illumination or the miniature anion-exchange centrifugation technique (MAECT), is more sensitive for detection of parasites than thick blood films. Enlargement of cervical lymph nodes is less pronounced in *T. b. rhodesiense* disease, and aspiration and examination of gland juice is of less use.

It is clearly of importance in a virulent infection such as *T. b. rhodesiense* to diagnose the disease as quickly as possible. Animal inoculations (0·5 ml to two mice), though sensitive, may require some time for the infection to show in the recipient animal. This involves the risk that CNS involvement could occur during the intervening period. Central nervous system involvement is detected by the presence of parasites in the cerebrospinal fluid after lumbar puncture. Centrifugation can be used to concentrate the trypanosomes if they are not found by direct examination.

Alternatively, the cerebrospinal fluid (CSF) may be inoculated into animals. The elevation of the cell count above 5/mm^3 or protein levels above 25 mg per cent (determined by the Sicard Cantaloube tube method) indicate CNS involvement. However, trypanosomes have been found in CSF when cell count and protein levels are below these levels. The choice of treatment is dependent on the stage of the infection; Suramin is effective in the early stages, Mel B being necessary if the CNS is involved. If the infection is at a very early stage a chancre may be present at the site of the bite and trypanosomes may be found in the chancre fluid. This lesion usually subsides within 2–3 weeks.

Parasitological diagnosis: Trypanosoma brucei gambiense

This organism is not easily found in the blood of man; thick blood films may reveal the parasite but the most common method of diagnosis, which was the basis of surveillance strategy for many years, is palpation of the cervical lymph nodes and subsequent lymph gland aspiration of those with enlarged glands. Aspirates are examined for parasites by the surveillance teams in the field and lumbar puncture is performed on those infected to determine the stage of infection. The criteria for late-stage CNS involvement are the same as for *T. b. rhodesiense*. Clinical suspects who are negative parasitologically are given lumbar punctures, for in advanced *T. b. gambiense* sleeping sickness parasites are frequently difficult to detect in the blood or lymph-gland juice. Central nervous system changes are regarded as indications for treating the patient for sleeping sickness even if parasites cannot be detected by direct examination, centrifugation of CSF or inoculation.

The inadequacy of the above parasitological techniques of diagnosis has stimulated trials of microhaematocrit centrifugation and examination of the buffy coat, either directly with a long working distance objective lens or after breaking the capillary tube under dark ground illumination; and of the miniature anion-exchange centrifugation techniques (MAECT) as concentration methods. These methods efficiently separate and concentrate parasites from larger volumes of blood than are used for thick blood films. Both have advantages but are more time consuming than serological techniques (see below). The MAECT is being developed for field use and the extra expense and difficulty is justified by the increased sensitivity of the test. The parasitaemia in *T. b. gambiense* infections is known to fluctuate daily, parasites being almost if not completely absent on some occasions, but relatively easy to detect on others.

Animal inoculation can be carried out and the usual method is the inoculation of blood or CSF into susceptible animals. However, *T. b. gambiense* is of low virulence even to susceptible animals such as nursling rats, the multimammate rat *Mastomys natalensis*, or guinea pigs and rabbits (intratesticular inoculation). Some of these techniques, though sensitive, are not suitable for use in the field and can only be carried out in laboratories where facilities are available. Because of the general insensitivity of direct and indirect parasitological techniques, serological techniques are important adjuncts to diagnosis.

Serological diagnosis

Serological diagnosis is of value in epidemics of *T. b. rhodesiense* infection, but is of greatest value for rapid screening of populations in areas endemic for *T. b. gambiense*. It has been extensively used, in particular in Zaire, Congo and the countries of Central and West Africa. However, it must be remembered that serological diagnosis of sleeping sickness presents some problems. The techniques demonstrate the presence of antibodies rather than parasites and repeated exposure to bites of *Glossina* and inoculation of animal trypanosomes, though non-infective to man, may mean antibodies to trypanosomes are present in the absence of active infection. Secondly, techniques such as IFT or IgM may not give immediate results and reference to a central laboratory may be necessary; this necessitates a return visit by the team to collect suspects for detailed parasitological examination by which time they may have "disappeared". Hence there is a need for on-the-spot diagnosis to ensure the maximum number of suspects are identified and treated.

The first successful serological technique was the detection of raised IgM levels in serum of suspects. Specific anti-IgM serum is incorporated into agar gel and discs of filter paper impregnated with the patients' blood are laid on the gel; after 48 h on the gel the discs are removed and the gel is washed in saline; after drying, the gels can be stained and the diameter of precipitation zones measured. Samples with zones greater than 4 mm are positive; control negative and positive samples should be carried out at the same time.

The indirect fluorescent antibody test using parasites of the subgenus *Trypan-*

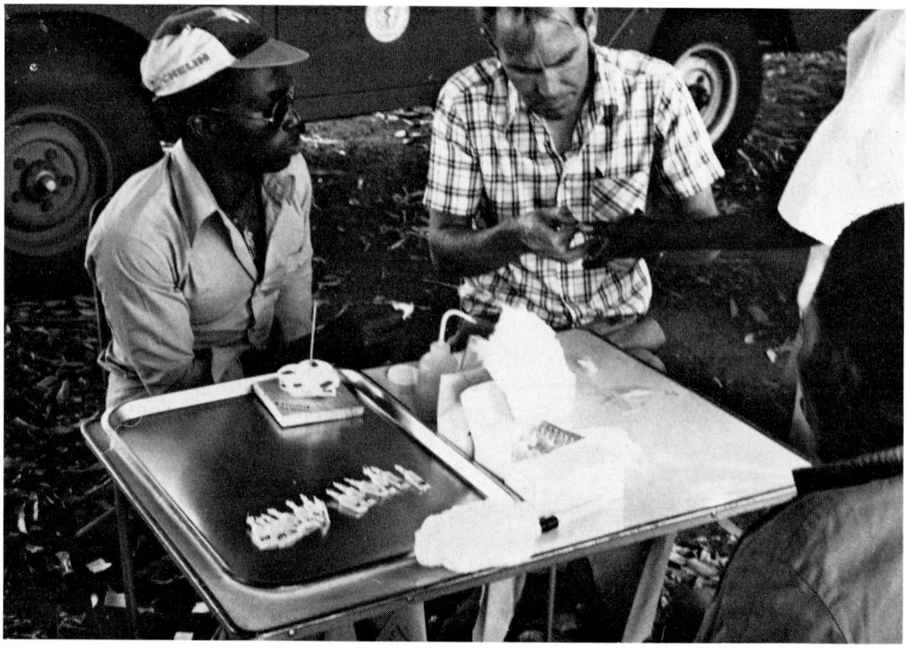

Figure 40. Taking blood by finger prick onto filter paper for later serology by indirect immunofluorescence test.

ozoon as antigen on slides is widely used. Blood can be obtained by finger prick and dried on filter paper for transportation to a central laboratory (figure 40). Filter paper discs with a phosphate buffered saline (PBS) solution or serum itself are incubated on the slides, which are then washed with PBS and incubated with fluorescein labelled antihuman serum for 30 minutes. Examination is then carried out under a fluorescent microscope and a brilliant fluorescence is considered positive; again known control positive and negative sera should be available for comparison. Other techniques which have been used over recent years are enzyme linked immunosorbent assay, a haemagglutination test in capillary tubes using antigen-sensitized human erythrocytes, latex agglutination tests and capillary flocculation tests.

The capillary haemagglutination test which has been developed for human trypanosomiasis allows on-the-spot diagnosis, but perhaps the most rapid and practical serodiagnostic test is a card agglutination test for trypanosomiasis (figure 41), which allows the results to be obtained within ten minutes of the addition of plasma, serum or blood itself to a plasticized card to which is also added a drop of antigen (defined antigenic type, formalin fixed, Coomassie blue stained trypanosomes). A positive result is indicated by blue staining of coarse agglutinated particles. The antigen is prepared using the common antigen type of *T. b. gambiense* occurring locally over a wide area. This test offers possibilities for use on a large scale as it is simple to use, requires no centrifugation and provides

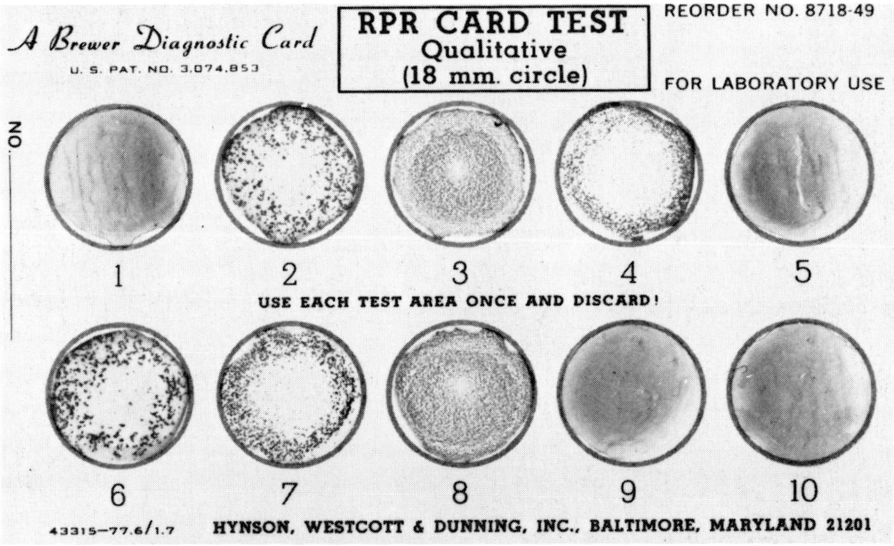

Figure 41. Examples of CATT results.
Spots 1 to 5: screening of 5 sera (dilution 1:4); 1 = −, 2 = + + +, 3 = +, 4 = + +, 5 = −.
Spots 6 to 10: titration of a positive serum (dilutions 1:4 to 1:64); 6 = + + +, 7 = + +, 8 = + (endpoint), 9 = −, (10) = −.
Courtesy of Dr N. van Miervenne and *Annales de la Société belge de Médecine Tropicale.*

results within 10–15 minutes, thus removing the problems of retracing suspects. The development of test kits and large-scale evaluation of this technique is in progress.

Clinical features

The symptomatology of a patient may aid in diagnosis, but vigorous attempts should always be made to identify the parasite itself. The chancre is the first symptom of the disease but is rarely seen in *T. b. gambiense* infections. The chancre is a rubbery, tender swelling occurring at the site of the bite. This is followed within weeks or months by an irregular intermittent fever; usually more intense in *rhodesiense* disease; lymphadenopathy occurs more frequently in *gambiense*. The patient complains of general malaise such as headache, pains in joints, loss of weight and pruritus (itching). Oedema of the face is a frequent sign; anaemia may be present, particularly in *T. b. rhodesiense*. Symptoms and signs associated with nervous system involvement are varied: in the early stage irritability and insomnia occur, but in advanced disease epileptic attacks, maniacal behaviour, somnolence and coma are typical. Patients are frequently misdiagnosed as psychiatric cases and if they escape treatment by traditional practitioners they may end their lives in mental hospitals. Damage to the heart, more common with *T. b. rhodesiense*, causes abnormalities in its rhythm, rate and in the blood pressure; X-rays may demonstrate hypertrophy of heart muscle. These cardiac changes may cause death. An enlarged spleen occurs in some cases. Abnormalities of the reproductive system occur such as impotence in males; ammenorrhoea, infertility and increased abortion rates have been reported in females. The complex pathology of the disease can cause disorders in other systems such as the digestive, endocrine, renal and respiratory systems as well as the liver. The immunosuppressive action of the parasites is probably the cause of secondary infection commonly resulting in pneumonia, a frequent cause of death. Reduced capacity to ventilate the lungs through central nervous system pathology can lead to a deterioration in respiratory function.

Pathology and pathogenesis of sleeping sickness

Relatively few autopsies have been carried out on sleeping sickness cases and the pathological description of the disease is based on relatively little material. The most significant pathology in the initial stage is an increase in the B lymphocytes which results in lymph-node enlargement. The meninges are also infiltrated with lymphocytes and there is a chronic progressive meningitis with the invasion of the brain with plasma cells which form characteristic morula cells (of Mott) associated with the blood vessels of the brain; the infiltration of the brain later produces neuronal degeneration. Cellular infiltration also occurs in the heart muscle. Damage to blood vessels may occur in man as a result of the release of pharmacologically active peptides — kinins — which increase vascular permeability.

The pathology in man may be due to the parasite's production of toxins. Toxic metabolites of the aromatic amino acids tyrosine, tryptophan and phenylalanine may either act directly or indirectly through immunological mechanisms. These substances (indole acids) can mimic anaesthetics in experimental animals producing damage to blood vessels, somnolence, temperature changes, haemolysis and immunosuppression. The role of these toxins in the pathogenesis of the disease in man is currently being elucidated. Most of the pathological changes observed in man with sleeping sickness are likely to be due to immunopathological reactions. Trypanosomes induce autoantibody production (antibody against human tissues), which may result in haemolytic anaemia and the observed cardiac and neural pathology. Immune complexes (between antigen and antibody) are deposited in organs and are found in sera, but not in CSF, of sleeping sickness patients; these antigen–antibody complexes could play a vital role in organ pathology. However, the most likely cause of sleeping sickness pathology is due to lymphocyte malfunction. Production of a B-cell mitogen by the trypanosomes appears to cause proliferation of B cells, which infiltrate the brain. The proliferation of these cells could explain elevated IgM and autoantibody production. If the stimulus to this proliferation is sustained, B cells become depleted, explaining the immunosuppression observed in trypanosomiasis including sleeping sickness. However, the mechanism by which B lymphocytes could cause the observed pathology in the brain and heart remains to be demonstrated.

Treatment

The treatment of sleeping sickness in man has always presented serious problems for the medical officer. This is due largely to the toxicity of the available drugs and the need to hospitalize patients during treatment. Extensive and careful nursing (including supplementation of diet) and regular follow-ups to check for relapse are also essential. The inability of some otherwise effective trypanocidal drugs to penetrate the blood–brain barrier requires the use in late stage sleeping sickness of arsenical compounds which have been found, even when administered under the most careful circumstances, to produce mortalities of around 5–10 per cent. This makes it all the more important to confirm the diagnosis, preferably parasitologically. Treatment is not justified on the basis of symptoms alone except in epidemics with numerous late cases. Diagnosis involves lumbar puncture; if the numbers of cells are elevated above 5 / mm^3 and the protein levels are above 25 mg per cent despite the apparent absence of parasites, then treatment with arsenicals should be commenced.

Schemes of treatment vary, but that recommended by the World Health Organisation ('WHO Expert Committee Report 1979', *WHO Technical Report Series 635*) for the early stage (no CNS involvement) in adults is as follows. Treatment on day one, 0·25 g of Suramin; day three, 0·5 g; day five, 1·0 g. This last dose is given again on days 11, 17, 23 and 30. Suramin should be used with care in areas where onchocerciasis is prevalent, as serious reactions can occur in onchocerciasis patients treated with a full course of Suramin. A test dose of 0·2 g is sometimes given before undertaking a full course.

Treatment of late stage disease can be accompanied by the use of corticosteroids to reduce complications, and parasites in the blood are first eliminated by two injections of Suramin (0·5 g) on days one and three. Three courses of Melarsoprol are then given at weekly intervals. The doses are increased for each course; Melarsoprol treatment requires close supervision which must be maintained for up to ten days after the last injection. Melarsoprol is given by intravenous injection, taking care that the drug does not leak into the surrounding tissues as the drug is carried in the highly irritant propylene glycol. In children where it may be difficult to find veins for Melarsoprol inoculation, a water-soluble compound Trimelarsen (Mel W) is given. This is effective against *T. b. gambiense* but the results against *T. b. rhodesiense* disease are inconclusive.

Mass chemoprophylaxis with the aromatic diamidine pentamidine (Lomidine), has been employed for sleeping sickness control. It is not used in areas of *T. b. rhodesiense* and should only be employed where workers are at special risk and where all the population can receive treatment at intervals not less frequently than every six months. The drug is given intramuscularly at dosages of 3–4 mg/kg body weight and patients should remain lying down after inoculation for a short time. Pentamidine prophylaxis may in fact sometimes suppress parasitaemia below the threshold of detection without effecting a cure.

EPIDEMIOLOGY

Trypanosoma brucei rhodesiense

The pattern of cases of this form of human trypanosomiasis indicates an infection acquired by man as a result of his intrusion into a cycle normally involving only flies and game animals. In the endemic situation sporadic cases are found among those members of the population whose activities bring them into contact with the savannah woodland habitat of the tsetse flies of the *Glossina morsitans* group, which normally feed on game animals. These patients are usually adult males indulging in hunting, honey and beeswax gathering and fishing, or who become infected during migration or local travels, or who farm on the edge of game and fly infested bush. Infection in man results in an acute disease so that he is usually not fit enough to work during the febrile periods when he is most infective to the fly. This is in distinct contrast to *T. b. gambiense* sleeping sickness and means that man–fly–man transmission is rare unless flies are present close to his home. However, should peridomestic transmission occur, then a man–fly–man cycle can ensue, resulting in an epidemic. This is marked by an increased number of cases in females, the elderly and children, who are usually less likely to be exposed in the endemic situation as they stay in the proximity of their homes.

It is apparent that local African populations may indeed have some resistance to *T. b. rhodesiense* through frequent exposure to fly bites as repeated inoculations of non-man infective organisms certainly induce antibody formation. It has been observed that European tourists infected with *T. b. rhodesiense* have a more rapid course of infection than Africans. Death in some European cases has occurred two weeks after known infection.

The traditional assumption that the *G. morsitans* group flies are the only vectors of *T. b. rhodesiense* sleeping sickness was abandoned when *G. fuscipes* was identified as a vector in Alego, Kenya. Here peridomestic transmission occurred when the riverine fly spread from the lakeshore to homesteads surrounded by *Euphorbia* vegetation. Similarly, infection was transmitted to fishermen along the shores of Lake Victoria by *G. fuscipes* and along streams in Ethiopia by *G. tachinoides*. Normally, however, *G. morsitans*, *G. pallidipes* and *G. swynnertoni* are the vectors.

Periods of drought tend to increase the number of cases owing to the search for fertile land and water in hitherto unoccupied areas. Increased hunting and gathering at these times results in greater contact between man and savannah species of flies.

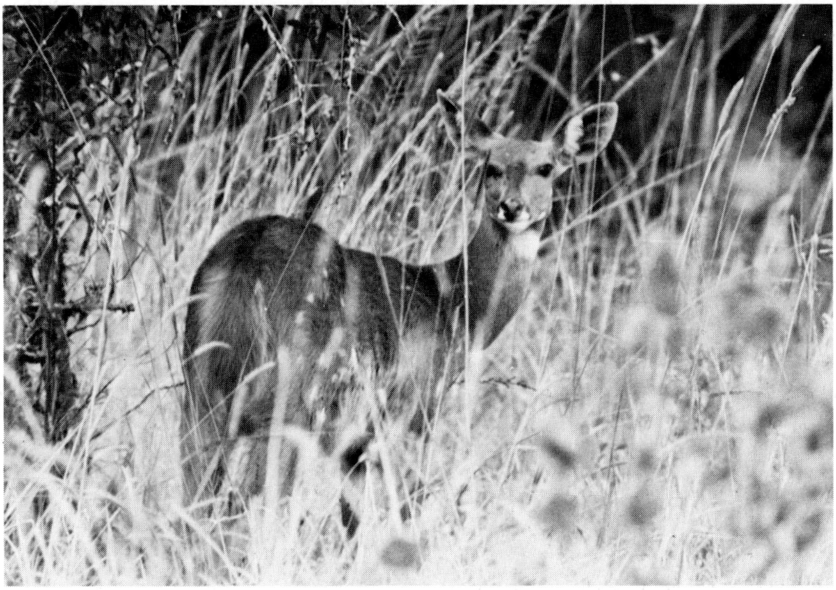

Figure 42. A female bushbuck, *Tragelaphus scriptus*. This species is known to harbour trypanosomes infective to man in East Africa. It has also been found infected with *T. brucei* in Upper Volta.

Courtesy of Dr M. Coe.

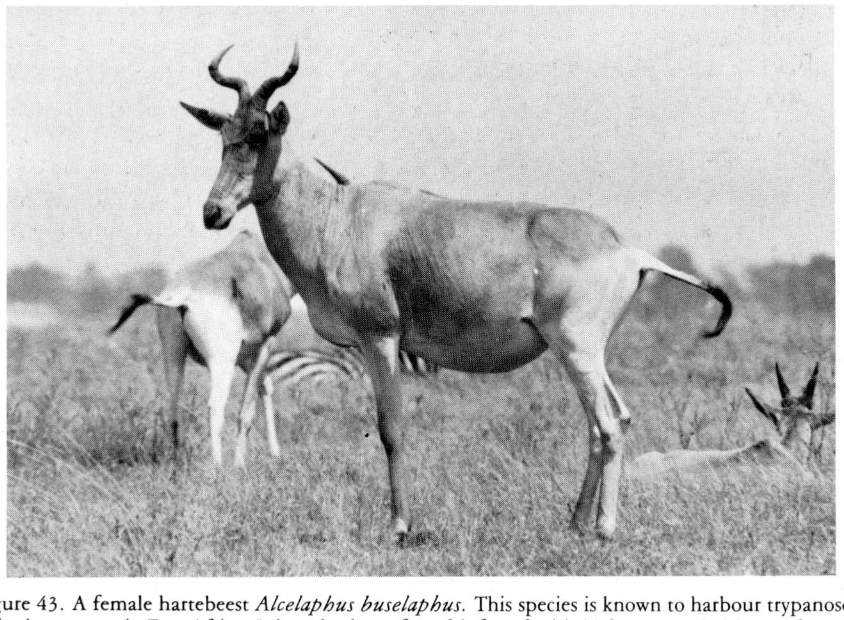

Figure 43. A female hartebeest *Alcelaphus buselaphus*. This species is known to harbour trypanosome infective to man in East Africa. It has also been found infected with *T. brucei*, probably *gambiense*, in Upper Volta.

Courtesy of Dr M. Coe.

These patterns of infection indicated that *T. b. rhodesiense* sleeping sickness is a zoonosis. The identification of *T. b. rhodesiense* depends on demonstrating its infectivity to man. To prove its zoonotic origin organisms derived from game and domestic animals were inoculated into volunteers during the late 1950s and 1960s. This practice has happily ceased. The wild animal species known to date to harbour *T. b. rhodesiense* are the bushbuck *Tragelaphus scriptus* (figure 42), the hartebeest *Alcelaphus buselaphus* (figure 43), the lion *Panthera leo* and the hyaena *Crocuta crocuta* (figure 44). It is suggested that carnivores are infected by the contamination of oral mucous membranes when eating infected wild herbivores; they are rarely bitten by *Glossina*. Cattle, like man, are also secondary hosts of *T. b. rhodesiense*.

Biochemical taxonomy and the blood incubation infectivity test (BIIT) have demonstrated that isolates from reedbuck and sheep may be infective to man and isoenzyme analysis has shown that an isolate from giraffe has similar characteristics to those from man with *T. b. rhodesiense*. Thus the range of potential hosts of man-infective forms may be wider than initially anticipated.

The concept of 'sustained triple contact' between man, game and fly has been evoked as necessary for transmission of endemic *T. b. rhodesiense*. Recent ideas suggest local focality of *T. b. rhodesiense* infections within the home range of individual bushbuck; the intrusion of man into these 'hot-spots' brings him into contact with the local bushbuck–fly–*T. b. rhodesiense* cycle, increasing his risk of

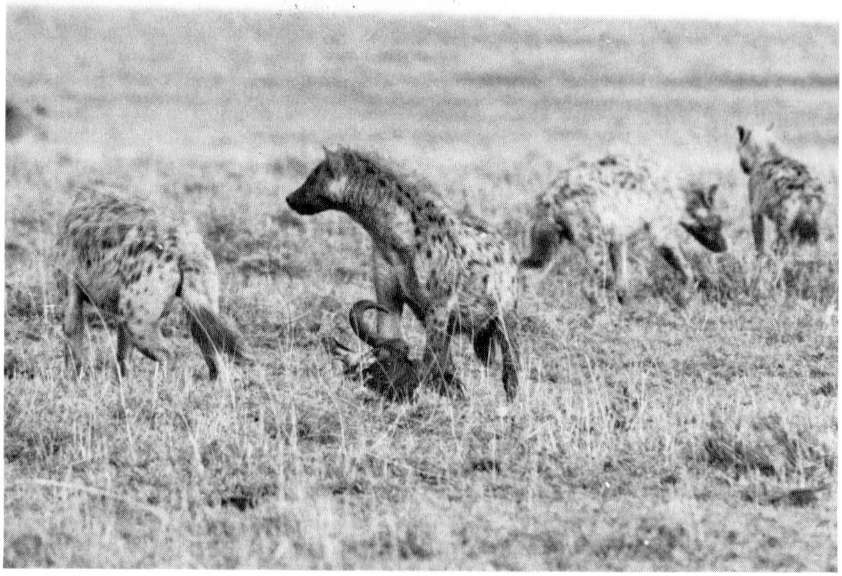

Figure 44. The spotted hyaena *Crocuta crocuta* which is frequently found infected with trypanosomes, acquired through eating infected herbivores as *Glossina* rarely feed on carnivores.

Courtesy of Dr M. Coe.

becoming infected. Bushbuck are secretive animals living in dense thickets, often close to human habitation, where they may be responsible for peridomestic cycles of infection; especially as they are also the preferred hosts of *G. pallidipes*. However, symptomless human carriers of *T. b. rhodesiense* are occasionally found in some areas such as Zambia, indicating the possibility of man–fly–man transmission.

Trypanosoma brucei gambiense

The success of surveillance and treatment in the control of the disease and the ability of a person infected with the disease to work and travel during the early stages when parasites are present in the blood as well as the long duration of the infection suggest that the epidemiology of *T. b. gambiense* is normally adequately explained by a man–fly–man cycle. The potential longevity of the infection is illustrated by a known carrier who has remained symptomless with parasites in her blood for 23 years since leaving Africa.

Transmission of the disease takes place at points of intimate man–fly contact (figures 45 and 46). Such points in the northern Guinea savannah are usually watering points, crossing points on rivers and streams where man and flies congregate in the dry season due to the low humidity elsewhere and man's continual need for water. *Glossina* have little alternative but to feed on man in this situation; this contrasts with the situation in the forest zone or in riverine habitats,

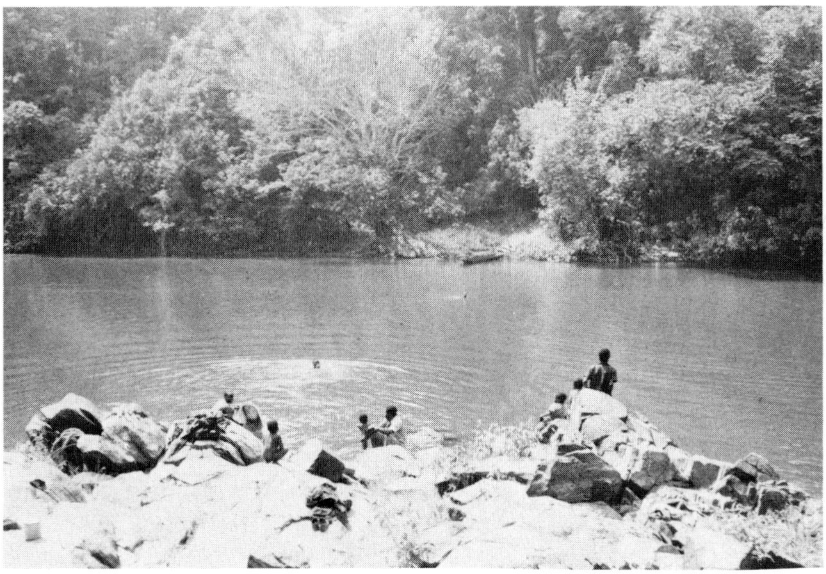

Figure 45. A point of man–fly contact, showing riverine vegetation in the background habitat of *G. palpalis* group flies. Washing and water collecting activities of the inhabitants of adjacent villages provided food for flies and show the potential of the point for transmission; Bouaflé, Ivory Coast.

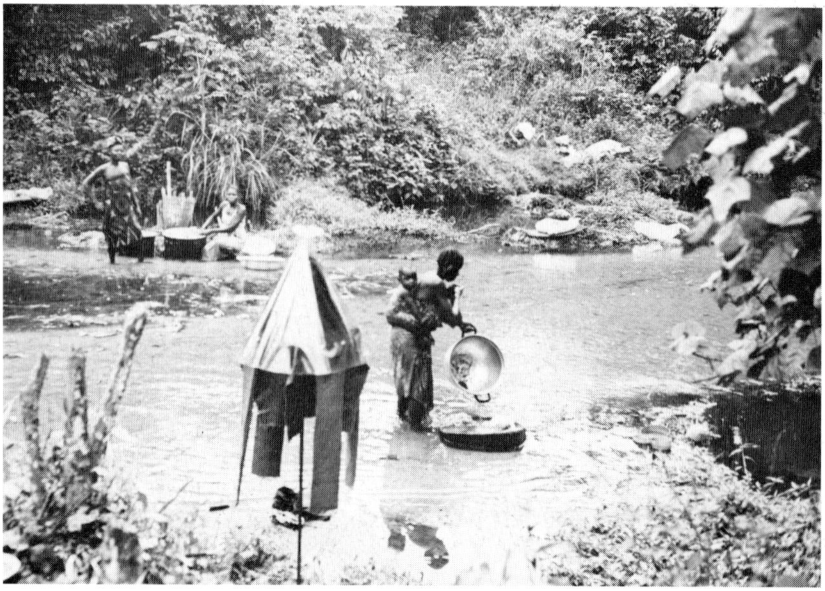

Figure 46. A washing area in a river in the Congo where villagers are protected by monoconical traps (foreground) impregnated with deltamethrin on four royal blue banderolles attached to clear plastic cone by metal studs.

along the Gambia River for example, where contact between man and fly is less intimate and the flies have the opportunity to feed on hosts other than man (figures 47 and 48).

However, despite the general acceptance of the importance of intense man–fly contact in *T. b. gambiense* sleeping sickness transmission, unanswered questions remain. Endemic foci, the so-called hardcore or residual foci, which repeatedly yield a few cases during surveys and from which epidemics probably arise, are difficult to explain. Therefore the existence of animal reservoirs of *T. b. gambiense* has been suggested. Recent studies in Ivory Coast and Liberia have shown that many pigs and dogs are infected with zymodemes identical or similar to those isolated from man. Some Upper Volta isolates from game animals, particularly from kob and hartebeest, are also closely similar or identical to human isolates.

Earlier studies of the possibility of an animal reservoir of *T. b. gambiense* were hindered by the ethical consideration of using humans as volunteers and the absence of other reliable methods for distinguishing these parasites from *T. b. brucei*. There was, however, evidence that dogs could be a source of infection to man. In addition, some human isolates have been cyclically transmitted through goats and sheep without losing their infectivity to man over some 20 passages. The importance of such sources of infection in the overall epidemiology requires further study.

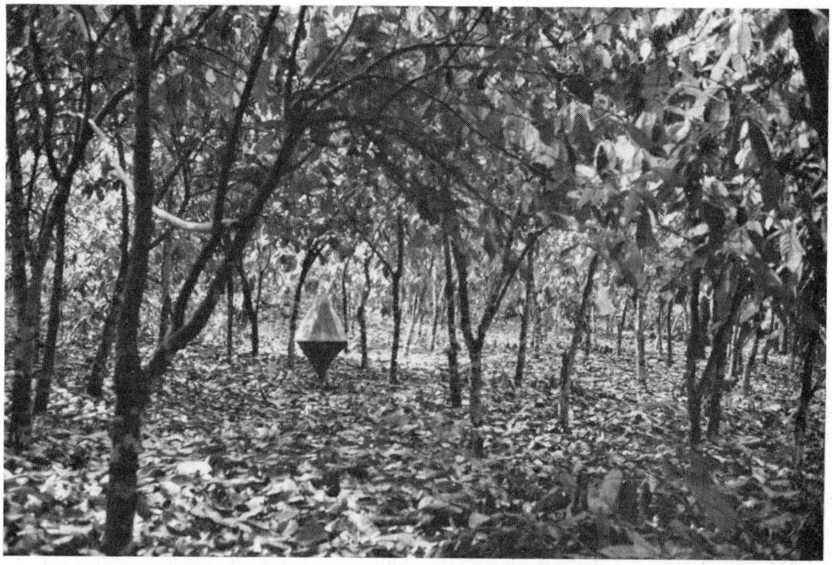

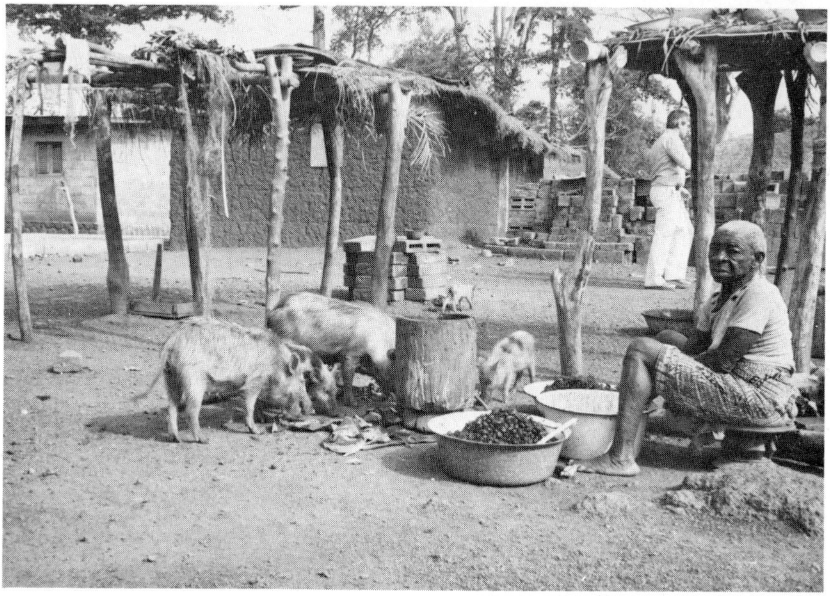

Figures 47 (top) and 48 (bottom). Sleeping sickness in Ivory Coast. A biconical trap in cocoa and coffee plantations; such plantations surround villages where pigs are in close contact with man and *Glossina*, which feed predominantly on pigs bred in peridomestic habitats.

As with *T. b. rhodesiense* the disease is most prevalent in those whose activities bring them into frequent contact with the fly, for example, farmers with land adjacent to the riverine forest, fishermen, or women who fetch water.

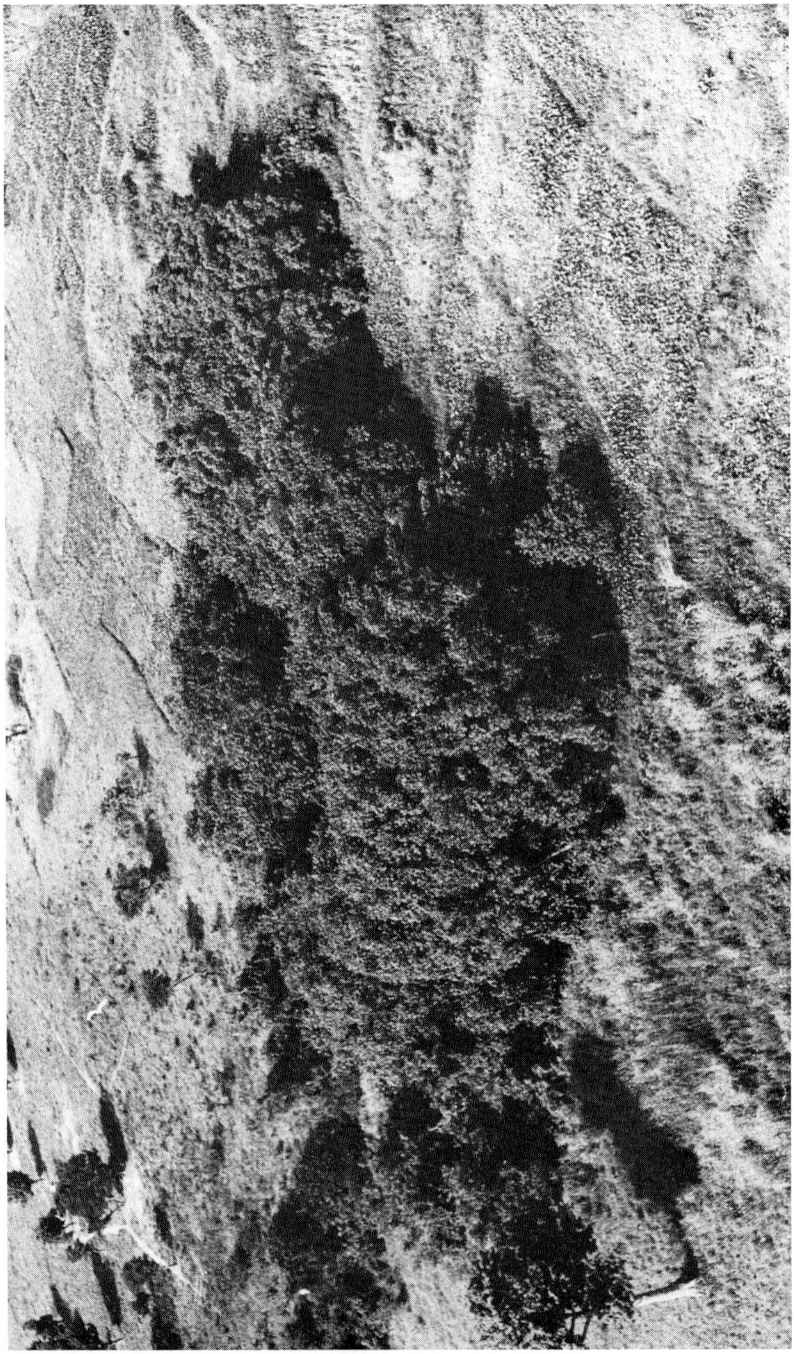

Figure 49. An aerial photograph of dense vegetation preserved in an area of cultivation (and such isolated pockets are sacred groves found in Ivory Coast and Upper Volta) where *Glossina palpalis* can survive and transmit sleeping sickness; near Korhogo, Ivory Coast.

Generally the ratio of infected males to females is 2:1 or 3:1, but the incidence among females may increase during peridomestic transmission. The grouping of cases within some villages can be explained by multiple probing of infected flies, or mechanical transmission. Congenital transmission from mother to offspring has been reported.

The chronicity of *T. b. gambiense* sleeping sickness means that its distribution through the endemic areas is enhanced by travel. Road barriers at which travellers are subjected to parasitological examination have recently been instituted in Ivory Coast. Apart from diagnosing trypanosomiasis patients, they help control the dispersal of the disease. Significantly, many of the patients in the recent Ivory Coast epidemic are immigrant workers who have acquired the infection in forest-edge plantations, and who, although resident in Ivory Coast, return annually to visit families in neighbouring countries such as Mali and Upper Volta. The ability of those infected to work and travel is of major significance in the spread of the disease.

VECTORS OF AFRICAN HUMAN TRYPANOSOMIASIS

Trypanosoma brucei rhodesiense

This disease is usually transmitted by *Glossina* species which inhabit the woodland savannah grasslands of East Africa (Table 9). The species and subspecies most commonly involved in transmission to man are *G. morsitans morsitans*, *G. m. centralis*, *G. pallidipes* and *G. swynnertoni*. However, the possibility exists that other species transmit the disease (e.g., *G. brevipalpis* and *G. longipalpis*). The riverine species *G. fuscipes* (a member of the *palpalis* group) has been identified

Table 9. Vectors of *Trypanosoma brucei rhodesiense*.

Species	Distribution	Habitat	Preferred food hosts
G. morsitans	Botswana, Ethiopia, Rwanda, Tanzania, Uganda, Zambia, Zimbabwe	Mopane and Miombo woodland savannah, low humidity	Suids (warthog), bovids (buffalo), bushbuck, eland
G. pallidipes	Ethiopia east of longitude 20°E, Kenya, Tanzania, Uganda, Zambia, Zimbabwe	Grassed woodland and thicket	Bushbuck, some suid meals
G. swynnertoni	Kenya, Tanzania	Grassed woodland and thicket	Warthog, giraffe

as a vector of epidemic *T. b. rhodesiense* in Kenya, where it became closely associated with man and was found breeding peridomestically.

Trypanasoma brucei gambiense

The chronic disease is transmitted by members of the *G. palpalis* group of flies (Table 10). These species inhabit predominantly riverine (riparian) vegetation associated with drainage lines, rivers and more permanent bodies of water such as lakes (lacustrine vegetation). These flies are less tolerant of low humidity than the *G. morsitans* group vectors of *T. b. rhodesiense*. Where vegetation encroaches on villages in areas of high humidity in the forest–savannah zones, flies may become peridomestic, for example, *G. tachinoides* in south-east Nigeria. *G. fuscipes* can invade villages along euphorbia hedges from its lakeshore habitat. *G. tachinoides* is the species most tolerant of the lower humidities. However, flies are usually found within riverine vegetation and only seek food outside in the adjacent savannah as they disperse more widely in the wet season. Riverine tsetse feed predominantly on reptiles, bovids and primates (presumably man), and occasionally on suids.

Table 10. Vectors of *Trypanosoma brucei gambiense*.

Species	Distribution	Habitat	Preferred food hosts
G. fuscipes	Central Africa: shores of Lake Victoria	Lacustrine, riverine vegetation	Reptiles, bovids, primates
G. palpalis	West Africa: Senegal – Cameroon	Lacustrine, riverine vegetation	Reptiles, bovids, primates suids
G. tachinoides	West Africa: Guinea – Central African Republic	Lacustrine, riverine vegetation	Primates, bovids, reptiles suids

CONTROL

Control of human trypanosomiasis is dependent on its epidemiology. It is unfortunately probable that neither *T. b. rhodesiense* nor *T. b. gambiense* disease can ever be eradicated. Thus control implies a continuing financial commitment to maintain the prevalence of disease at a reduced level tolerable to the local population and the national health authorities, and which reduces the likelihood of devastating epidemics. Authorities must adopt an attitude of continued awareness of the risk; a relaxation in that attitude and neglect of surveillance in countries with *T. b. gambiense* could have consequences similar to what happened in Zaire after 1960, in southern Sudan during the civil disturbances of the early 1970s or in Uganda in 1979–1981.

Trypanosoma brucei rhodesiense

The zoonotic origin and acute nature of endemic *T. b. rhodesiense* sleeping sickness means that specific control measures are generally not practicable. Most diagnoses are made in permanent medical centres, and no surveillance is practised except during epidemics. Large-scale vector control of savannah fly populations is not justified because of the costs involved. Removal of the reservoir, though it has served as a means of control of the animal disease in the past, is unacceptable for aesthetic and ecological reasons and because of the value of wildlife as an economic resource to many African countries. Without treatment the disease is usually fatal, but case detection and treatment is particularly important in epidemics involving man–fly–man transmission so as to reduce the reservoir in man. This may be accompanied by vector control by insecticide treatment of bush if resting sites of flies can be found and places of transmission identified. Prevention of contact between man and fly was the basis of the success of preventing the spread of the disease in Tanzania in the early part of the century where agricultural development of cleared zones followed by settlement removed both the fly and the game on which it feeds.

Trypanosoma brucei gambiense

The extensive low endemicity in permanent residual foci, the chronic nature of the disease, man's ability to continue to work and travel and thus infect more tsetse, and the danger of sudden epidemics mean that surveillance followed by treatment is the main basis of control of *T. b. gambiense* sleeping sickness.

Originally, specific sleeping sickness surveillance teams were developed to find cases and organize their removal for treatment at suitable centres. However, surveillance for sleeping sickness is now undertaken by polyvalent medical teams, responsible for a variety of diseases in addition to sleeping sickness, and there has been a diminution of diagnostic expertise and a reduction of time allocated to sleeping sickness itself.

The regular surveillance of exposed populations once or twice a year permits recognition of early infection by blood and by lymph gland examination of patients with enlarged lymph glands. On-the-spot diagnosis is preferable as the delays which occur in some serological surveys (e.g. by IFT) necessitate a return some weeks later. Consequently, a high proportion of suspects may be lost. These individuals provide the opportunity for further transmission to flies, and hence perpetuate the disease in that community. Control relies on the elimination of the main reservoir of the disease, i.e., infected man. Although in some areas it is likely that animal reservoirs exist, the effectiveness of case finding and treatment over many years indicates the importance in epidemics of man–fly–man transmission.

On-the-spot serological tests such as the card agglutination test for trypanosomes (figure 41, p. 111) provide hope for a more rapid and sensitive survey technique, where suspects identified during the visit of a surveillance team can be taken immediately to a fixed medical centre for parasitological diagnosis and, if necessary, treatment. Medical surveillance teams also have an important function in following up cases already treated to ascertain whether relapses have occurred. Barriers at road junctions or other strategic points have been introduced in some areas for the detection of infection in travellers to reduce the likelihood of the spread of disease.

Pentamidine has been used in the past as a prophylactic, to prevent infection in persons at risk, for example, tin miners in Nigeria. However, the duration of the effectiveness is not known and, although the effect is said to last for six months, more frequent inoculations are desirable. There are also reports of resistance to Pentamidine. Six-monthly treatment of exposed populations and case detection is administratively difficult. A serious danger is that Pentamidine may suppress an existing infection below patency, without cure, permitting invasion of the central nervous system.

Prior to the advent of insecticides the destruction of the habitat of *Glossina* provided an effective means of vector control, which at least reduced transmission at places of man–fly contact. This was carried out by mechanical or manual bush clearing and was repeated when required to prevent regrowth of the habitat; for the control of riverine fly the water sources were usually cleared for variable distances either side of locations where man acquires the infection.

The earliest method of insecticide application against *Glossina* was the application of DDT by knapsack sprayers (figure 50), or crudely from aircraft, to riverine and woodland vegetation. Increased ecological knowledge, particularly from studies on the resting sites of *Glossina*, has enabled a more selective and economic approach to the application of insecticides to be adopted. Only certain parts of the vegetation need be sprayed as it is assumed that if a proportion of the known resting sites are sprayed with residual insecticide then each fly is likely to contact the sprayed site before the insecticide has lost its efficacy. *Glossina palpalis* and *G. tachinoides* are known to rest within a metre of the edge of the water on twigs, creepers and low branches in riverine vegetation rarely above 1–2 m in height.

Groundspray application of residual insecticide to resting sites of riverine flies is clearly a most effective method of reducing transmission at places of intense man–fly contact. Insecticide application by fixed-wing aircraft has been employed for the control of animal trypanosomiasis in East and Central Africa, using aerosol application of low doses of endosulfan (figure 51). This may have had an effect on the transmission of *T. b. rhodesiense* in Zambia and in the Okavango Delta area of Botswana, but the operations were not specifically designed for human sleeping sickness control.

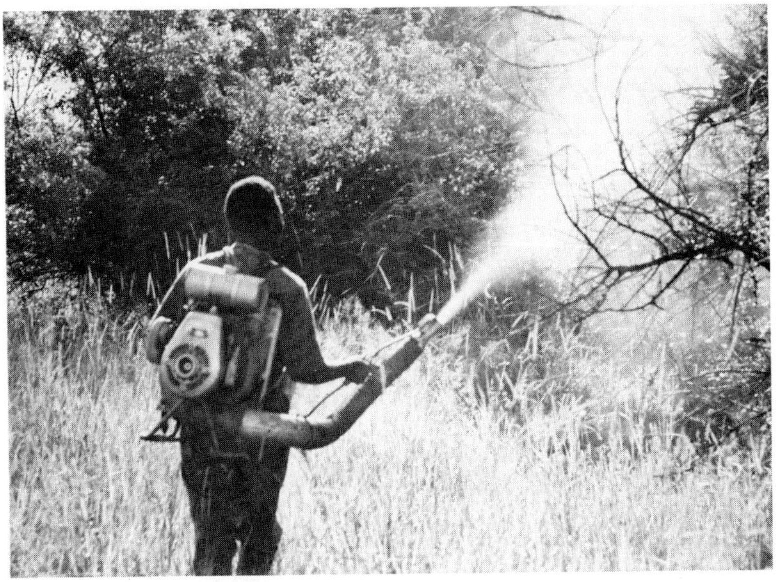

Figure 50. Spraying thicket vegetation with a motorized mistblower which produces a fog of small droplets.

Courtesy of Dr D. A. T. Baldry.

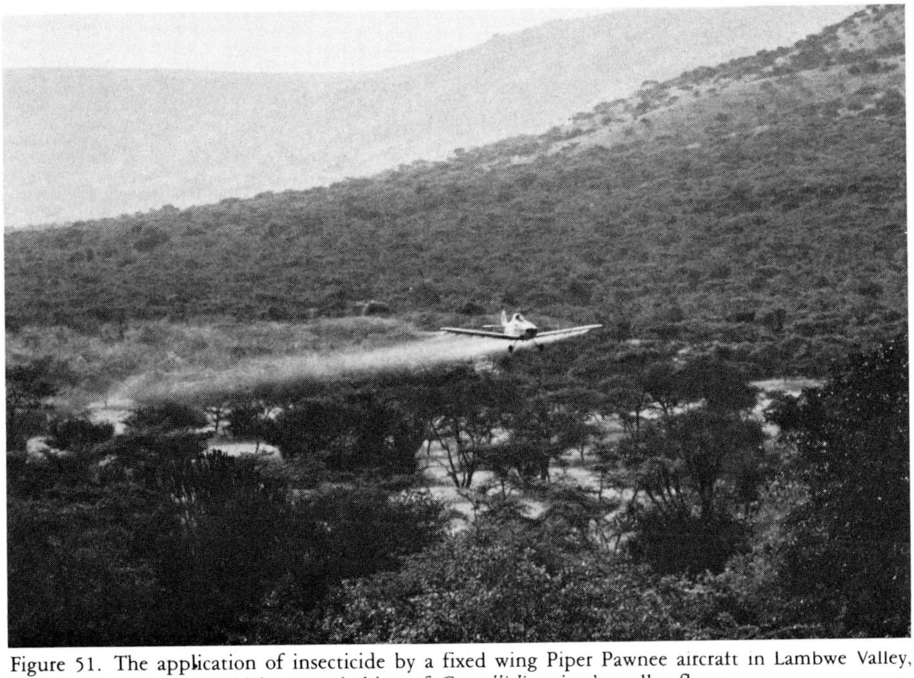

Figure 51. The application of insecticide by a fixed wing Piper Pawnee aircraft in Lambwe Valley, Kenya. Note the dense thicket type habitat of *G. pallidipes* in the valley floor.

Courtesy of Dr D. A. T. Baldry.

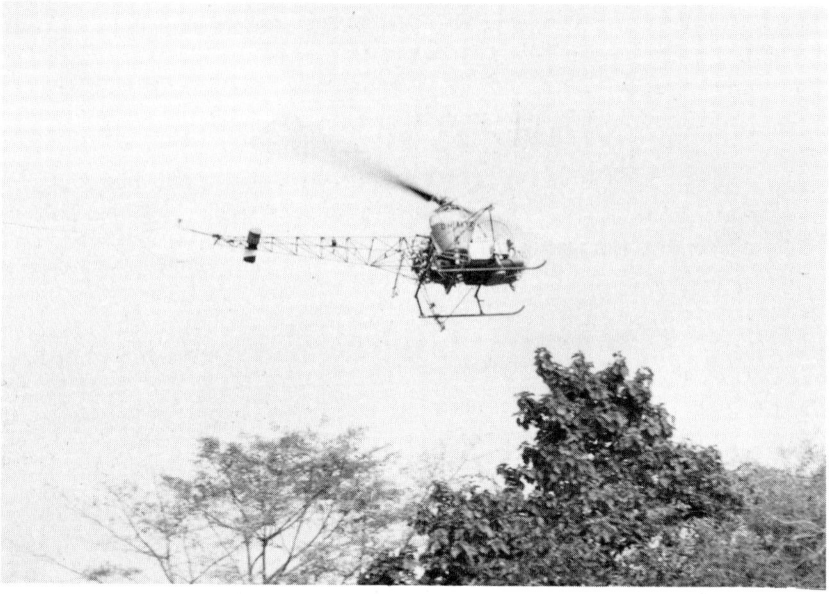

(a)

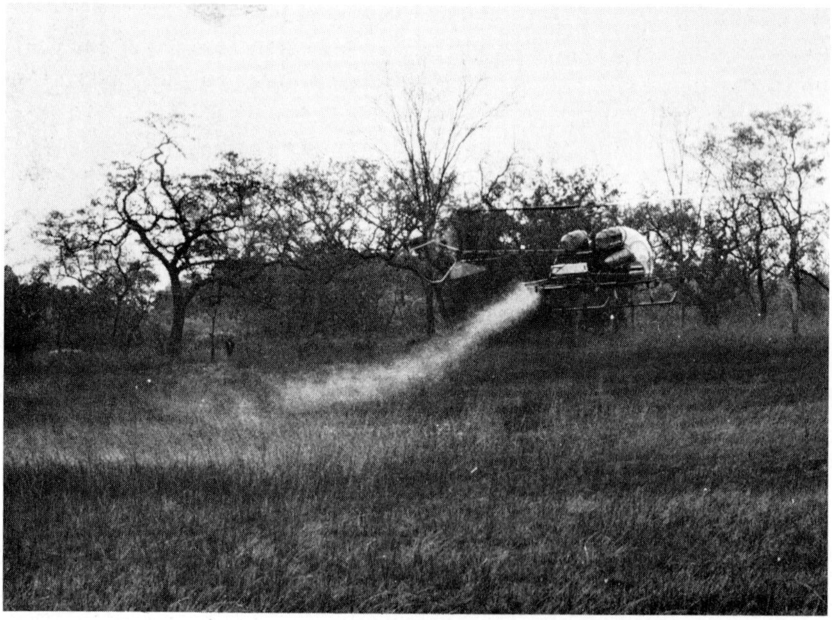

(b)

Figure 52. (a) A Bell 47 G 4A helicopter spraying a riverine habitat. (b) The same helicopter demonstrates unilateral spraying using only one side of the boom and shows the sideways movement of droplets and downdraft suitable for spraying riverine habitats.

The successful use of helicopters for application of the residual insecticides DDT, dieldrin and endosulfan in the control of woodland and riverine *Glossina* in Nigeria prompted a feasibility study of aerosol application by helicopter in Upper Volta (figure 52). Aerosol application had to be carried out over a two-month period, in 5–6 cycles at the low dosages (10–20 g/ha endosulfan) which are non-residual. The aim of the technique is to provide a less polluting method of application which can be used in emergency situations such as sudden epidemics. The technique is not applicable to the control of endemic disease. Studies on the effects of the insecticide on *Glossina* populations are now accompanied by studies on the effects on non-target organisms, which are particularly important with endosulfan as it is highly toxic to fish. The newly introduced synthetic pyrethroids are highly toxic to Crustacea.

The insecticides currently available for tsetse control are DDT, dieldrin, endosulfan and the synthetic pyrethroids. The latter, although expensive, are highly effective, permethrin being the least irritant and of lowest mammalian toxicity. The choice of insecticide depends largely on cost, supply, and importance of environmental considerations. As yet no reports of insecticide resistance in *Glossina* have occurred.

The use of simple community level methods of tsetse control have recently been advocated, particularly ones which are cheap, reduce transmission and involve community participation. Methods undergoing trials include the use of insecticide impregnated screens, biconical traps and tyres around villages, and the incorporation of spraymen, normally employed for crop spraying, into a programme of residual insecticide application to resting sites at points around villages where transmission is likely to occur. Methods such as this can play an important role in disease control in epidemics when it is important to reduce the level of transmission as a matter of urgency.

The Island of Principe was freed of human trypanosomiasis and the vector, *Glossina palpalis*, was eradicated by the use of sticky boards carried on the backs of plantation workers. Similarly, in Zaire over 30 000 *Glossina* were captured by villagers who were paid the equivalent of 5 US cents per fly caught. Such simple methods may be highly effective, and given the motivation and confidence of the population and administrative support, they may succeed where more expensive vector control activities could fail.

Much effort and energy has been expended in developing the sterile male release technique for the control of the vectors of animal trypanosomiasis. At present the use of this technique is not feasible, cost-effective or relevant for human trypanosomiasis control. In the longer term an integrated control programme incorporating sterile-male release *may* have a role in the programme for animal trypanosomiasis control. However, it must be remembered that it is a monospecific technique compared with insecticides. The original population is usually reduced by 90–95 per cent using non-residual insecticide application (e.g., endosulfan) so that sterile males can finally flood the remaining population. An uninterrupted supply of sterile males may be required over a period of several

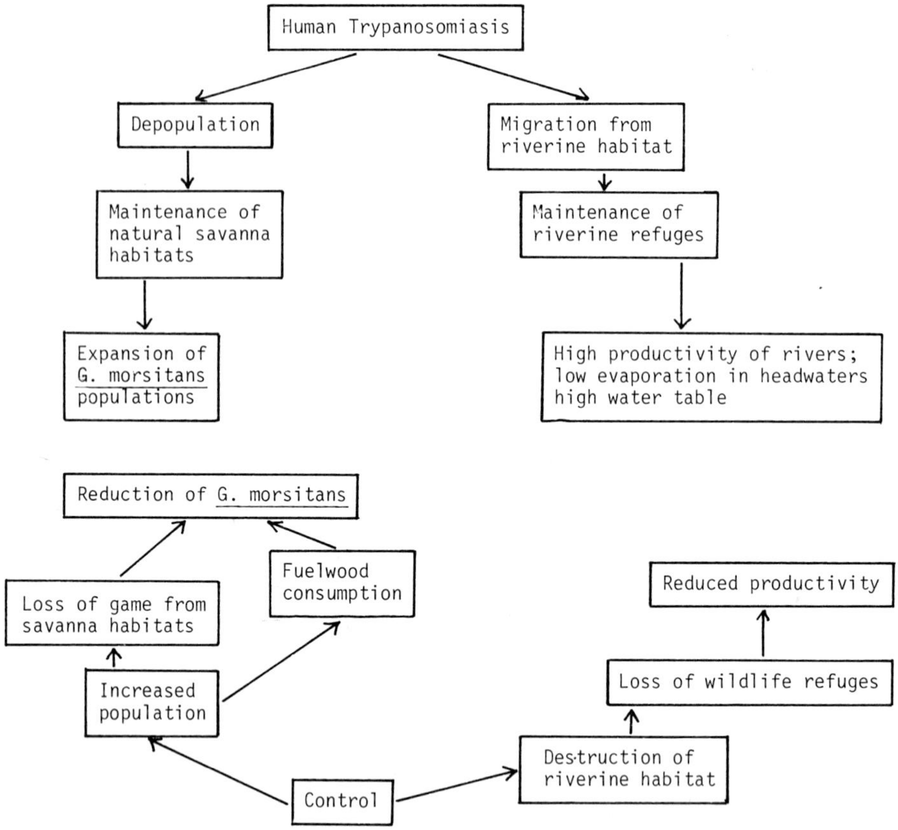

Figure 53. A summary diagram of ecological relationships in human trypanosomiasis.

years and it must also be recalled that some important vector species of *Glossina* (e.g., *G. pallidipes*) are not easy to breed in the laboratory. Figure 53 summarizes some of the consequences of human trypanosomiasis and its control.

Chapter 4. African Animal Trypanosomiasis

> "Trypanosomiasis is probably the only disease which has profoundly affected the settlement and economic development of a major part of a continent".
>
> F. A. O.

INTRODUCTION

The pathogenic trypanosomes of domestic livestock in Africa are recognized as the most economically important of all trypanosomes. This was reinforced by a resolution of the 1974 World Food Conference which mandated the Food and Agricultural Organisation of the United Nations to launch "as a matter of urgency" a control programme. Thus the disease was accorded a high priority by both scientists and politicians. Although there is controversy about the ecological wisdom of controlling these diseases, there is no doubt that the grasslands of Africa could support enormously increased livestock populations.

Around 7–10 million km^2 of Africa are infested with tsetse and this land has an average carrying capacity of 20 cattle/km^2. Thus the capacity of such land is at least 140 million head of cattle, and at present only approximately 20 million cattle are raised in tsetse infested areas. Within the infested zone the extra 120 million head of cattle could result in an increased meat production of 1·5 million tons at a value of approximately US$ 750 million per annum (1978 prices). Alternatively, an additional 150 million sheep and 250 million goats could be raised. The extra cattle production would not only reduce dependence in some countries on imported meat but increase nitrogenous content of soil, make available more draught animals and raise the nutritional levels of the community. The rate of deterioration of marginal tsetse-free rangeland might also be reduced. In this chapter we describe the biology of the trypanosomes which are of most importance in the pathology of livestock, namely *T. vivax* and *T. congolense*.

Although *T. brucei* is frequently found in livestock, it is not such an important pathogen and, in view of its close relationship with the human pathogens it is not dealt with specifically in this chapter. The importance of game animals in the epizootiology of trypanosomiasis is also discussed, as are the porcine trypanosomes.

DISTRIBUTION

Subgenus *Duttonella*

T. (Duttonella) vivax
T. (Duttonella) uniforme

The trypanosomes of the subgenus *Duttonella*, the principle pathogen of which is *T. vivax*, are distributed throughout the tsetse belt where they are parasitic in domestic livestock and game animals. *T. vivax* is also commonly found outside the tsetse belt as it is more readily transmitted mechanically by other biting flies (such as *Tabanus*).

A trypanosome very closely related to *T. vivax* is *T. uniforme*; this has been accorded a separate specific status although some authors have expressed doubts about its validity. *T. uniforme* has been recognized in Angola, Uganda and Zaire, but no records appear to exist from West Africa; it was initially described from bovines but it has been recorded from game animals also.

Subgenus *Nannomonas*

T. (Nannomonas) congolense
T. (Nannomonas) simiae

T. congolense, like *T. vivax,* is distributed throughout the zone of *Glossina* infestation in sub-Saharan Africa. *T. congolense* seems less easily transmitted mechanically than *T. vivax* and is therefore confined to zones where *Glossina* exist. *T. congolense* is found in domestic bovines and game animals.

A second member of the subgenus, *T. simiae*, is an important pathogen of pigs in some areas and is normally found in wild suids throughout Africa.

Subgenus *Pycnomonas*

T. (Pycnomonas) suis

This is a rare and little-known trypanosome which is found in domestic and wild suids; records of this parasite have been from Burundi, Tanzania and eastern Zaire; there is no information on its occurrence elsewhere in Africa.

MORPHOLOGY AND CHARACTERIZATION

Subgenus *Duttonella*

T. vivax (figures 54 and 55) was named because of the vigour of its activity under the microscope when examined in fresh preparations. The parasite moves rapidly across the field of view. The trypanosomes are 18–31 μm in total length (a free flagellum of 3–5 μm with a body length of around 15–26 μm). The related organism *T. uniforme* is smaller but possesses the same general features. The subgenus *Duttonella* is characterized by a large kinetoplast usually situated close to the posterior end. There is a degree of dimorphism, some forms being club-shaped posteriorly while others are more slender. There is also a free flagellum, in contrast to *Nannomonas* organisms. Multiplication is by equal longitudinal binary fission, usually in the bloodstream. Three separate zymodemes have been identified from cattle in Nigeria showing variations in alanine aminotransferase (ALAT) and ASAT enzymes, and other enzyme variants have since been demonstrated. However, the problems of studying *T. vivax*, due to the general lack of infectivity to rodents, indicates that more studies are required to enable

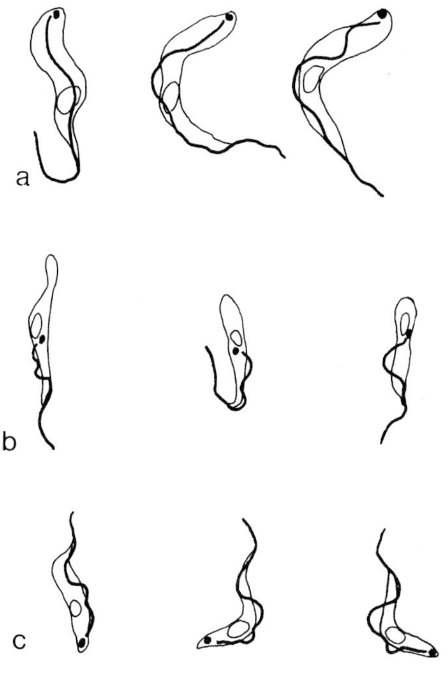

Figure 54. *T. vivax,* subgenus *Duttonella* (× 1300).
Row a, blood stream forms of *T. vivax*.
Row b, epimastigotes of *T. vivax* from the proboscis of a fly.
Row c, metacyclic trypomastigotes of *T. vivax* from the hypopharynx of *Glossina*.

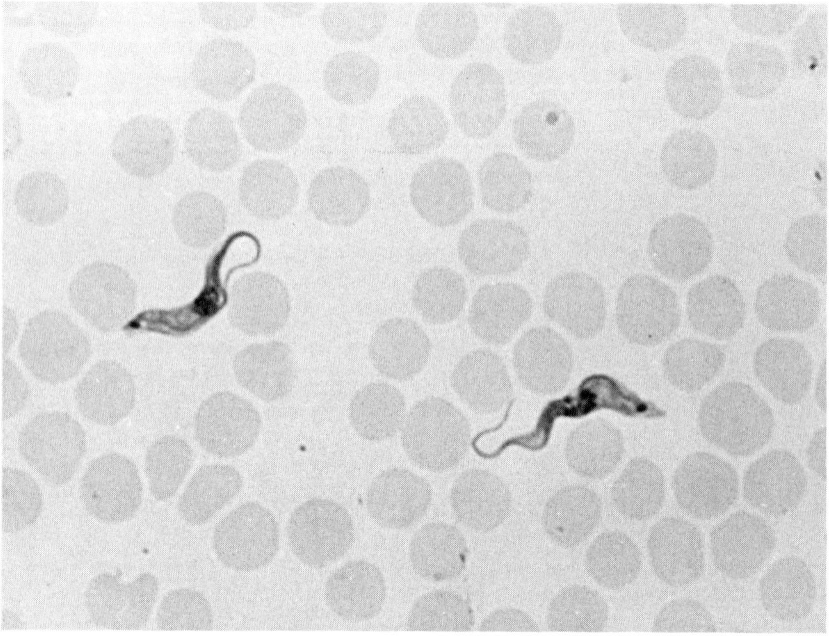

Figure 55. *T. vivax* in ox blood from Mauritius (× 1600).

full parasite characterization and elucidation of the inter-relationships between the African tsetse-transmitted stocks and those from outside Africa (see Chapter 5).

Subgenus *Nannomonas*

The trypanosomes of this subgenus have a range in total length of 8–24 μm. There is no free flagellum at any stage in the life cycle, an unusual characteristic; the flagellum thus terminates at the anterior end of the parasite. The posterior end of the body is usually rounded but can be slightly pointed in longer parasites. The medium-sized kinetoplast is usually in a marginal and sub-terminal position. *T. congolense* is one of the smallest trypanosomes with a mean length of 12–17 μm (figures 56 and 57). *T. simiae*, the porcine trypanosome, is more pleomorphic in its characteristics and the mean length is 15–19 μm, slightly longer than *T. congolense*. *Nannomonas* trypanosomes are very active in fresh blood films but do not tend to move far across the microscope field. They also demonstrate agglutinating properties by tending to adhere to each other as well as to host tissue *in vivo*. Reproduction is by longitudinal binary fission.

Recent isoenzyme studies have demonstrated that polymorphism of *T. congolense* exists in at least West Africa. Enzyme variation occurs in ALAT and such variation has been associated with *T. congolense* isolates from savannah and

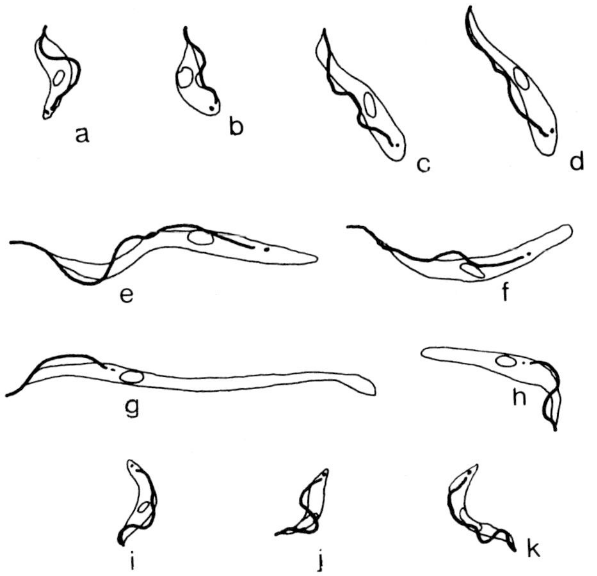

Figure 56. *T. congolense* and *T. simiae*, subgenus *Nannomonas* (× 1300).
a and b, Blood stream forms of *T. congolense*.
c and d, Blood stream forms of *T. simiae*.
e and f, Procyclic trypomastigotes of *T. congolense* from the midgut of *Glossina*.
g and h, Epimastigotes of *T. congolense* from the proboscis of *Glossina*.
i–k, Metacyclic trypomastigotes from the hypopharynx of *Glossina*.

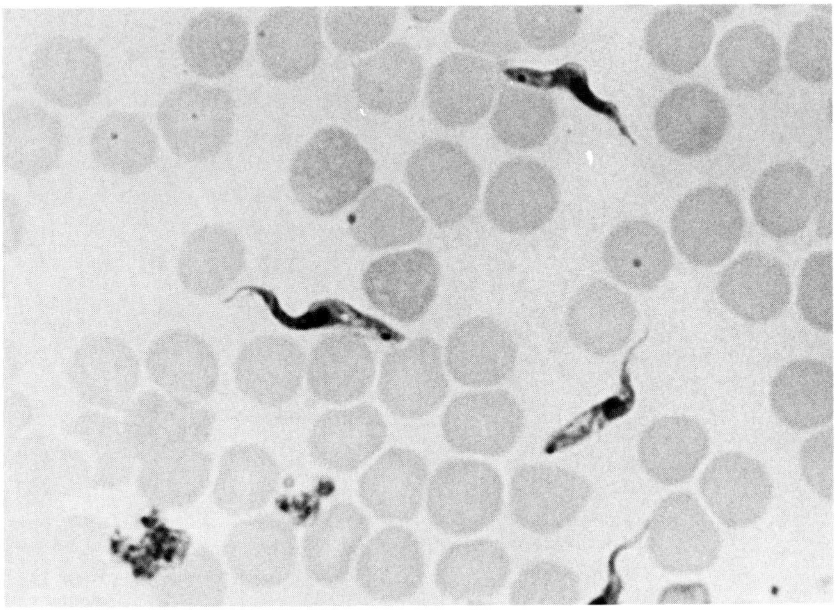

Figure 57. *T. congolense* in mouse blood (× 1600).

forest sources. The relationship between *T. congolense* zymodemes and *T. simiae* remains to be elucidated. The earlier suggested differentiation of this subgenus between *'T. congolense'* and *'T. dimorphon'* could have a basis which can be detected by enzyme electrophoresis.

Subgenus *Pycnomonas*

This subgenus is represented by *T. suis* which is a short, stout monomorphic trypanosome whose movement in wet films is said to be as a 'leaf agitated in a light wind' (translation). There is a free flagellum, a small subterminal kinetoplast, and the normal length of the body is 9–19 μm with a mean around 15 μm. Division in the blood is by longitudinal binary fission. The stoutness of the body has lead to suggestions that some forms resemble sphaeromastigotes. There is no information on enzymic characterization of this rare parasite.

LIFE CYCLES IN THE VECTOR

Subgenus *Duttonella*

All *Glossina* species are capable of acting as vectors of *Duttonella*. The life cycle of *T. vivax* is the simplest of the Salivaria trypanosomes as the whole cycle of development is confined to the tsetse proboscis, without any stage of development in the midgut or salivary glands. Infections in the proboscis are initially established on the labrum where epimastigotes form rosettes firmly attached to the cuticle lining the food canal. These epimastigotes measure 16–35 μm in length. A high proportion of the food canal is colonized with these flagellates, some of which detach and invade the hypopharynx. Some rosettes are found in the hypopharynx, but it is here the epimastigotes transform into trypomastigotes, the fully transformed ones being the infective metacyclics capable of initiating an infection of the mammalian host. Metacyclic trypanosomes of *T. vivax* measure 14–16 μm in length, and, unusually for metacyclics, they do not reaquire a surface coat.

The time of development of *T. vivax* in *Glossina* varies with temperature. At 22°C, 12–13 days must elapse between the infective feed and the production of metacyclic trypanosomes capable of infecting mammals, whereas at 29°C the cycle can be completed in five days. Infection in the fly can persist throughout its life. The relative simplicity of the life cycle of *T. vivax* is believed to be a reason for the relatively high infection rates observed both in the field and under experimental conditions compared with infection rates observed in the subgenera *Trypanozoon* and *Nannomonas*. *T. vivax* has been found capable of infecting over 70 per cent of *Glossina* under optimum laboratory conditions and field infection rates of *T. vivax* usually exceed 10 per cent and often 50 per cent. There is no relationship between the age of the fly and its susceptibility to *T. vivax* infection as there is in *Trypanozoon* species; presumably also due to the localization of the parasites in the proboscis. A high pupal incubation temperature is said to induce a high infection rate in teneral adult *Glossina* fed on an infected animal.

The localization of cyclic development of *T. vivax* in the proboscis of *Glossina* and in no other vector is curious in view of the likely similarity in other haematophagous arthropods to the conditions which pertain in what is essentially a cuticular tube. The reason for the selectivity of *T. vivax* to development in this site only is unknown.

T. uniforme has been little studied, but what information is available confirms that development is also restricted to the proboscis and that infection rates are of the same order as in *T. vivax*. However, little is known about the relationship between the duration of the cycle and temperature of fly maintenance.

T. vivax is a common parasite of bovids and rarely infects suids. Both in West and East Africa infection rates of *T. vivax* decrease as the percentage of blood meals taken by *Glossina* from Suidae increases.

Subgenus *Nannomonas*

T. congolense and *T. simiae* have similar life cycles in the *Glossina* species in which they develop. Although not completely refractory to infections with the subgenus

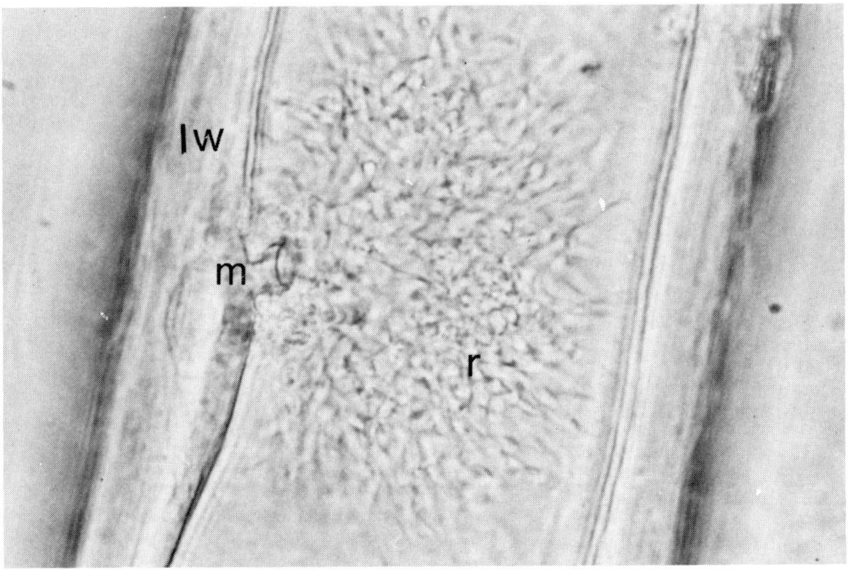

Figure 58. A photomicrograph of the labrum of a *G. morsitans* infected with *T. congolense*. Note the rosette, r, of trypanosomes which occupies a large part of the section of the food canal. The parasites are associated with a mechanoreceptor, m, on the wall of the food canal; lw = labrum.

Courtesy of Dr I. Maudlin.

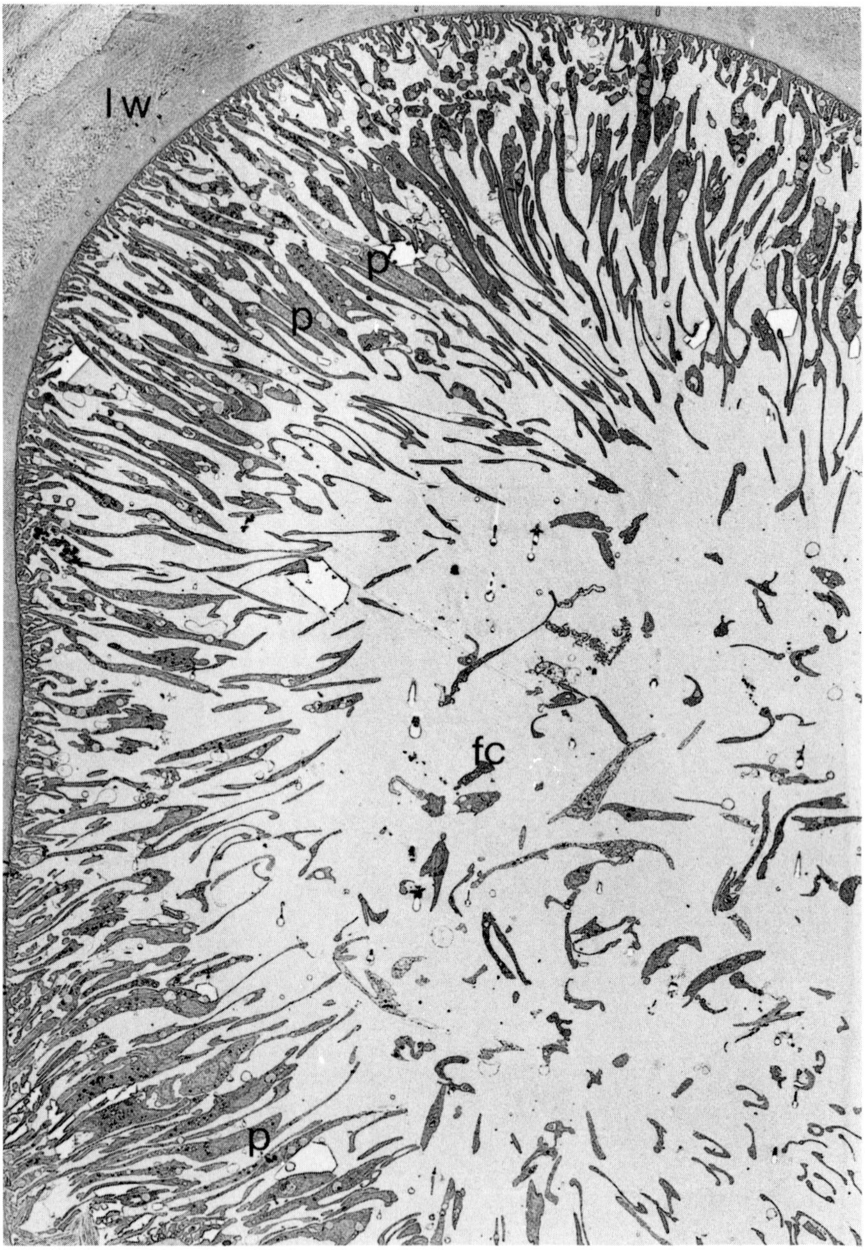

Figure 59. A section of *T. congolense* infected labrum of *Glossina m. morsitans*. Note the complete parasitization of the wall of the labrum, lw (× 1900).

Courtesy of *Acta Tropica* and Thevenaz and Hecker.

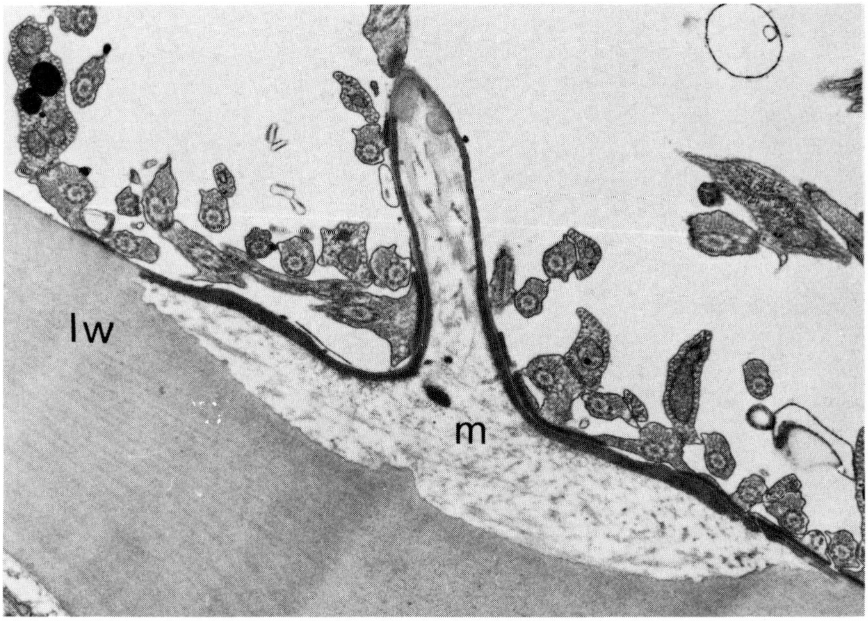

Figure 60. A section of labrum of *Glossina m. morsitans* infected with *T. congolense*. The parasites are attached to a mechanoreceptor, ml; lw = labrum wall (× 15 000).

Courtesy of *Acta Tropica* and Thevenaz and Hecker.

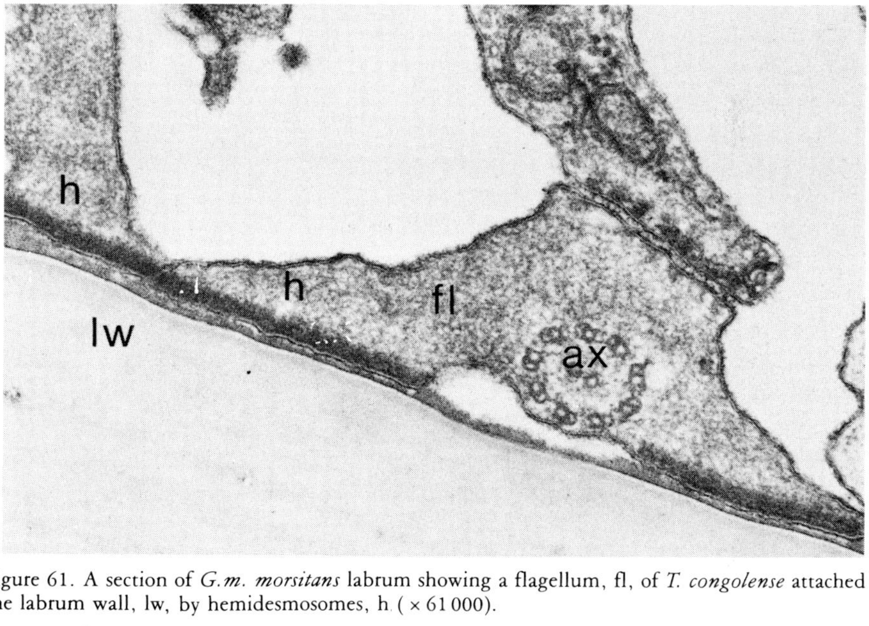

Figure 61. A section of *G.m. morsitans* labrum showing a flagellum, fl, of *T. congolense* attached to the labrum wall, lw, by hemidesmosomes, h (× 61 000).

Courtesy of *Acta Tropica* and Thevenaz and Hecker.

Nannomonas, *G. palpalis* group flies are much less susceptible than other members of the genus, for example, *G. morsitans* and *G. fusca* group flies. The life cycle of *T. congolense* in *Glossina* involves both a midgut and a proboscis stage. The infection rates of *T. congolense* in *G. morsitans* in the field and laboratory are intermediate between those of *Trypanozoon* and *Duttonella*. Infection rates in the laboratory of up to 30 per cent can be obtained in *G. morsitans,* the high infection rates being achieved when the pupal incubation temperature is high. Infection rates in the wild are variable, and of the order of 5–15 per cent.

Initial development takes place in the endoperitrophic space of the posterior midgut where elongated trypomastigotes 40 μm in length multiply before moving to the ectoperitrophic space. *T. congolense* has also recently been found within the epithelial cells of the midgut. The trypomastigotes re-enter the endoperitrophic space by penetrating the soft peritrophic membrane in the proventricular region, and then move anteriorly to the proboscis. Here they transform to epimastigotes and attach to the walls of the food canal (figures 58–61). Parasites attach to mechanoreceptive sensilla in this site affecting the probing behaviour of the fly. The epimastigotes, which measure 14–36μm in length, multiply in colonies or rosettes. The rosettes gradually colonize the labrum and enter the hypopharynx where metacyclic trypanosomes (9–11μm in length) resembling small bloodstream forms are produced. These are infective to mammals.

The life cycle of *T. congolense* in tsetse requires a minimum of 12 days but takes longer at lower temperatures. About 25 per cent of flies remain infected and infective throughout life. The life cycle and infection rate of *T. simiae* in *Glossina* is similar to that of *T. congolense*; cyclical development takes 16–25 days and infection rates in the laboratory were between 0 and 8·6 per cent in *G. m. submorsitans* and less in *G. tachinoides* (1·6–6·3 per cent). Recent studies indicate that the susceptibility of *G. m. morsitans* to *T. congolense* is genetically determined through the female line.

The inverse relationship between infection rates of *T. vivax* and the percentage of *Glossina* blood meals derived from Suidae is not found in *T. congolense* whose infection rates in *Glossina* remain approximately the same whether blood-meal sources are predominantly Bovidae or Suidae.

Subgenus *Pycnomonas*

T. suis has been little studied. However, its life cycle in *Glossina* is similar to the subgenus *Trypanozoon*. Trypomastigotes occur in the midgut and migrate via the proventricular region and proboscis to the salivary glands. Metacyclics occur in the hypopharynx. The development cycle takes 28 days and infection rates of 1–2 per cent are reported; flies remain infected throughout their life.

Subgenus *Trypanozoon*

The life cycle of this subgenus has been described in Chapter 3 (pp. 101–107). The *Trypanozoon* parasites of animals have a similar life cycle to those infective to man.

Other Trypanosomes in *Glossina*

In addition to the Salivaria trypanosomes which develop in the midgut, proboscis and salivary glands, the crocodile trypanosome *T. grayi* also develops in *Glossina*. Although this organism is not a pathogen, it is mentioned here as its presence may be recorded during dissection of *G. palpalis* group flies as riverine tsetse flies; *G. palpalis* subspecies, *G. tachinoides* and *G. fuscipes* take blood from crocodiles and monitor lizards. *T. grayi* develops in the midgut and hindgut of *Glossina* and heavy infections result from the attachment of several layers of parasites to the wall of the gut. Transmission of *T. grayi* to crocodiles is by contamination as a result of crushing flies or the deposition of faeces on or around the mouth. Experimental infection rates are around 17 per cent; when crocodiles were more common, wild caught flies had infection rates of 11 per cent. The level of parasitaemia in the crocodile is very low; monitor lizards are probably also infected with *T. grayi*-like organisms. *Glossina palpalis* group are also occasionally infected with a haemogregarine, *Hepatozoon pettiti,* which develops in the haemocoele of flies.

HOSTS OF AFRICAN ANIMAL TRYPANOSOMES

General considerations

The salivarian parasites described here have an extremely wide host range and all the large African game mammals show varying degrees of susceptibility to *Duttonella, Nannomonas* and *Trypanozoon*. The subgenus *Pycnomonas,* however, appears to be confined to domestic pigs and wild suids. Table 11 indicates the wide host range of these trypanosomes in African mammals. To date, no pathogenic trypanosomes have been recorded from primates other than man, Chiroptera (bats), insectivores, lagomorphs or rodents. The only naturally infected non-mammalian vertebrate host recorded to date is a single chicken in Ivory Coast infected with *Trypanozoon*; the significance of this finding is not yet known. Table 11 does not indicate the percentage infection rates or the levels of parasitaemia recorded, because in most cases the information is limited.

There is a relationship between the frequency of infection and the attractiveness of a host to *Glossina*. For example, although zebra are recorded as having been infected with three subgenera of Salivaria, they are normally not infected with trypanosomes as they are rarely bitten by *Glossina*. On the other hand, carnivores (lion and hyaena) are also rarely bitten by *Glossina* but may

Table 11. Host distribution of some salivarian trypanosomes in African animals.

Host	Common name	'T. Vivax' *Duttonella*	'T. congolense' *Nannomonas*	'T. brucei' *Trypanozoon*
Proboscidae				
Loxodonta africana	African elephant		+	+
Perissodactyla				
Equus sp.	Zebra	+	+	+
E. asinus	Donkey	+	+	+
E. caballus	Horse	+	+	+
Artiodactyla				
Aepyceros melampus	Impala	+	+	+
Alcelaphus buselaphus	Hartebeest	+	+	+
Bos indicus	Zebu	+	+	+
B. taurus	Domestic cattle	+	+	+
Camelus dromedarius	Two humped camel		+ (*simiae*)	+
Capra hircus	Domestic goat	+	+	+
Cephalophus spp.	Duiker	+	+	+
Connochaetes gnou	Wildebeest			+
Damaliscus korrigum	Topi	+	+	+
Gazella sp.	Gazelle	+	+	
Giraffa camelopardalis	Giraffe	+	+	
Hippotragus equinus	Roan antelope	+	+	+
Kobus spp.	Waterbuck	+	+	+
Ourebia ourebi	Oribi	+	+	+
Phacochoerus aethiopicus	Warthog	+	+ (*simiae*)	+
Potamochoerus porcus	Bushpig		+	
Redunca spp.	Reedbuck	+	+	+
Sus scrofa	Domestic pig	+	+	+
Sylvicapra grimmia	Duiker	+	+	+
Syncerus caffer	Buffalo	+	+	+
Taurotragus oryx	Eland	+	+	+
Tragelaphus scriptus	Bushbuck	+	+	+
T. strepsiceros	Kudu	+	+	
Carnivora				
Crocuta crocuta	Spotted hyaena	+	+	+
Panthera leo	Lion	+	+	+
Canis familiaris	Domestic dog	+	+	+

have high infection rates as the result of oral infection from eating infected prey. The levels of parasitaemia in many species of game are extremely low and many can be detected only by subinoculation of blood into susceptible rodents; this is likely to result in a heavy selection of *Nannomonas* and *Trypanozoon* infections due to the relative insusceptibility of rodents to *Duttonella* (*T. vivax*). Although stocks of *Nannomonas* and *Trypanozoon* species can be maintained in rodents and by cryopreservation, the subgenus *Duttonella* has to be maintained in cattle, sheep and goats, except for some strains of Nigerian origin which have been adapted to grow in mice and which maintain their infectivity to *Glossina*. However, mouse–*Glossina*–mouse transmission of these *T. vivax* isolates is difficult. In view of the insensitivity of blood film examination as a diagnostic method, it is likely that many infections were undetected in past surveys, most of which relied solely on this technique.

Trypanosomes in wildlife

The game animals of Africa form an enormous reservoir of pathogenic trypanosomes. Their importance as reservoirs is emphasized by the successful control of cattle trypanosomiasis by selective shooting of game in certain areas of Africa, notably Uganda and Zimbabwe. Happily this method of control has been abandoned as it is recognized that the African game animals represent a vast economic resource, in terms of tourism and possibly in meat production, as well as their ecological importance in maintaining stability in ecosystems. Although many species of game are infected there are certain *Glossina*–game relationships which are of prime importance in trypanosomiasis epidemiology and epizootiology. The identification of such relationships has resulted largely from blood-meal identification techniques which have enabled recognition of the specific hosts of *Glossina*.

Certain species and groups of *Glossina* are extremely catholic in their tastes; the most notable group being the *G. palpalis* group. Even so, certain populations may take a high proportion of blood meals from only one host species. For example, peridomestic *G. palpalis* and *G. tachinoides* populations in Ivory Coast and Nigeria, respectively, feed mainly on pigs, while in other areas they may feed on reptiles, man or bushbuck, depending on the availability of food.

The bushbuck is a preferred host of *G. pallidipes* and is recognized as an important reservoir of *T. b. rhodesiense*. Bushbuck densities are high in '*G. pallidipes* thickets' in Kenya and Uganda, but bushbuck are preferred even when the density of alternative hosts is greater. The bushbuck has a restricted home range resulting in microfoci of infection associated with the thicket edges. Man encountering such a microfocus is exposed to a high risk of infection from infected *G. pallidipes*; hence the concept of 'hot spots' of disease. Other species of game, such as buffalo and roan antelope, though less important in the maintenance of infections because of their wider home range, may disperse the parasites to other areas. Warthogs (*Phacochoerus aethiopicus*) are favoured hosts of the *G. morsitans* group, both in East and West Africa.

Trypanosome infection rates of game animals are highly variable; available figures suggest that the approximate overall infection rates of some of the more common game animals with salivarian trypanosomes, in tsetse areas are as follows: lion and hyaena, 70 per cent; waterbuck, 50 per cent; kudu, 45 per cent; reedbuck, 44 per cent; giraffe, 35 per cent; and eland and bushbuck, 30 per cent. The prevalence in zebra is low (6 per cent). Buffalo, bushpig, duiker, hartebeest, warthog and roan antelope have 10–15 per cent infection rates. Variations between different parts of Africa are likely and the figures are also dependent on the trypanosome detection techniques employed. The bovids are also infected with *T. theileri*-like trypanosomes of the subgenus *Megatrypanum*. These parasites are occasionally seen in blood films but are more likely to be detected by cultivation; their host range, vectors and the taxonomic relationships between *Megatrypanum* from the variety of infected hosts remain to be elucidated.

Trypanosomes are not usually pathogenic to game animals and secondary infections are probably the prime cause of pathogenicity. By suppressing the immune response they may render the host incapable of keeping a previously cryptic trypanosome infection in check. Experimental infections cannot give a true indication of parasite behaviour in wild hosts since capture and captivity can cause unnatural stress. However, in captive bred bushbuck a chancre may develop at the site of the bite of infected tsetse as in cattle and man. Autopsied game animals have shown mild encephalitis and mycocarditis associated with *T. brucei*. *T. congolense* lesions in lion are reported to be similar to those observed in cattle. Significant trypanosome associated pathological lesions have also been observed in impala, Thomson's gazelle and hartebeest. There are reports of mixed infections in game animals and it seems that infection with *T. brucei* predisposes animals to subsequent infection with other subgenera. It seems in cattle, for example, that *T. brucei* is the first species to be observed in the blood, but this is then replaced by *T. vivax* and *T. congolense*.

There are likely to be many factors which influence the prevalence of trypanosomes in game animals. Some of these are related to *Glossina* biology and there is evidence of innate resistance to infection in animals. The impala is able to twitch its skin preventing tsetse bites, and oryx are said to spear the insects with their horns. 'Stress', such as drought or concurrent infection which may lead to immunosuppression, could increase susceptibility to trypanosomiasis. Mechanical transmission of trypanosomes by flies such as *Tabanus* or *Stomoxys* may be important in game herds or where animal density is sufficiently high to allow an interrupted feed to be continued on a second host.

Trypanosome infection in game has been studied using blood from animals either fatally shot or, as is more common now, immobilized by anaesthetic darts. The latter allows sufficient time for blood to be taken, and an antidote is then given to allow the animal to recover. Immobilization techniques are highly specialized and require veterinary expertise; the major problems are the assessment of the anaesthetic dosage required to bring down an animal in a short time and getting close enough to it to ensure the dart reaches a suitable muscle. This problem is difficult in dense vegetation as immobilization is not immediate and animals may be difficult to follow after darting.

Epizootiology of animal trypanosomiasis

The study of the dynamics of transmission of disease among animals is known as epizootiology. The analysis of the many factors likely to affect prevalence of infection, incidence of new infection or the severity of the disease is a complex but stimulating activity which involves consideration of many interacting disciplines. To date mathematical models are, at best, crude approximations. The most important consideration relates to the level of infection in flies, to the density of the fly population and the susceptibility of hosts. Recent studies of animal as well as human trypanosomiasis indicate that there is a simple linear relationship between the apparent density of *Glossina* vectors and the incidence of trypanosomiasis in animals. This observation, if confirmed as being widely applicable, will simplify the assessment of trypanosome risk or challenge. In the past, challenge has been described as 'light', 'medium', or 'heavy' without exact quantitative definition of the terms, except in relation to apparent density of *Glossina* as determined from data collected during flyrounds. The linear relationship between fly density and incidence may be distorted if trypanosome infected individual flies behave differently from non-infected flies and probe and feed more frequently.

The complex inter-relationships which determine infections in flies, domestic animals or wild animal hosts are show in Table 8 (p. 107). This attempts to include all the factors which may influence infection but others may be identified at a later date. The factors outlined affecting the infection rate in populations of flies ot the likelihood of an individual fly becoming infected must be regarded as separate from trypanosome risk or challenge. This term has had a variety of definitions. Initially it referred solely to the abundance of tsetse on the basis of their apparent density, i.e., the number of invective bites per unit time. Indices of transmission and challenge have also been used to enable workers to assess the risk to cattle populations or the frequency with which to use drugs, for example, the Berenil Index.

The epizootiology of animal trypanosomiasis is influenced by many host determined factors. Factors contributing to the complex epizootiology of animal trypanosomiasis include intraspecific host variation in response to infection, variation in *Glossina* host preferences, and the seasonal migration of both game and domestic animals — in relation to availability of pasture or water or to avoid fly belts.

TREATMENT AND PATHOLOGY

Drug treatment of animal trypanosomiasis

Several drugs are available for the treatment of trypanosomiasis infected animals. Some drugs can also be used as prophylactics. However, for efficient treatment of large numbers of cattle it is normal practice that the whole herd is treated as soon as some of the animals show clinical symptoms. Details of the available drugs and their veterinary use are given in Table 12. These drugs have been in use for three decades during which time no new compounds have been introduced. However, substantial resistance has developed to all of the available drugs except Berenil, which seriously complicates prophylaxis and treatment — especially of relapse infections. Drug resistance is stable and transmissible through *Glossina*. Control is dependent on the use of five compounds; these are homidium (Ethidium), quinapryamine (Antrycide), diminazene (Berenil), pyrithidium (Prothidium) and isometamidium salts (Samorin). Suramin is used for the treatment of *T. evansi* in camels (see Chapter 5 p. 158) and *T. brucei* in horses.

The wide availability of trypanocidal drugs in Africa and their frequent misuse, particularly through underdosing, possibly due to underestimation of the weight of the animal, has contributed to the development of drug-resistant strains. In addition, there is cross-resistance between some drugs, although fortunately to date no cross-resistance between isometamidium (Samorin) and diminazene (Berenil) has been reported. The risk of drug resistance can be minimized by alternating the use of these two drugs. Other causes of resistance may be the lack of dispersal of a drug from the site of inoculation, the use of preventive drugs in curative treatments, and infrequent or irregular preventive treatments. It is also important to ensure that drugs are freshly made up and not kept in solution longer than necessary. There is evidence from studies on *T. brucei* in mice that the phenomenon of drug resistance may have been mistaken in the past for parasite breakthrough due to parasites in sites of the body inaccessible to drugs; such sites have been identified as the brain and choroid plexus in

Table 12. Drugs available for the control of African animal trypanosomiasis.

Drug	Trade Name	Chemotherapeutic (C) or prophylactic (P)
Homidium bromide	Ethidium	C
Homidium chloride	Novidium	C
Diminazene aceturate	Berenil	C
Isometamidium chloride	Samorin	C/P
	Trypamidium	C/P
Suramin		C
Pyrithidium bromide	Prothidium	P
Quinapyramine sulphate	Antrycide sulfate	C
Quinapyramine chloride + sulphate	Antrycide prosalt	P
Suramin–quinapyramine capsule		P

Trypanozoon-infected mice, but have not yet been satisfactorily identified in livestock infected with *T. vivax* and *T. congolense*, if indeed they exist.

Prophylactic drugs should be used with caution and for specific purposes such as protection of cattle passing through tsetse-infested areas to slaughter, or of animals living on ranches.

Animals should be monitored for some time after treatment for toxic side effects, and the site of inoculation well massaged to aid dispersion of drug. Animals to be used for meat should be given the drug in musculature which has no economic value because of the risk of iatrogenic necrotic foci and tissue discoloration.

Pathology of trypanosomiasis in livestock

The different pathogenic trypanosome species generally produce the same complex of symptoms and thus the description is applicable to them all unless otherwise stated. The earliest sign of trypanosomiasis following infection is a local reaction at the site of the bite, but this is rarely seen in natural infections. These sites contain foci of trypanosomes in the dermal collagenous connective tissue which persist, in the case of *T. congolense*, for 1–3 weeks after infection. Initially, infiltration of polymorphonuclear leucocytes occurs; these are later replaced, as the reaction declines, with macrophages and plasma cells. The dominant feature of trypanosomiasis in cattle is anaemia and, although other organisms (*Babesia, Anaplasma* and *Theileria*) cause anaemia, the severity is greater in trypanosome infections than in other diseases. The anaemia has two phases: an acute haemolytic phase associated with rising parasitaemia, and a chronic phase associated with declining parasitaemia. During the latter phase there is a packed cell volume (PCV) of 22–27 per cent, depending on the breed of animal, compared with a normal PCV of 35 per cent. Not all animals survive the acute stage of the disease. Several mechanisms have been proposed to account for this anaemia, between which interaction is likely: haemolysis, immunoglobulin complex formation on RBCs leading to erythrophagocytosis by macrophages, and increased RBC fragility as a result of the fever. A haemorrhagic syndrome occurs in some *T. vivax* infections. The rapid recovery of an infected animal after treatment demonstrates that the parasites themselves cause the anaemia.

Adult cattle undergo weight loss and young animals have a reduced growth rate. Infected cattle (figure 62) are dull, lose their appetite and have difficulty keeping up with the herd. Anaemia can be detected by paleness of the conjunctivae, and the lymph nodes and spleen are enlarged. The gross anaemia, together with myocarditis and increased vascular permeability, results in cardiac failure, frequently in the first years of life; however, recovery does occur, particularly in tolerant breeds.

Organ and tissue damage of liver, heart, kidney and skeletal muscle is common, and there is perivascular oedema and infiltration predominantly of

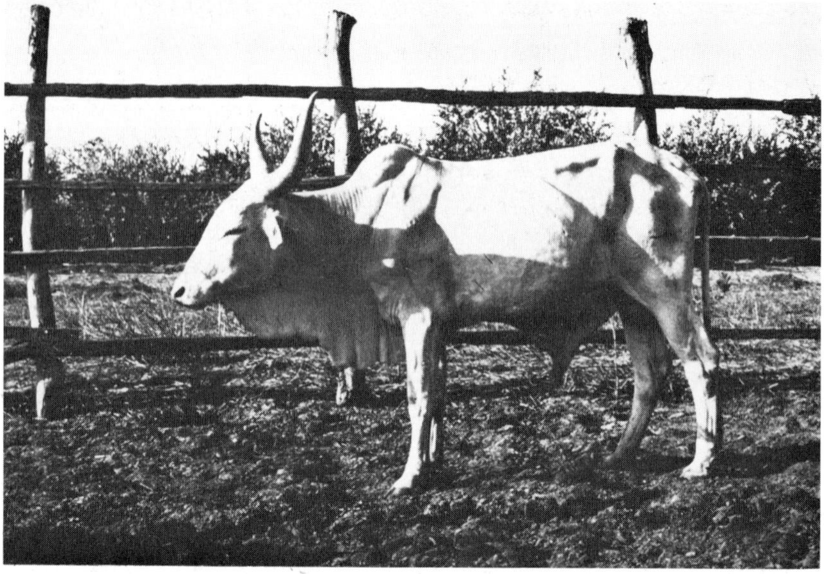

Figure 62. A zebu suffering from chronic trypanosomiasis (*T. congolense*). Courtesy of Dr M. Murray.

small lymphocytes. The heart is usually affected in trypanosomiasis; cellular infiltration occurs and there is severe damage to and degeneration of myocardial fibres. Chronically infected animals show immunosuppression associated with depletion of lymphoid cells, but in the acute stage of the disease the lymph nodes and spleen are filled with proliferating germinal centres. Necrotic foci are found in the brain, heart and skeletal muscle. There is strong evidence of immunosuppression in cattle infected with trypanosomes as there is a ten-fold reduction in the capacity to respond to other antigens. This is clearly highly relevant to the success of vaccination campaigns (against, for example, rinderpest or foot and mouth disease) in areas of endemic trypanosomiasis. The reproductive system is frequently affected and 'abortion storms' and infertility are common in herds in areas of high trypanosome challenge.

Testicular damage also occurs, affecting sperm viability and thus fertility. The central nervous system is also affected, and cattle with *T. b. rhodesiense* have been shown to have a histopathological picture similar to that observed in late-stage sleeping sickness in man.

Although trypanosomes are frequently regarded as blood parasites there is much evidence to show that the *T. brucei* subgroup trypanosomes particularly are also found in the tissue spaces. *T. vivax* and *T. congolense* are usually regarded as being parasites of the circulation, although *T. vivax* has an extravascular phase.

There is good evidence that increased vascular permeability is brought about by the release of pharmacologically active substances — kinins — as a result of trypanosome infection. *T. congolense* produces an inflammatory permeability factor as well as attaching itself to and damaging the microvasculature.

The pathogenesis of trypanosomiasis has been the subject of much speculation. However, recently several biologically active trypanosome metabolites have been incriminated in the pathology. These 'toxins' include metabolites of aromatic amino acids, B-lymphocyte mitogens, haemolysins and platelet aggregating factors as well as 'factors' causing immunosuppression, inflammation and complement activation.

Pathology in livestock involves the same complex of symptoms and a general description applies to the different trypanosomes in different breeds. It is apparent that the disease process which produces either death or chronic wasting in trypanosome infected animals is highly complex, involving a wide range of effects which interact *in vivo*, impinging on normal physiological and immunological processes.

Trypanotolerance

One method of reducing the effects of animal trypanosomiasis and increasing productivity of stock is to exploit the tolerance to trypanosome infection displayed by some breeds of cattle. Animals which display this characteristic are described as trypanotolerant and such breeds grow and survive in areas where *Glossina* transmitted trypanosomes occur and where other breeds cannot survive. Around 30 million sheep and goats and eight million cattle reside in areas of West and Central Africa where they are constantly challenged by trypanosome infected *Glossina*. The trypanotolerant cattle are mainly humpless taurine breeds (*Bos taurus*); there are three main groups, the N'dama, Muturu and Dahomey. The N'dama (figure 63) and Muturu breeds are the most common and have been introduced into other areas of Africa. Populations of cross-bred animals (with zebu, *Bos indicus*, figure 62) are found on the boundaries of the distribution of trypanotolerant breeds. Trypanotolerant cattle are smaller than the humped zebu (about half the weight); they are used by peasants for milk and in some areas as draught animals; tolerant breeds are not good milk producers however, and milking is detrimental to the calves. Young bulls are slaughtered at 18–36 months and cows when they are no longer productive. About 12 per cent of the herd is slaughtered annually, which is the same level as that for zebu cattle in the Sahel, but trypanotolerant animals weigh much less at slaughter. However, under conditions of trypanosomiasis challenge, trypanotolerant breeds gain weight whereas zebus lose weight. If additional stress is placed on trypanotolerant animals such as a severe dry season, they too will lose weight. Fertility of zebu is known to be affected by trypanosomiasis, and despite their trypanotolerance, N'dama females naturally infected with trypanosomes also have reduced fertility.

Sheep and goats are more numerous than cattle in areas of Africa where trypanosomiasis is found; indigenous sheep (Red Masai) and goats (Galla) have been

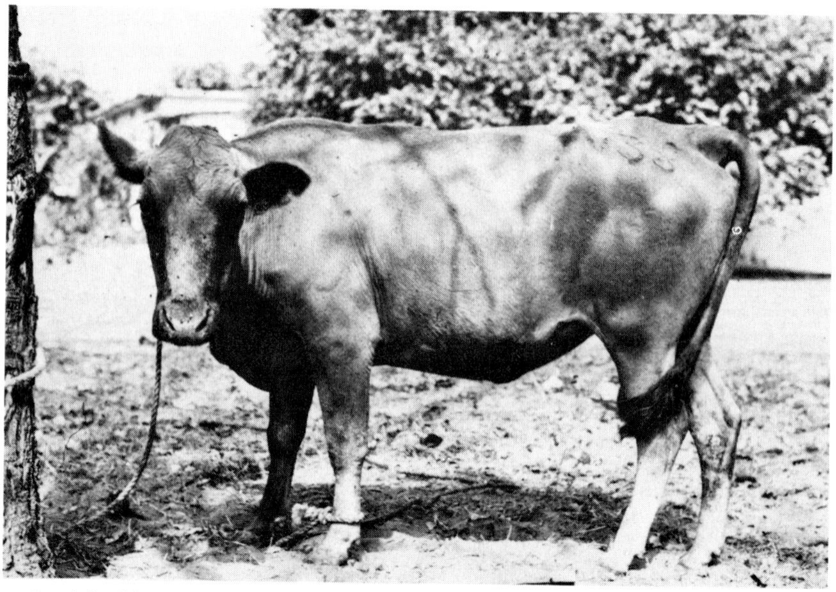

Figure 63. A healthy N'Dama (polled).
Courtesy of Dr M. Murray.

found more tolerant to experimental trypanosome infection than exotic breeds such as Saanen goats and Merino sheep. The inherent ability of game animals to resist virulent trypanosomes is also regarded as trypanotolerance. As with the trypanotolerant breeds of cattle, this can be broken down by stress conditions, such as lack of food or water and intercurrent infections. The finding, in mice, of a genetic basis of resistance to *T. congolense* infection suggests that tolerance in both cattle and mice is an incompletely dominant trait under polygenic control. The tolerance is associated with differences in the capacity of the immune system to respond to trypanosomes and the maintenance of high antibody levels over a longer period by tolerant animals. Biochemical differences have been found in the Y chromosome between N'dama and zebu, as well as haemoglobin differences. For example, pure N'damas have haemoglobin A only, whereas zebus have A and B and sometimes C. It has been noted that the PCVs of infected N'dama are higher than those of zebu, averaging 27 per cent compared with 22 per cent. The innate basis of tolerance has been confirmed by fly and needle challenge in the Gambia where, over a three-year period, 61 zebu cattle all died while only three of 60 N'dama kept under the same conditions did so. Parasitaemia levels were consistently and significantly lower in N'dama.

The phenomenon of tolerance to trypanosome infection is not absolute. Trypanotolerant breeds frequently exhibit parasitaemias and the maintenance of tolerance in the herd is dependent on regular challenge. There is also a dose dependent response; the more organisms are inoculated, the more severe the symptoms are. In addition, humped zebu animals are not completely sensitive, and exhibit levels of tolerance. Should trypanotolerance break down in N'dama, for example through intercurrent infections, poor management, massive challenge, work, pregnancy, lactation or poor nutrition, then clinical trypanosomiasis presents itself as in normally sensitive zebu stock. In an experimental situation where the levels of parasitaemia were higher in zebu than N'dama, the former showed a greater fall in PCV. Level of parasitaemia and PCV are dependent on the level of challenge. If N'dama receive a high dose of parasites they become as parasitized and anaemic as zebu receiving a smaller dose, indicating that tolerance is a relative rather than an absolute character.

Attempts have been made to increase the productivity of trypanotolerant stock by crossing with exotic European breeds while maintaining tolerance. Some success has been achieved in increasing milk production and growth rate to maturity using Jersey and Tarentais stocks.

The exploitation of trypanotolerance is underway in several African countries. This should result in methods of avoiding the worst effects of the disease and will be particularly valuable in areas where tsetse control is not feasible and where exotic breeds of cattle cannot survive. Trypanotolerant stocks are a viable economic proposition, thus the needs at present appear to be the conservation of those stocks, together with long-term breeding programmes and a better understanding of underlying mechanisms of trypanotolerance.

Economic implications of African animal trypanosomiasis

Animal trypanosomiasis has serious economic consequences, including the loss of meat and milk protein to the population, and a subsequent demand for imports of meat and dairy products; further, potential export earnings remain unrealized. Agricultural communities are denied the benefits of draught animals. In addition, concentration of cattle in marginal land results in overgrazing and subsequently in erosion. There are also the costs of treatment and the planning, execution and evaluation of vector control programmes.

However, although *Glossina* species, particularly *G. morsitans*, have made livestock development difficult in many areas, there is an alternative view, that these flies have been responsible for the preservation of natural resources. The exclusion of domestic livestock is held to have protected wild game which can be exploited, for food or for tourism. The exclusion by trypanosomiasis of cattle from marginal land has perhaps prevented further land degradation and desertification. This can be considered to balance the economic consequences of the disease outlined above.

The economic advantages of animal trypanosomiasis control include lower mortality and morbidity in livestock, increased productivity of both pastoral and agricultural communities, improved nutritional status of the population (particularly children), improvement in national balances of payments, reduced human trypanosomiasis as a result of vector control campaigns and the easing of population pressure due to increased availability of land for settlement and development. However clear these benefits may be the long term overall strategy must be designed to use land as effectively as possible after any control operation has taken place.

Tsetse can generally be viewed as a handicap to optimal land usage, but in certain areas tsetse eradication or control may not be appropriate. This is particularly true of mountainous or rocky areas, where there is the need for wildlife conservation, or those areas susceptible to degradation of vegetation and soil erosion. Balanced land-use planning should also take account of alternative and perhaps more economic uses of land where tsetse control would not be required, such as areas of forest for fuel and tree products, village pasture areas — as traditionally used for small ruminants — and areas suitable for a balanced

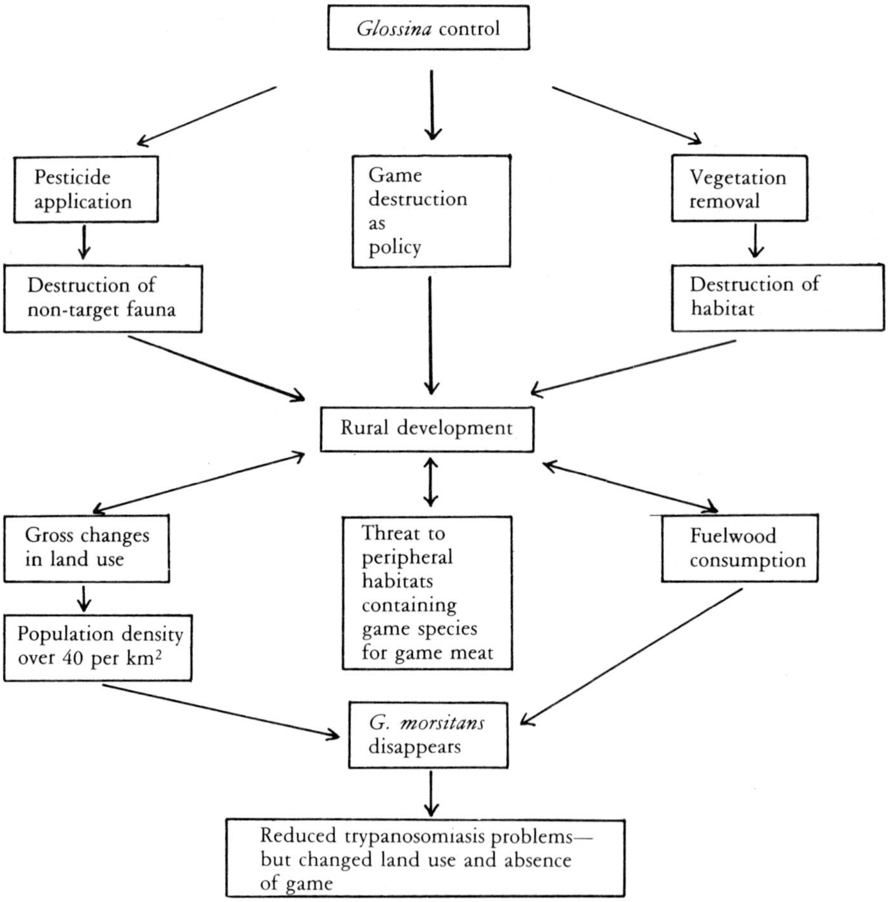

Figure 64. A summary diagram of ecological relationships in animal trypanosomiasis.

arable economy based on traditional crops. Human population pressure on infested land can in itself result in a reduction of *Glossina*, particularly of savannah species. A human population density of 40/km^2 is believed to be too dense for *G. morsitans* survival. Riverine tsetse can withstand this population pressure and associated traditional land use, as can other species of tsetse in such habitats as mango, sugar-cane, banana or coffee plantations. Figure 64 illustrates the interactions between the needs for control on one hand and conservation on the other.

The trends in meat production and human population between 1972–1974 and 1985 suggest that African countries will move from being net exporters of meat to net importers. The increase in demand is expected to exceed the increase in production. It is hoped that trypanosomiasis control will counteract this predicted deficit, thus favourably affecting the balance of payments. Extensive markets exist for sheep and goat meat in the Middle East, and with improved quality of meat products African countries could not only meet their own needs but also become important exporters of meat. However, the marketing system will have to be improved if African exporters are to compete with exporters from Oceania and South America.

The investment requirements for trypanosomiasis control/eradication have been estimated to be of the order of US$ 2–3 per hectare; giving an overall figure of US$ 2–3 billion at 1978 prices for all the infected areas. This would produce an estimated increase in beef protein production of 1·5 million tons per annum if the disease was fully controlled; however additional resources would be required to develop efficient marketing and distribution systems.

Chapter 5. Non–Tsetse Transmitted Trypanosomiases

INTRODUCTION

Although *Glossina* transmitted animal trypanosomiases are the most important economically there are large numbers of cases of trypanosomiasis in a variety of domestic animals outside the tsetse belt of Africa as well as in the Americas and Eurasia.

These are predominantly infected with trypanosomes of the subgenera *Trypanozoon* and *Duttonella*. There is no evidence of the extensive occurrence of infection of *Nannomonas* and *Pycnomonas* outside the zone of *Glossina* infestation. Among the *Trypanozoon*, *T. equiperdum* has become adapted to transmission at coitus; this organism is found only in equines. Those members of the subgenus *Trypanozoon* which have become adapted to non-cyclical modes of transmission have lost, generally speaking, the pleomorphism displayed by the cyclically transmitted *T. brucei* subspecies, and are monomorphic and occasionally dyskinetoplastic.

Dyskinetoplasty is the loss of the typical fibrillar rod-like DNA component of the kinetoplast; the kinetoplast–mitochondrial envelope remains intact but the DNA content is condensed to a compact mass of dense material and is replicated at division along with the acristate mitochondrial network. The reduction of the functional kinetoplast in these organisms led to the identification of a separate species of trypanosome which was permanently without a visible kinetoplast when examined in Giemsa stained preparations. These so-called 'akinetoplastic' stocks of monomorphic equine parasite were referred to as *T. equinum*, a separate species from *T. evansi*. They are now regarded as the same species. Dyskinetoplasty may also appear after treatment of *T. evansi* and other trypanosomes with Berenil or Prothidium.

TRYPANOSOMA EVANSI

This organism, described by Evans working in the Punjab of India, has the distinction of being the first pathogenic mammalian trypanosome to have been recognized. Evans attributed the disease of horses known locally as 'surra' to trypanosomes. The organism was later named *Trypanosoma evansi*. The early reports of this disease in camels and equines came from Asia, particularly southern Russia, Burma and India. Later reports of equine trypanosomiasis came from South America and of camel trypanosomiasis from Africa. This resulted in many different scientific names being allocated to non-tsetse transmitted *Trypanozoon* of South and Central America and Asia. It is now agreed that all these organisms are *T. evansi* although some 33 local specific names have been given to the disease it causes in various hosts. *T. evansi* trypanosomiasis is of great importance in those areas of the world with large camel populations as it causes serious morbidity and some mortality.

History records that *T. evansi* has considerably reduced populations of livestock. Well documented accounts indicate that in Central and South America during the latter part of the last century horses were decimated by what was known as 'mal de caderas'; in European Russia in the 1880s when surra spread from Asia it killed an estimated 70 per cent of camel stocks, and epizootics with high mortalities in Asia have continued to be reported from India, Malaysia and, most recently, Vietnam, where buffaloes are affected. In Africa, just north of tsetse belts, the prevalence of surra in camels is between 15 and 20 per cent but can rise to over 50 per cent in severe outbreaks, with grave implications for the economy of these already marginal zones.

Hosts

T. evansi is primarily an infection of equines (horses, asses and mules) and camels. However, other species, particularly cattle (South and Central America) and buffaloes (Asia), may be infected, and these can act as asymptomatic reservoirs. The capybara *Hydrochoerus*, ocelot *Felis pardalis*, deer *Odocoileus* and vampire bat *Desmodus* have also been identified as hosts in South America. In fact vampire bats can act as both hosts and vectors of *T. evansi* in the Americas.

In Africa and Asia, sheep, goats, deer and antelope are carriers of *T. evansi*. Although dogs are highly susceptible, the acute course of the disease disqualifies them as effective reservoirs. In Asia there are records of *T. evansi* from tigers, foxes, Indian elephants *Elephas maximus*, orang-utans *Pongo pygmaeus* and tapirs *Tapirus indicus*; thus the organism has an unusually wide host range. Laboratory models for *T. evansi* include dogs, rabbits, guinea pigs, rats, mice and the South American rodent, *Proechimys* (figure 86, p. 206).

Distribution and origin

T. evansi is widely distributed in the Old World tropics and neotropics. It is believed to have originated in Africa as a result of camels entering the tsetse belt and becoming infected with pleomorphic *T. brucei*; returning infected camels then became the source of infection for other camels as the disease was spread 'mechanically' by biting flies. Continuous non-cyclical transmission in the absence of *Glossina* resulted in the loss of cyclic transmissibility and in the development of monomorphism.

The movement of camels across the Sahara spread the disease throughout North Africa, and their use in Asia resulted in an eastward spread. The disease also occurs in the islands of Mauritius and Madagascar. It is believed that the Mauritius outbreaks of *T. evansi* originated in India. *T. evansi* in equines and bovines has an even wider distribution than in cameline hosts — the disease is found as far east as Indonesia and the Philippines and throughout the Middle East, the Indian subcontinent and into more temperate parts of Russia. *T. evansi* was also found in North America and Australia but has been eradicated from these areas. The organism is likely to have been imported into South America with the horses of the Spanish conquistadores, which came from enzootic parts of North Africa, or by the importation of cattle; neither equines nor bovines were indigenous to the neotropics. It is not known on how many occasions *T. evansi* was introduced to the New World. Following its introduction into a new area the disease is at first severe, causing enormous losses.

Morphology and characterization

In the bloodstream *T. evansi* usually occurs as monomorphic trypomastigotes 15–36 μm in length, with a mean of 24 μm. There is a small sub-terminal kinetoplast in organisms from populations which are not dyskinetoplastic. The morphology is therefore typically that of slender forms of other members of the subgenus *Trypanozoon*. Occasionally stumpy forms are observed, but the proportion of such forms is very low; posteronuclear forms have also been observed in some isolates. Division is by longitudinal binary fission. The morphology of *T. evansi* is similar throughout its known range.

Biochemical methods of characterization have revealed a remarkable isoenzymic similarity between isolates of *T. evansi* from South America and East and West Africa in ten enzyme systems examined. The implication is that *T. evansi* stocks are derived from a particular *T. brucei* zymodeme which has spread widely by mechanical transmission; what is recognized as *T. evansi* outside the distribution of *Glossina* may have differentiated on one occasion; alternatively only one '*T. brucei*' zymodeme may be capable of extensive mechanical transmission.

Transmission

No cyclical transmission of *T. evansi* occurs and the infection is transmitted between hosts by mechanical transmission effected by biting flies, particularly horse-flies (*Tabanus*) and stable flies (*Stomoxys*). This method of dissemination depends on the movement of a fly with trypanosome contaminated mouthparts to a new host within a short time, so the parasites in the mouthparts remain infective. Such transmission depends on an interrupted feed as it is necessary for the fly to continue to probe and feed when it has moved to another host. Thus the shorter the interval between feeds or attempted feeds the greater the chance of transmission. The abundance of tabanids is also important; there is an apparent link between the seasonal occurrence of outbreaks of *T. evansi* in camels in Sudan and that of the greatest abundance of tabanids, particularly *Tabanus taeniola*, during the rainy season. However, this species is present throughout the year ensuring transmission continues, albeit to a lesser extent.

Experimental studies have shown that *T. evansi* does not survive in the gut of biting flies, even in *Glossina*, being destroyed within hours of ingestion. *Stomoxys* are less efficient vectors of *T. evansi*, but may be important in stables where horses are confined.

In Central and South America vampire bats (*Desmodus rotundus*), which are obligatory blood suckers, become infected via the oral mucous membranes when feeding on *T. evansi* infected cattle. The infection can persist in bats for up to one month and may be fatal.

However, during this time, while biting at night, the bats transmit the infection from the oral secretions to new hosts. Vampire bats imbibe up to 50 ml of blood at a meal and a few parasites are usually present. Parasite numbers increase in the bats, making transmission at each subsequent feed more likely. Transmission of *T. evansi* to carnivores by their eating infected carcasses has also been demonstrated (as with *T. brucei*).

Tabanids as transmitters of *Trypanosoma evansi*

Tabanids lay their eggs on plants associated with or close to water. When the larvae hatch, they drop into the water or onto moist earth nearby.

The larvae are carnivorous and, after several months, they pupate in drier conditions along watercourse edges. When the adults emerge they remain in the shade, except when searching for food in the heat of the day. Only the females are haematophagous, taking up to 200 μl of blood in a meal, but they also need to imbibe water. Their flight range is around 1–3 km. Tabanids can be caught easily by Manitoba traps (conical traps with a black sphere at the base of the cone; figure 65). The distribution of surra in the neotropics and tropics seems closely associated with the ecology and distribution of tabanids.

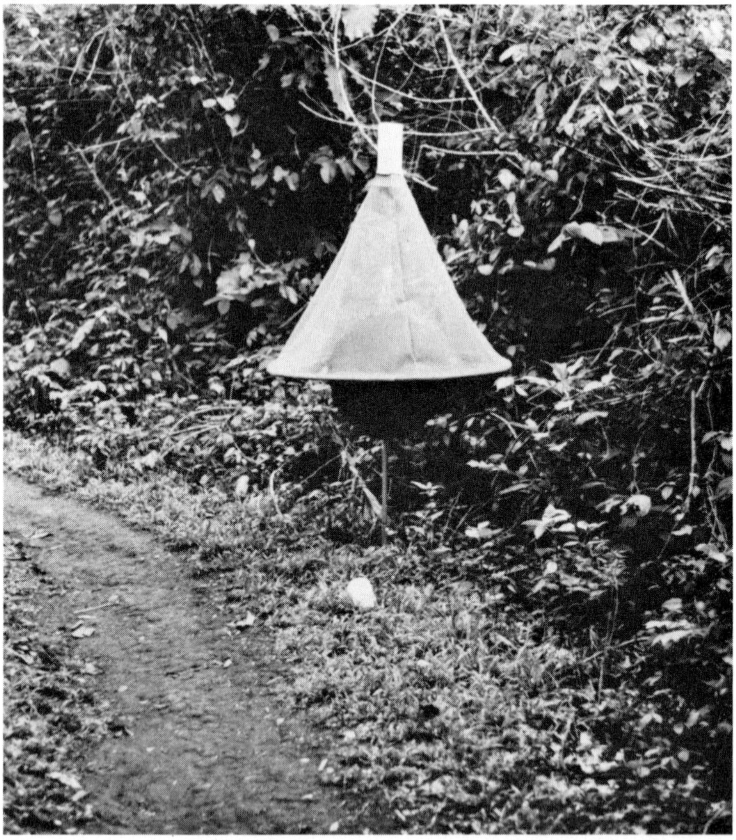

Figure 65. A Manitoba trap consisting of a black sphere with a white upper inverted cone. These traps can be used to collect tabanid populations which can transmit trypanosomiasis mechanically.

Courtesy of Dr L. Ryan.

Parasitological and serological diagnosis

Classical blood film preparations (thin, thick and wet) are of limited sensitivity for the detection of all trypanosome infections, and *T. evansi* is no exception. Concentration methods using microhaematocrit centrifuge or anion exchange columns which have been tested for cattle and human trypanosomiasis have not yet been applied extensively to *T. evansi*, though they would be expected to give greater diagnostic sensitivity.

Similarly, rat and mouse inoculation increases the numbers of animals found positive by approximately 50 per cent compared with blood film techniques. However, the use of such laboratory animals in endemic areas of camel trypanosomiasis for diagnosis is expensive and impractical in view of the time taken for the development of patent parasitaemia in rats (3–9 days) and mice(5–9 days). Various serological tests have recently been extensively evaluated. The difficulties of diagnosing *T. evansi* parasitologically led earlier workers to develop simple tests, applicable in the field, which detected an increased serum globulin. However, these tests are not specific for trypanosomiasis. They include the mercuric chloride, formol gel and thymol–turbidity tests. Such tests more frequently give false negative reactions than those which are designed to detect circulating trypanosomal antibodies.

These serological tests show a greater correlation with trypanosome infection in camels than do the tests for increased serum globulin. The indirect fluorescent antibody test (IFAT) and the enzyme linked immunosorbent assay (ELISA) have been developed and haemagglutination tests have been used in India.

The persistence of antibodies to *T. evansi* infections after chemotherapy may complicate serological results. However, the more sensitive tests indicate that the levels of circulating antibody tend to fall following drug treatment. Concentration methods for parasitological diagnosis together with IFAT and ELISA will improve the sensitivity and specificity of diagnostic surveys and it is important that these are applied in the enzootic areas.

Pathology and pathogenesis

The degree of pathogenicity of trypanosomiasis caused by *T. evansi* varies greatly over its very wide range. Environmental and host factors, such as other infections and 'stress', will undoutedly also affect the severity and outcome of the disease, as with *T. brucei*.

In camels the prepatent period is around seven days and clinical signs and symptoms are only evident after about one month when weakness, changes in coat condition and general loss of condition become apparent. Animals are reluctant to stand up and experience difficulty in walking. Abortion may occur in late pregnancy. There are recurrent bouts of fever. The disease can range either from being fatal within a few months to a symptomless carrier state. More chronic disease with animals surviving up to four years is known to occur, but spontaneous recovery is rare.

Similar symptoms are recorded from horses with *T. evansi* infection. They display anaemia, recurrent fever, oedema, coat changes, reluctance to walk and unsteady gait associated with muscular weakness. Urticarial plaques occur sporadically. In horses the infection may last up to four months before the animals succumb. Episodes of fever are associated with reduced appetite. Changes occur in the brain of animals which have been infected for several months. *T. evansi* causes histological changes in tissues of infected animals similar to those caused by *T. brucei*. Horses are generally more susceptible to *T. evansi* infection than donkeys, which seem to be capable of resisting the infection despite a high parasitaemia accompanied by an anaemia. After about one month trypanosomes can be detected only by animal inoculation. The symptoms of infection in donkeys are similar to but milder than those in horses. *T. evansi* also infects dogs and elephants, where symptoms are severe and the outcome is often fatal. Infections in cattle and pigs tend to be mild, like *T. brucei*. Sheep and goats can be infected, but the symptoms again are not as severe as in horses and camels.

Chemotherapy

Most of the usual trypanocides have been used for treating *T. evansi*. The type of drug to be used is dependent on the species to be cured and the levels of drug resistance in the region. Experimental studies of Mel B and tryparsamide in mice followed by the use of these drugs in equines showed that these arsenicals were effective against surra. Quinapyramine and diminazene (Berenil) are effective in bovines. The aminophenanthridium drugs have also been tested and isometamidium chloride (Samorin) is effective against *T. evansi* in dogs. Side effects prevent its regular use in camels, but it is of use if the parasites are resistant to Suramin. Quinapyramine–suramin complexes can be used for chemoprophylactic purposes giving 6–10 months protection to horses; however, this causes tissue necrosis at the site of inoculation. Isometamidium chloride will also confer a chemoprophylactic action of 2–4 months in livestock if given at 0·5–1·0 mg/kg deep intramuscularly.

Diminazene aceturate (Berenil) cures *T. evansi* in bovines at 8·0 mg/kg (the normal therapeutic dose is 3·5 mg/kg). However, a dose of 7 mg/kg of the drug is fatal to trypanosome infected camels. In equines a fatal cerebral reaction to Berenil can occur, but this is rare and local reactions at the site of intramuscular inoculation are more common. Trypanosome infected dogs can also succumb to Berenil with brain damage at the normal therapeutic dose. Tolerance to this drug is therefore variable between as well as within species.

Drug resistant *T. evansi* have been described from Sudan, India and the USSR, but in general Suramin-resistant stocks are sensitive to quinapyramine and isometamidium. However, the extent of resistance is ill-defined and constant vigilance is required on the part of the veterinary authorities.

TRYPANOSOMA EQUIPERDUM

T. equiperdum has the distinction of being the only trypanosome whose normal method of transmission is by coitus. The infection is restricted in nature to equines, in which it causes the disease dourine. It has been recognized for many centuries and, like *T. evansi,* it is widely distributed outside Africa which, in view of the morphology of the parasite, must have been its ancestral home. It has not been reported from West Africa, but is found in South Africa and Namibia. There are reports of the disease from North Africa, Europe, Asia, North and South America.

T. equiperdum is a tissue parasite and bloodstream forms are rarely observed, but such forms are important in the dissemination of the organism to different organs and the skin. *T. equiperdum* is morphologically indistinguishable from *T. evansi*, and pleomorphism has been reported occasionally. Multiplication is by longitudinal binary fission.

Transmission occurs during coitus as a result of the presence of trypanosomes in the seminal fluid and mucus exudate of the male genitals of stallions and the vaginal mucus of mares. Transmission to a healthy partner occurs by the establishment of parasites in the genital-tract mucus and between the epithelial cells. Later the parasites invade the subcutaneous tissues establishing oedematous regions, 'plaques', in the skin.

The mucous membranes of the eyes and nose of foals can be contaminated by vaginal discharge, and transmission to foals from udder lesions is also possible.

T. equiperdum is an extremely difficult organism to establish in laboratory animals such as mice and rats. The most successful method developed to date is the inoculation of rabbit testes with contaminated material from horses. The parasite can be maintained by serial intratesticular passage. Deer mice, *Peromyscus*, develop both acute and chronic infections. The infection can also be transmitted to ruminants which display mild clinical manifestations. Those laboratory strains which have been established in rodents display antigenic variation similar to other *Trypanozoon* stocks. However, few if any recent isolates of this organism are available.

Dourine, like other trypanosome diseases, varies in the severity of its clinical presentations. The initial sites of infection are the genitalia, which generally become oedematous within a short period of the infecting union. The infection spreads through the skin producing plaques which appear and regress. Parasites can be found in the exudate from these plaques. Anaemia and neurological symptoms occur later in the disease. Acutely infected animals die within months, but chronic infections may continue for several years and symptomless carriers are found. Stallions usually die from dourine, but the disease is less severe in mares. There is a less severe course of disease in wild or semi-wild horses as well as in donkeys and asses. Foals may display a protective immunity if born to infected mares.

Prevention of the spread of dourine is dependent on the rigidity of the control measures imposed on the importation of equines.

Another factor which influences the spread of the disease is the level of awareness in breeding establishments of the symptoms of the disease. Compulsory slaughter of infected stallions and mares will clearly eliminate the disease as no insect vector is involved in its transmission, thus eradication is possible. Use of serological techniques for screening stallions is also of use. Parasitological diagnosis is, however, difficult as trypanosomes are scanty. Direct examination of scrapings of genital mucosa and the fluid contents at the border of the urticarial skin plaques may show parasites, but repeated examination may be necessary to confirm parasitologically the aetiology of the clinical symptoms.

Suramin and quinapyramine are effective against dourine at the dose rates used for equines infected with *T. evansi*. However, if eradication is a national policy, test and slaughter is considered to be the most appropriate remedy.

TRYPANOSOMA VIVAX

This organism, most frequently associated with *Glossina* transmitted animal trypanosomiasis in sub-Saharan Africa, has been found outside the zone of *Glossina* infestation, where it is transmitted non-cyclically by other species of biting flies. The movement of African cattle to the Caribbean, South America and Mauritius resulted in the dissemination of *T. vivax* where it has persisted in local cattle populations, except in Mauritius where it was eradicated.

The morphology, methods of diagnosis and treatment of *T. vivax* are similar inside and outside the zone of *Glossina*. The dissemination and establishment of *T. vivax* outside the *Glossina* belt is due to the ease with which it can be transmitted mechanically. The dependence on non-cyclical transmission, as for example in tsetse-free zones in sub-Saharan Africa, results in the loss of infectivity to *Glossina*. In the neotropics *T. vivax* is transmitted by Tabanidae and *Stomoxys*. Attempts to demonstrate cyclical transmission of *T. vivax* by other haematophagous arthropods in the New World have not been successful to date.

It appears that in Mauritius *T. vivax* in bovines was symptomless, but the same strain in sheep and goats was fatal. Variations in *T. vivax* pathogenicity also occur in South America where in Brazil, the disease has passed virtually unrecognized for many years, whilst in Venezuela acute infections with 30 per cent mortality have been described. Similar variation in pathogenicity of *T. vivax* occurs within its distribution in *Glossina* infested zones. Biochemical characterization of mechanically transmitted *T. vivax* should provide interesting information about their origins. However, the problems of the general insusceptibility of laboratory animals to *T. vivax* remains serious.

Chapter 6. Chagas' Disease and Trypanosomiasis outside Africa

CHAGAS' DISEASE

Introduction

Chagas' disease was named after Carlos Chagas who described the causative organism, *T. (Schizotrypanum) cruzi*, in 1909. The parasite differs markedly from the African trypanosomes. In addition to trypomastigotes in the blood, which do not divide, there are pseudocysts in the tissues containing masses of amastigotes. Most of the pathology is the result of the effects of these pseudocysts on their muscle host cells. Transmission to man is by contamination and not by the bite of the vector, which is a bug. Controversy surrounded the initial description of the disease and it was not until the 1930s that its real significance and the value of Chagas' work were fully appreciated. It was only after this period that the achievement was accorded the credit it deserved, but regrettably in the interim Chagas was vilified for his work and his beliefs. Chagas described the organism responsible and the vector bugs, identified one of the reservoir hosts and suggested some of the clinical symptoms associated with the disease. The organism has also been named *Schizotrypanum cruzi* but *Schizotrypanum* has now been relegated to the subgeneric status following the revision of mammalian trypanosome taxonomy. The designation *Trypanosoma (Schizotrypanum) cruzi cruzi* for the organisms which infect man, with the addition of a subspecies name, has recently been proposed; biological (host range) and biochemical (isoenzyme, DNA density) differences between human isolates and those from South American bats have been identified and these latter stocks are designated *T. (S.) cruzi marinkellei*. Morphologically similar but biochemically different parasites also occur in Old World Chiroptera (bats).

The species *T. (S.) dionisii* and related parasites are used for laboratory studies as they are regarded as safer to handle than *T. cruzi* which is still virtually incurable.

T. cruzi is unusual among pathogenic trypanosomes as it is transmitted by contamination, the life cycle in the insect vector being confined to the gut of triatomine bugs. Chagas recognized that these bugs, known in South America as 'barbeiros', were common in human habitations and were haematophagous. Chagas was also familiar with the increasingly widely recognized role of insects in the transmission of other diseases such as malaria, relapsing fever, plague and African sleeping sickness. He also knew of the transmission of mammalian trypanosomes such as *T. lewisi* by fleas. He thus believed that the epimastigotes he found in the guts of barbeiros would be either monoxenous flagellates or a stage in the life history of a mammalian trypanosome. Chagas was also familiar with a monkey (*Callithrix*) trypanosome, *T. minasense*. However, in some monkeys which had been in contact with triatomine bugs he found an entirely different trypanosome which was characterized by a large kinetoplast close to the posterior end of the organism. This finding was followed by his examination of the blood

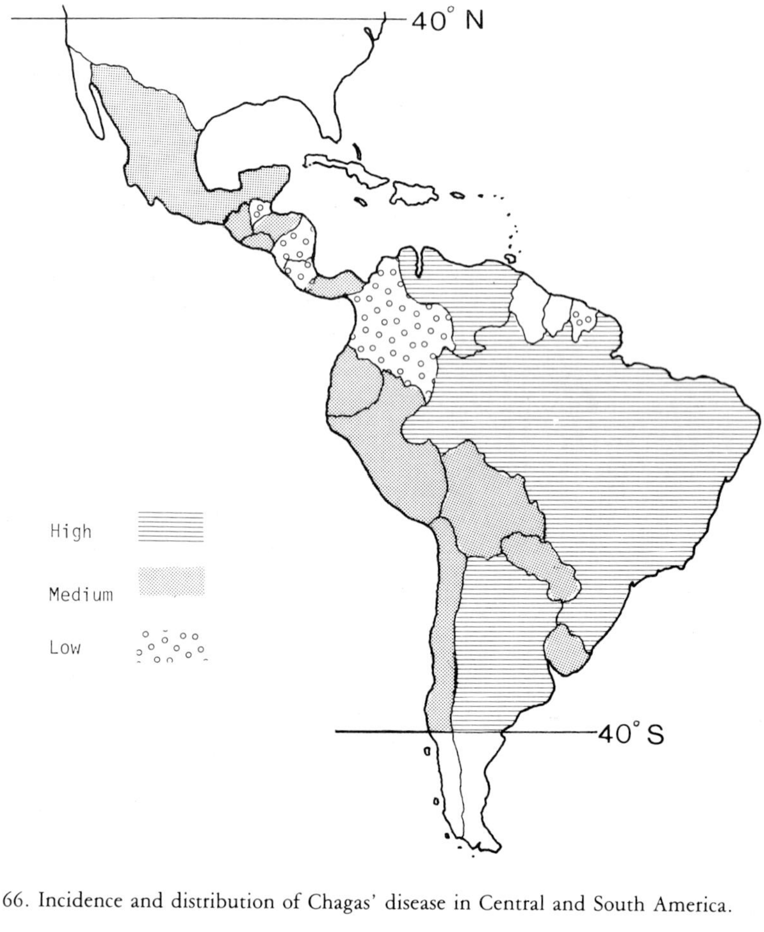

Figure 66. Incidence and distribution of Chagas' disease in Central and South America.

from a febrile child from a home where a large population of triatomines was known to occur. Trypanosomes of the same morphology with a large posterior kinetoplast were found in the blood of the child. Chagas named the organism *Trypanosoma cruzi* after Dr Oswaldo Cruz, the director of the Manguinhos Institute in Rio de Janeiro where Chagas worked.

There is no doubt however that spectacular symptoms of *T. cruzi* were recognized by many travellers, explorers and missionaries in South America before Chagas' discovery of the causative organisms. A chronic disease known as 'bicho' in American texts occurred in areas where triatomines are now known to occur. The first description of symptoms was as early as 1587 and other accounts of the so-called mega condition of the oesophagus and colon and swollen eyelids (Romana's sign) appear repeatedly in the old texts. The megacolon condition, however, was usually believed to be the result of worms, probably the whipworm *Trichuris* and the pinworm *Enterobius*.

The World Health Organisation estimated in 1980 that 35 million people were exposed to infection. This estimate was based on the distribution of the vector. A recent review suggested that 13–14 million people were infected and it is unlikely this figure has fallen. Thirty per cent of infected persons may have electro-cardiographic alterations indicating myocardial damage and up to 60 per cent of people in rural populations may be seropositive for *T. cruzi*.

Chagas' disease is thus recognized as being one of the most important causes of morbidity and mortality in South and Central America. There are no entirely suitable drugs to cure the chronic condition; the vectors are relatively insusceptible to organochlorine insecticides and alternatives are expensive to purchase and apply; continued poor housing conditions in the lower socio-economic groups provide excellent bug habitats. These factors combine to suggest that the disease will remain a problem in these regions for many years to come.

Distribution

T. cruzi is found widely between latitudes 40°N and 40°S in South and Central America and some of the southern states of the USA (figure 66). It has been identified in mammalian hosts as far north as Maryland; the southern limits of its distribution are in Argentina and Chile. Parasitologically confirmed autochthonous cases have been found in every South and Central American country; there is doubt about its status in Belize, Guyana, Suriname and the Caribbean Islands. *T. cruzi*-like infections in mammals exist in these latter areas and there is some serological evidence that man is infected, but this requires confirmation. *T. cruzi*-like organisms do occur in some Caribbean Islands and the southern USA, but parasitological proof of human infection is lacking. Cases of human disease are not usually found further north than Mexico. Animal infections of *T. cruzi*-like organisms are more widespread than the human disease and have been found in all South and Central American countries. This may be due to the habits and ecology of the bugs and their association with reservoir animals rather than man.

The organisms

T. cruzi-like organisms have a highly characteristic morphology in the blood stream of the mammalian hosts (figure 67). They are usually found as C- or S-shaped organisms in thin blood films; they have a large kinetoplast situated close to the pointed posterior end. They measure around 20 μm in length (range 12–30 μm), have a free flagellum 2–11 μm in length and an undulating membrane. They never divide as trypomastigotes in the blood. The parasites in the bloodstream of mammals infected with species of the subgenus *Schizotrypanum* are morphologically indistinguishable. This gives problems in distinguishing between organisms which have significance as parasites infective to man and causing human disease, and those that are only infective to animals and have no significance as a public health problem.

Recently, however, the isoenzyme electrophoresis techniques have enabled the morphologically indistinguishable organisms to be separated by biochemical characteristics as with the other subgenera of mammalian trypanosomes. These techniques, when applied on a large scale to many isolates from man, mammalian hosts and bugs, have provided a much clearer picture of the epidemiology of the disease and parasitology of the subgenus.

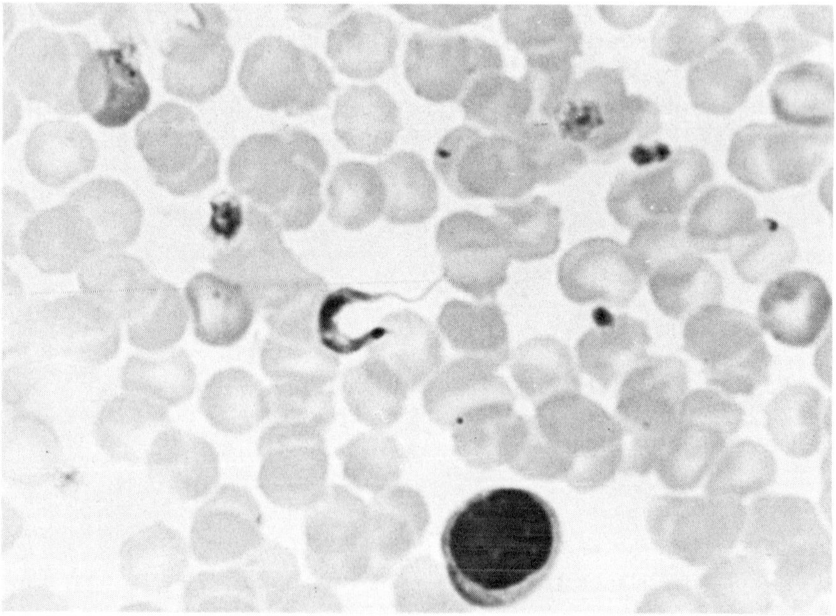

Figure 67. *T. cruzi* in mouse blood (× 1600).

Isoenzyme studies of isolates of the subgenus *Schizotrypanum* are made on lysates of culture forms. Cultures are maintained in diphasic blood agar media or in monophasic liquid media. Initial isolation is usually by xenodiagnosis or cultivation and then inoculation of susceptible experimental animals such as mice.

Studies on cultured isolates from a variety of sources have indicated that, as previously believed, there are sylvatic and domiciliary cycles of distinct zymodemes of *T. cruzi*-like organisms. Further, as referred to above, the parasites isolated from man have been compared with isolates from other sources such as New and Old World bats and have been shown to have different isoenzymes as well as other biochemical characteristics.

Analysis of over two hundred *T. cruzi* stocks isolated from different localities and habitats in Bahia State, Brazil have shown that sylvatic mammals and triatomines can harbour parasites infective to man. Z1 and Z3, the sylvatic zymodemes from Brazil, are more frequently isolated from sylvatic sources however; Z1 is found in some domestic localities in Venezuela. The opossum *Didelphis* (figure 69), is a major source of zymodemes Z1 and Z3 associated originally with the armadillo *Dasypus* and its associated bug *Panstrongylus megistus*. Z2 has not yet been identified with a sylvatic source, being primarily associated with the domestic transmission cycle. Recent studies have shown that the sylvatic zymodemes Z1 and Z3 are more frequently associated with patients with acute Chagas' disease. Zymodeme Z2 was found in domestic situations in acute and chronic cases with cardiac and digestive symptoms. This zymodeme also

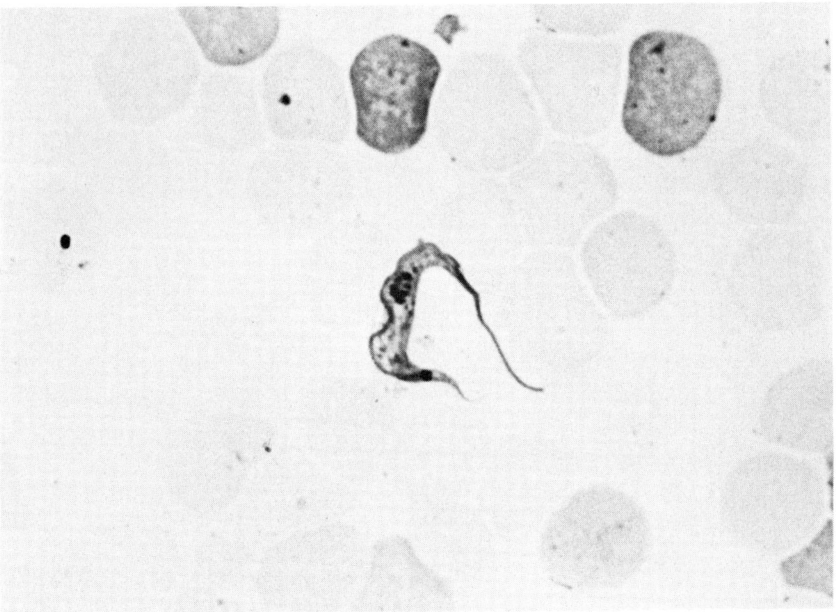

Figure 68. *T. rangeli* in mouse blood (× 1600).

has a restricted geographical distribution. There appears to be a correlation between clinical symptoms and the zymodeme with which a patient is infected. In Venezuela, endemic Chagas' disease is due mainly to Z1 and megasyndromes do not occur; however, in central and eastern Brazil Z2 (not found in Venezuela or the Amazon Basin) was found in most patients and is commonly associated with the megasyndromes.

Some *T. cruzi* stocks have been shown to be polymorphic, particularly during the early phases of parasitaemia, although bloodstream forms of *Schizotrypanum* have generally been regarded as monomorphic.

The predominance of slender forms early in the parasitaemia and their subsequent disappearance from the blood has suggested that these forms are better capable of penetrating cells of normal hosts to give rise to reproductive pseudocysts. Slender forms are also believed to be more sensitive to the host's immune response. Experimental studies seem to confirm that slender forms have greater penetrative ability in tissue, and stumpy forms are those infective to bugs.

T. cruzi has no division stages in the mammalian bloodstream. Multiplication by equal binary fission always occurs intracellularly by amastigotes (2·4–6·5 μm in diameter) and epimastigotes (6–15 μm in length) (figure 70), in pseudocysts in several cell types, particularly cardiac muscle cells (figure 71), smooth muscle cells,

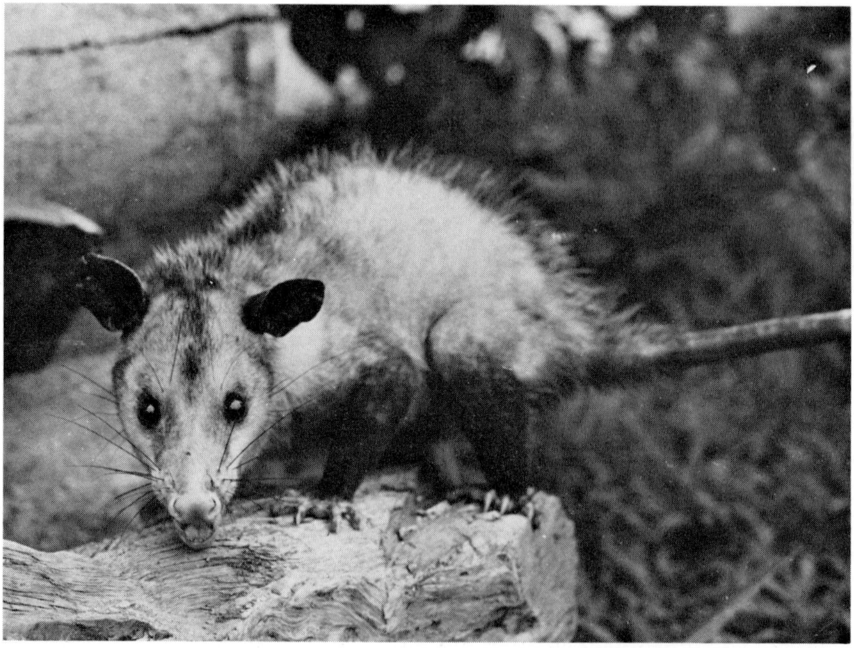

Figure 69. An opossum (*Didelphis*), reservoir host of *T. cruzi*.
Courtesy and copyright of Dr W. Petana.

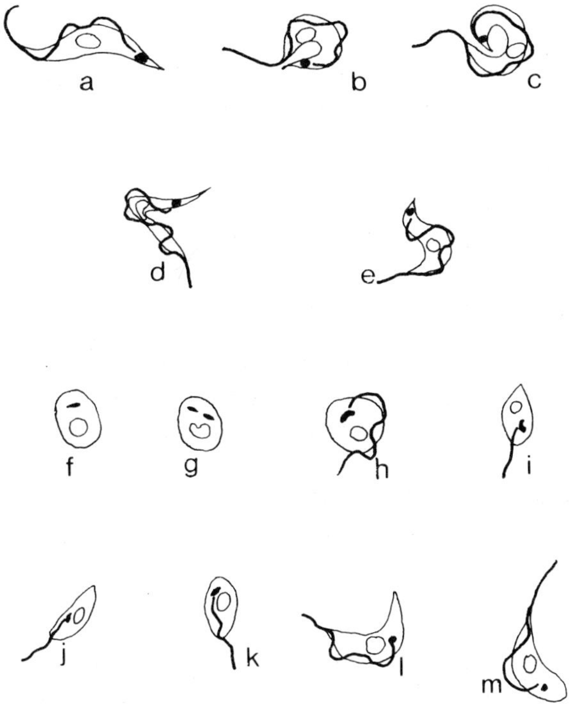

Figure 70. *T. cruzi* stages in mammalian hosts (× 1300).
a–e, Blood stream forms of *T. cruzi*.
d, Long slender forms of early parasitaemia, possibly a penetrative form which enters tissue.
e, Stumpy forms found in chronic parasitaemia.
f–g, Amastigotes from a heart tissue smear of a pseudocyst, g–dividing.
h, Sphaeromastigote from heart tissue.
i–j, Epimastigotes from heart tissue.
k–m, Transitional forms in the process of developing into blood stream forms from epi- and sphaeromastigotes in heart tissue.

the autonomic nervous system and the mononuclear phagocytic cells. The reproductive cycle is synchronous and is of about 5 days duration. When the pseudocysts rupture amastigotes, sphaeromastigotes and epimastigotes transform to trypomastigotes and pass into the bloodstream. These are the forms circulating in the blood but they are still able to reinvade tissue cells. In chronic *T. cruzi* trypanosomiasis the stumpy forms are characteristic and are believed to be more infective to triatomine bugs; there is evidence that parasites in the blood in the acute phase of the infection infect vectors less easily. In chronic Chagas' disease immunosuppression results in recrudescence of a parasitaemia.

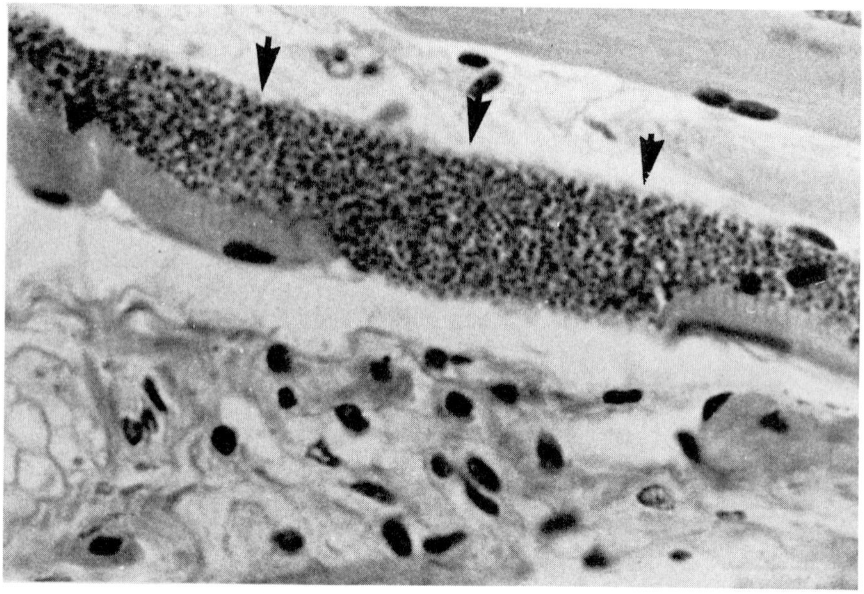

Figure 71. Pseudocyst (arrowed) in cardiac muscle which is packed with amastigotes of *T. cruzi* (× 2000).

Courtesy and copyright of Dr W. Petana.

Life cycle in the vector and transmission

It is thought that the life cycle of *T. cruzi* is similar in all the species of bugs which can act as vectors, producing infective metacyclic parasites in the rectum. The transformation of stumpy trypomastigotes to epimastigote and sphaeromastigote organisms occurs in the midgut. The small epimastigotes (10–20μm) which are preceded by promastigote-like forms multiply profusely by binary fission and thus form a reservoir of parasites maintaining the infection in the bug. Longer epimastigotes of 35–40μm pass posteriorly to the rectum where transformation to mammal infective metacyclic trypomastigotes occurs (figures 72 and 73). These long epimastigote parasites in the rectum adhere to the epithelium of the rectal gland, sometimes in more than one layer, giving a hairy appearance to the epithelium. Metacyclic parasites are produced from epimastigotes via sphaeromastigotes and are usually free in the rectal lumen. Metacyclics do not divide, are 17–22μm in length and highly active. The duration of this stage of the life cycle is 6–15 days depending on the stage of the bug which ingests the parasite and the temperature at which the bug lives.

There are no stages outside the gut in *T. cruzi* and up to 100 per cent of bugs which feed on a parasitaemic host can become infected. It is considered that the local species of domiciliary bug is likely to be the most susceptible to that particular stock of organism. It has been shown that the susceptibility of *Rhodnius*

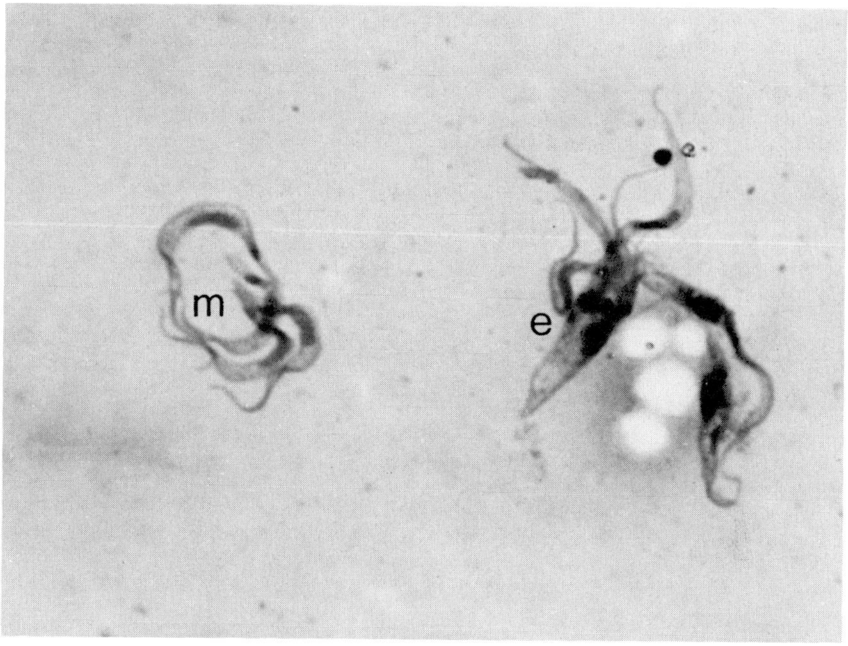

Figure 72. Metacyclic trypanosomes, m, and epimastigotes, e, in a Giemsa stained smear of the gut contents of an infected bug (× 3000).

Courtesy and copyright of Dr W. Petana.

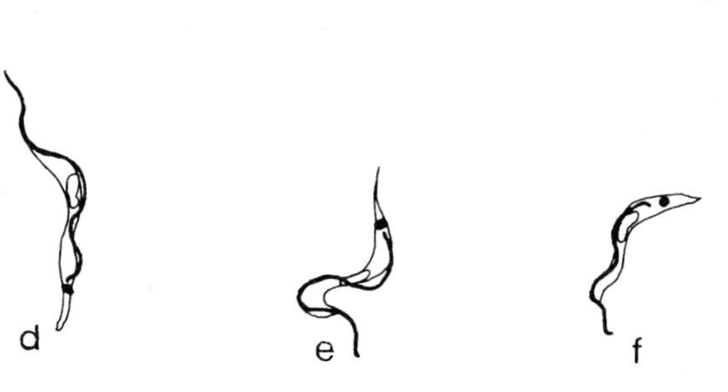

Figure 73. *T. cruzi* stages in the vector triatomine (× 1300).
a–c, Epimastigote stages in the intestine.
d–f, Metacyclic trypanosomes found in the rectum and voided in faeces after the bite and which are infective to man.

prolixus to *T. cruzi* is a quantitative characteristic under polygenic control, nearly all bugs being capable of acquiring infection. Once a bug is infected it remains so for the duration of its life. *T. cruzi* has not been observed to have any adverse effect on bugs. Infection rates of bugs in the wild always vary with the origin of the insects and whether their preferred food source is infected.

Transmission of Chagas' disease is by contamination of patients by metacyclic forms passed in the faeces. Faeces from bugs are deposited after feeding and the time between engorgement and defaecation has an important bearing on the efficiency of a bug as a vector. If a bug defaecates during or soon after feeding (figure 74) the likelihood of the infective forms being deposited on the skin of the host is higher than if defaecation occurred after the bug had moved from the host. Although other arthropods have been infected experimentally, and some such as the bed bugs *Cimex* and ticks have been found naturally infected, they are not epidemiologically of any importance. In *Rhodnius prolixus* early instar nymphs may suck blood and haemocoelic fluid from a recently engorged bug; this has been demonstrated in the laboratory, but the importance of these methods of infection of bugs remain to be evaluated in nature. This phenomenon has recently been re-examined in *R. prolixus* and described as 'hygroklepty' (fluid theft), as the terms cannibalism and coprophagy, used previously, are inappropriate.

The metacyclic forms deposited on man in bug excreta can penetrate mucosal

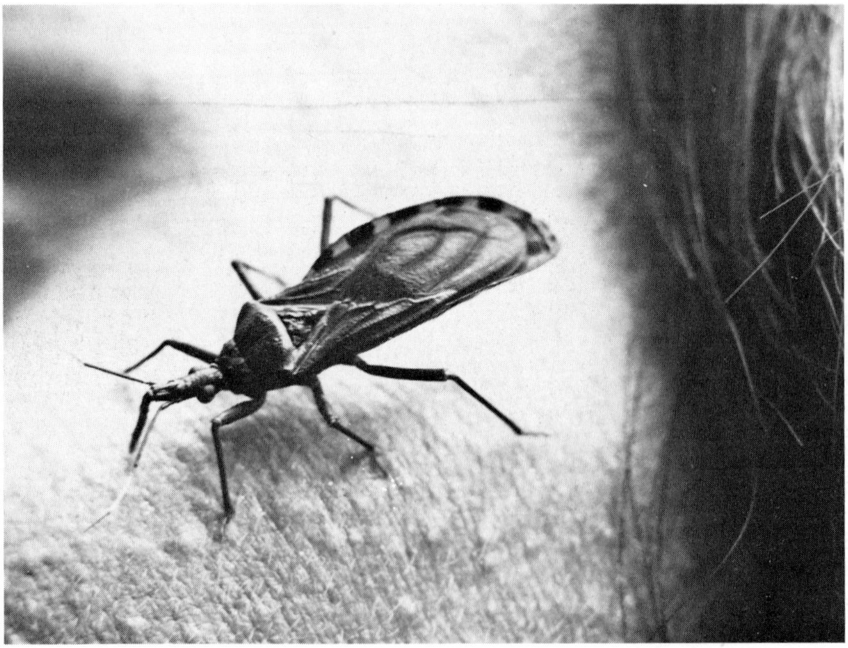

Figure 74. *Triatoma dimidiata* feeding on the face of a man (×2·5). Courtesy and copyright of Dr W. Petana.

surfaces or wounds (especially those resulting from the bite). There is limited evidence that metacyclic trypanosomes can penetrate unbroken skin. However, the severe pruritus caused by the bite of the bug and the subsequent local urticaria and erythema with the normal response of man of scratching will increase the likelihood of infection. The local reaction of the eye (Romana's sign) is associated with contamination of the conjunctiva. Histamine has been isolated from bug saliva and faeces, and anticoagulants and haemolytic factors from saliva. Immediate reactions, which are species specific, occur which are indicative of previous exposure to bites. Delayed reactions appear when no sensitization has occurred. Infection through the oral mucosa when bugs have bitten the face is also possible. Indeed, the infection of many reservoir hosts by eating bugs is likely; rats, mice and opossums consume bugs avidly under laboratory conditions and infection could also be acquired as a result of grooming when the fur is contaminated with faeces.

Over 90 species of triatomines have been found naturally infected with *T. cruzi*; 36 of these are associated with human dwellings (figure 75). There are only about 10 species, however, which are important epidemiologically as vectors of human disease. The ability of these species to invade human habitations from their original sylvatic habitats must be regarded as an important feature of the

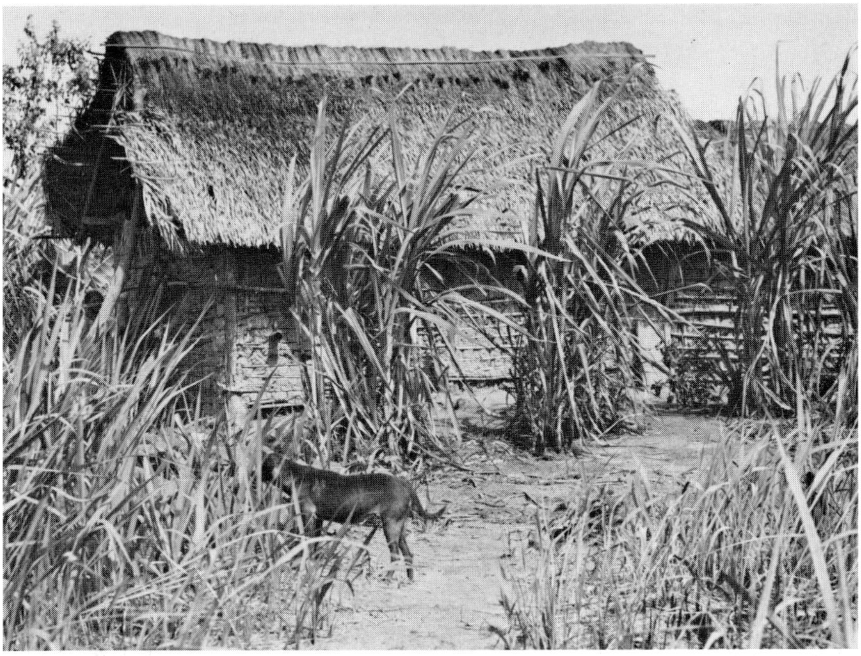

Figure 75. Rural housing in Central America showing roofing and walls of a dwelling which provide ideal habitats for the vector bug. The dog in the foreground is a reservoir host of *T. cruzi*.

Courtesy and copyright of Dr W. Petana.

dissemination of the disease to man. Bugs can also be transported in luggage, and therefore human movement is of considerable importance in spreading vectors as well as disease. The most important bugs which live in close contact with man are species of the genera *Panstronglyus* (*P. megistus*), *Rhodnius* (*R. prolixus* and *R. pallescens*) and *Triatoma* (*T. infestans, T. dimidiata* and *T. sordida*). Most of these bugs have both domestic and sylvatic habitats and are known to be efficient vectors of *T. cruzi*; no true sylvatic habitat is known for *T. infestans*.

Reservoir hosts

It is recognized that two main categories of reservoir of *T. cruzi* exist — the domestic reservoirs and the sylvatic reservoirs. Thus Chagas' disease is a zoonosis. Examples of the former group are dogs, cats, rats, guinea-pigs and mice. The link between the domestic cycle and the sylvatic cycle could be man (e.g. forestry workers), who may become infected by a sylvatic parasite, the opossum *Didelphis* (figure 69, p. 166) which maintains a parasitaemia throughout its life and is a highly adaptable animal, or bugs which, having been initially infected in the forest, enter houses attracted, for example, by lights.

Sylvatic hosts of *T. cruzi*-like organisms include around 150 species or subspecies from the mammalian orders Marsupialia, Chiroptera, Rodentia, Lagomorpha, Edentata, Carnivora and Primates.

Attempted experimental infection of man is clearly not an appropriate technique for determining if such organisms are infective to man. Hence if an isolate from a reservoir produces infection in laboratory mice, has parasites of typical morphology, amastigotes in tissues, grows in cultures and infects triatomine bugs, then such an organism can be justifiably regarded as *T. cruzi*. Isoenzyme techniques are becoming increasingly useful in parasite identification and these will, as they have in African trypanosomes, increasingly provide data of epidemiological importance. Important sylvatic reservoirs are the opossum *Didelphis*, the anteater *Tamandua*, the armadillo *Dasypus*, various genera of bat (e.g., *Glossophaga*, *Carollia*, *Desmodus*) and the primates *Aotus*, *Saimiri* and *Ateles*. In the USA *T. cruzi*-like organisms are recorded in feral mammals, particularly the wood rat *Neotoma*, opossum *Didelphis*, skunk *Mephitis*, racoon *Procyon*, armadillo *Dasypus*, ring-tailed cat *Bassaricus* and squirrel *Ammospermophilus*. There are, however, three types of transmission cycle, the purely sylvatic or enzootic cycle, which relies on purely sylvatic bugs, the overlapping or linking cycle between the sylvatic and domestic cycles where the vector species are common to both cycles, and the non-overlapping cycles of both sylvatic and domestic transmission with distinct sylvatic and domiciliary bug vectors. This classification, however, is simplified, as under normal circumstances the ecological conditions vary considerably due to human activities with resultant disturbances which will affect vector and reservoir host distribution and behaviour.

In their natural habitats the sylvatic reservoir hosts are usually associated with particular species of triatomine bug which live in close association with the burrows or nests. Examples of such associations are: *Panstrongylus geniculatus* which lives in armadillo burrows, *Triatoma gerstaekeri* and *T. lecticularius* in the lodges or nests of the wood rat *Neotoma* and the squirrel *Ammospermophilus*, and *Cavernicola pilosa* which is a triatomine frequently associated with roosting sites of bats such as caves or hollow trees. Other sites where triatomines are found are under stones, in the axils of bromeliads, in palm-tree crowns or birds' nests in association with various vertebrates which inhabit these sites.

Other methods of transmission of *T. cruzi*

Although man is usually infected by contamination with faeces from bugs containing metacyclic trypanosomes it has been demonstrated conclusively that he can become infected in other ways. One important transmission mechanism is in blood transfusion; this is prevented by inclusion of 1:4000 Gentian violet in donor blood and storing for 24 hours at 4 °C prior to transfusion, which kills the parasites without affecting the quality of the blood. Testing blood in banks in endemic areas by serological techniques has demonstrated the extent of this problem, particularly in cities where poverty may force migrants from rural areas to sell their blood.

Transmission across the placenta has been confirmed, and rates of transplacental transmission are around 1–3 per cent of births in endemic areas. Transmission from mother to infant can also occur as trypanosomes have been found in the milk of lactating mothers as well as in experimentally infected animals. However, protection from infection may be provided by anti-*T. cruzi* antibodies in the milk.

There have also been suggestions that transmission to man can result from contamination of food by infected bugs. It has been demonstrated that cats can become infected by eating infected mice, so oral infection of man through contaminated uncooked food is a possibility. Suggestions that transmission can occur as a result of coitus requires confirmation, but *T. cruzi* has been observed to concentrate in the male reproductive organs. The epidemiological importance of these unusual methods of acquisition of Chagas' disease in man remains to be evaluated.

Parasitological diagnosis

Parasitological diagnosis of Chagas' disease is dependent on demonstration of the organism directly or indirectly. The direct method is by the examination of blood films. Thick blood films are essential because of the low parasitaemias found in chronic infections; parasites are easier to find in acute infections. Centrifugation methods such as the microhaematocrit technique are not as yet extensively used.

Indirect methods of parasitological diagnosis involve xenodiagnosis using laboratory colonies of susceptible triatomines. The species most frequently used are *Triatoma infestans*, *Rhodnius prolixus*, *Dipetalogaster maxima* and *Panstrongylus megistus*. Batches of 20 clean, laboratory bred fourth or fifth instar bugs are fed on the suspect and after around 3–4 weeks their faeces are examined for the presence of flagellates. Recently, first and third instar *D. maxima*, the largest species of triatomid, have been recommended, as larger numbers can be employed. This is curious as this bug is found only in Baja California, Mexico and its susceptibility contradicts the view that local vectors are best for xenodiagnosis. If flagellates cannot be found in the faeces the bugs can be dissected. The bugs are able to develop infections of *T. cruzi* on ingestion of very small numbers of parasites. Indeed, when several bugs in a batch are fed on a suspect sometimes only a small proportion become infected, demonstrating that the parasitaemia was too low for all the bugs to ingest parasites, despite the relatively large quantities of blood ingested. The normal blood meal is 200–500 mg, while over 1000 mg has been recorded. The examination of pooled faeces from a large batch of bugs may improve sensitivity. An alternative to xenodiagnosis is to inoculate a quantity of blood from a patient into culture tubes (usually blood agar slopes) and allow 2–3 weeks for the infection to develop. A series of 4–6 culture tubes is usually used per suspect; around 0·2 ml of blood can be inoculated into each tube and the cultures are maintained at 25 °C. The majority of authors who have compared haemoculture and xenodiagnosis using bugs believe the latter is the more sensitive method.

Animal inoculation of blood can also be used as a diagnostic method. However, xenodiagnosis and culture diagnostic methods are slow in producing a result and thus for surveys parasitological techniques have largely been replaced by serological ones.

Serological diagnosis

A wide variety of serological techniques are available for the detection of antibodies to *T. cruzi* in the blood of patients with Chagas' disease. The complement fixation test (CFT) is the best studied; the most promising antigens are benzene treated culture forms of *T. cruzi* or a protein fraction of lyophilized parasites. The indirect fluorescent antibody test (IFAT) is highly sensitive and gives an early indication of infection by detecting IgM anti-*T. cruzi* antibodies characteristic of early infections. The test can be carried out using eluates of dried blood from filter paper on freeze dried or formalized antigen. The results of CFT and IFAT tests correlate well.

Immunoperoxidase tests are an alternative to immunofluorescence and do not require a fluorescent microscope. Haemagglutination tests (HA) have been used and have the advantage that they are easy to perform, can be read by eye and produce results in 1–2 hours on microplates using, if necessary, eluates of dried blood on filter paper. Erythrocytes are sensitized with *T. cruzi* as the antigen and are treated with tannic acid. Other agglutination tests which are available are the direct agglutination of trypsinized epimastigotes and the parasite disintegrated rapid flocculation test. These tests are used routinely to check potential employees in South America. Serologically positive individuals have a markedly reduced opportunity for employment despite the fact that a large number of such people will never develop clinical symptoms.

The enzyme linked immunosorbent assay (ELISA) and complement enzyme linked immunosorbent assay (CELISA) have been evaluated. The latter technique showed significant correlation with the CF test with sera from Chagas' disease patients, but not with indirect haemagglutination or IFAT results.

Immunological aspects of Chagas' disease pathology

The role of the immune response in acute and chronic Chagas' disease has been intensively studied, permitting a better understanding of the gross pathological features of the disease, such as cardiomyopathy and the formation of megoe-sophagus and megacolon (figure 76). The acute disease seems to be a direct consequence of invasion and multiplication of the parasites; however in the mega

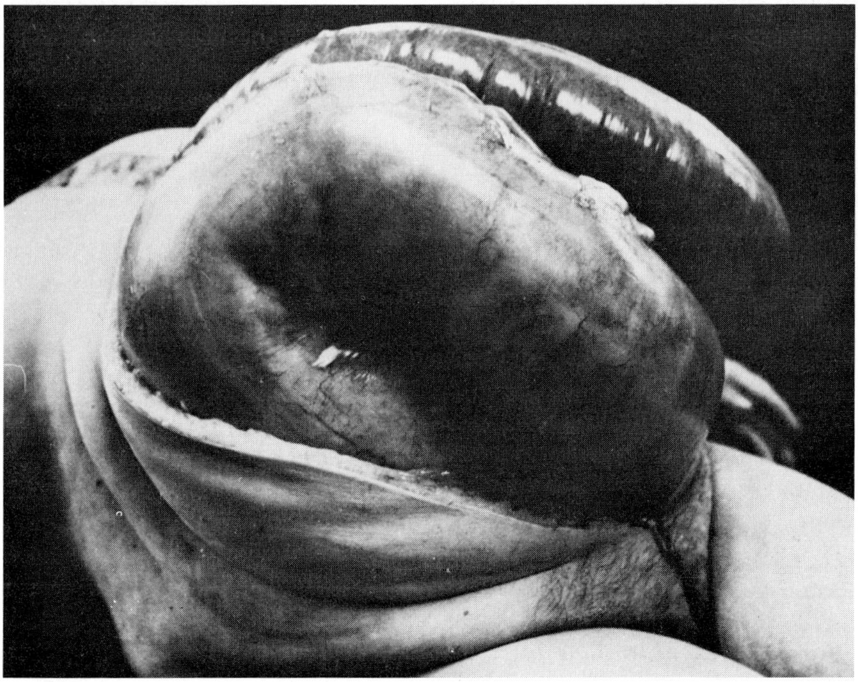

Figure 76. Post-mortem of a patient with megacolon.
Courtesy and copyright of Dr W. Petana.

syndromes destruction of parasympathetic, sympathetic and peptidergic nerve elements and ganglia with lymphocyte infiltration have been observed; in addition cardiac denervation has been postulated as a mechanism of the cardiomyopathy. There is evidence, from immunological studies, of autoimmune tissue destruction during both acute and chronic disease.

Reduced levels of vasoactive intestinal polypeptides and other gut hormones were demonstrated in Chagas' disease patients compared with controls, indicating that the disease causes local neuropathology and damages endocrine producing cells of the gut.

The ability of the host to resolve the acute infection is related to specific immunological mechanisms of antibody production and cell mediated immunity and a non-specific macrophage activity which combine to reduce the numbers of circulating parasites. The importance of the cell mediated immune response is shown by demonstrating the ability of passively transferred lymphocytes from infected rats and mice to produce resistance in recipients subsequently exposed to infection. *T. cruzi* can survive and multiply in the cytoplasm of macrophages, but previously sensitized macrophages can kill parasites even if the sensitization is by unrelated stimuli. However, the cell mediated and humoral responses do not kill all the parasites and some survive to reside in tissues, allowing the chronic condition to supervene.

Recent *in vitro* studies have shown that parasite antigens can bind to muscle and nerve cells, thus providing a stimulus for attack of the bound sites by cytotoxic T-lymphocytes. This work supports the view that the pathology of *T. cruzi* is related to the autoimmune destruction of tissues. Autoantibodies to endocardium, vessels, skeletal muscles and peripheral nerves have been detected in sera from Chagas' disease patients using immunofluorescent techniques.

Chemotherapy

No really satisfactory drug is available for the treatment of chronic Chagas' disease. Only two drugs — Lampit, a 5-nitrofuran, and Rochagan, a benznidazole — have undergone extensive clinical trials and are marketed for the treatment of Chagas' disease. Lampit seems effective in the acute stages of the disease but its ability to destroy intracellular stages of *T. cruzi* in chronic cases at tolerable doses remains in doubt. Under appropriate conditions a 90 per cent cure rate has been claimed, but the drug must be administered under medical supervision and a 120-day course of treatment is required if a satisfactory cure is to be obtained.

As with African human trypanosomiasis there seems to be little difficulty in clearing parasites from the blood; it is the tissue stages which seem capable of avoiding chemotherapeutic attacks in Chagas' disease as is the case with the forms in the CNS in late stage African trypanosomiasis. In Chagas' disease, however, unlike the latter, intracellular forms develop almost immediately, and thus complete cure, in the absence of a drug which can satisfactorily penetrate the pseudocysts, is unlikely.

Several groups of compounds have been found to have activity in mice or other experimental animals, or clear the blood of parasites, only for a subsequent parasitaemia to develop; some have been tested in man with disappointing results.

The cost of developing drugs which can be registered for use in man is a major inhibiting factor in the search for trypanocides. However,the market situation suggests that the development of an effective compound against Chagas' disease would probably repay investment. Unfortunately the main compounds which indicate activity are nitro-compounds which may show inherent properties of mutagenicity and carcinogenicity in later tests. Another group of promising compounds, the 8-aminoquinolines, are relatively toxic and are sometimes associated with teratogenicity.

Vaccination prospects

As man and animals have a capacity to develop resistance to acute infections of *T. cruzi* it is hoped that eventually a vaccine for use in man will be developed. Such a vaccine should produce a sterile immunity to break the cycle of transmission. The development of a non-living vaccine, preferably with well defined antigenic components, would ameliorate the clinical conditions, thus preventing disease. The use of killed vaccines is indicated as preferable to living vaccines as live attenuated organisms could cause infection. A further reason for optimism is the absence of antigenic variation, at least in the blood stream stage of *T. cruzi*, as far as our knowledge extends to date. In addition to this, large quantities of material can be grown in culture, in particular the insect stages. Thus a large number of experiments have been carried out using a variety of experimental designs to determine the most appropriate stage to be used, the most appropriate method of killing the parasites, the possibility of using living non-pathogenic agents such as *Leptomonas* species or bat trypanosomes to induce a protective immunity and, finally, the best adjuvant.

The methods of killing parasites which have been studied include irradiation, ultrasonication, freeze-thawing, formalin treatment and agitation with glass beads. Protection was obtained using repeated injections of *T. cruzi* which had been grown in monkey kidney cell cultures and irradiated with 150 kilorads. Protection has also been achieved using a subcutaneous injection of freeze-thawed or formalin killed cultured epimastigotes with Quillaya Saponin as an adjuvant. Other adjuvants tested to date for inclusion in vaccines are *Bordetella pertussis* and *Corynebacterium parvum*. Handicaps in the development of these vaccines for use in man are the presence of an endotoxin-like material in *T. cruzi* and the lack of knowledge about the pathogenesis of chronic Chagas' disease. It is possible that vaccination could increase the severity of the chronic stages through antigens in *T. cruzi* cross-reacting with, for example, nerves and the heart. Autoimmunity induced in this way is believed to be responsible for the pathology in the chronic disease. The repeated immunization with subcellular fractions of *T. cruzi* produces pathology in rabbits similar to that found in Chagas' disease, giving cause for disquiet unless candidate antigens are well defined. However, success has recently been reported in the vaccination of mice with a glycoprotein of molecular weight around 90 000 daltons, which is present throughout the life cycle of the parasite and which does not undergo antigenic variation. Vaccinations with such a protein with adjuvant protect mice against a lethal dose and are not associated with autoimmune antibodies. This method of vaccination would clearly have advantages over whole organism vaccines if a suitable adjuvant for human use was available.

Control

Unlike African trypanosomiasis, untreated Chagas' disease is not inevitably fatal and many chronic sufferers with mild or no overt symptoms survive in endemic areas of South and Central America. Although it has been shown to be of value in the treatment of acute Chagas' disease, Lampit requires a long period of treatment (up to 120 days) and it is recognized to be less effective in the chronic stage of the disease. Thus, chemotherapeutic control by the treatment of infected individuals or chemoprophylaxis is clearly not feasible, particularly in view of the estimates of up to 14 million cases.

The main emphasis has therefore been on vector control, but there have been some setbacks. The use of chlorinated hydrocarbons in antimalaria campaigns where house spraying was carried out was reported to have reduced numbers of domiciliary bugs. However, triatomines have never been susceptible to low enough doses of DDT for this to have a significant effect and the continuous use of organochlorine compounds as residual insecticides is under review. Alternative insecticides such as organophosphorus compounds, carbamates and synthetic pyrethroids are being evaluated. Argentina is using malathion in its vector control operations. Spraying against triatomine bugs is conducted by knapsack spraying equipment inside houses. In some regions, however, the spraying programmes result in one species of bug declining but being replaced by other species. The ideal attribute of an insecticide and its applications are: ability to penetrate creviced walls, long-term residual effect on surfaces, a capability to destroy eggs and avoidance of development of resistance. The recrudescence of bug populations after insecticide application has been suggested as being due to the destruction of their natural predators and parasites. The so-called third generation pesticides are currently being tested. These include compounds such as pheromones, attractants and insect growth regulators; their use, together with natural pathogens and modifications in house construction, constitutes the application of concepts of integrated pest control and management to the problem of Chagas' disease. Juvenile hormone analogues have been tested as control agents on the development of the fifth instar nymphal stages, but their practical use seems limited due to their effectiveness over a short period. Juvenile hormone analogues or mimics will prevent the acquisition of adult characteristics when applied to fifth instar nymphs, as would the application of juvenile hormone itself: precocenes — plant derived compounds — mimic *anti*-juvenile hormone activity and shorten the life of bugs producing so-called sterile 'adultoids' with little vectorial capability.

Recent work has suggested that biological control of triatomines in humid conditions could be possible using the mermithid nematode *Neoaplectana* which invades by penetrating all instars of bugs and could be applied by spraying or by introducing infected cockroaches into homes. Predators or parasitoids of triatomines have been documented, but little is known of their role in controlling populations. Spiders are known to prey on bugs; mites have been found to infect triatomines and can destroy laboratory colonies rapidly. Parasitic Hymenoptera of the genus *Telenomus* are a natural enemy of triatomines. This wasp has a wide distribution, although it shows geographical variations in physiology and behaviour as well as in its ability to parasitize different bug species. Percentage infection of the eggs of triatomines in nature is of the order of 10–25 per cent. Cockroaches, predatory bugs and ants are also known to feed on triatomines. The human trypanosome *T. rangeli* is known to be pathogenic to *Rhodnius prolixus* and is recognized as a factor in controlling populations in the wild; another flagellate, *Blastocrithidia triatomae,* has also been recognized as a pathogen of *Triatoma infestans*.

Although these predators, parasites and pathogens could play a role in an integrated control of triatomines, the most likely method of reducing disease prevalence in the endemic areas is by the improvement of housing conditions. The association of the domiciliary vectors of Chagas' disease with inadequate and poorly constructed dwellings has been known for many years. Studies indicate a correlation between the infection rate as determined by serology and the quality of the housing, particularly the wall and roof structures. In one study two-thirds of seroreactive children lived in mudstick houses with local roofing materials and over 90 per cent of *P. megistus* infestation occurred in this type of house. Materials — substances such as concrete, tiles or corrugated iron — clearly reduce the habitat available for the bugs — cracks and crevices in walls and roofs. The long-term objective of house construction in brick or concrete would play a considerable part in reducing transmission; however, these materials are relatively expensive and at present soil–cement mixtures, wall plaster and polyester or epoxy materials are alternatives to reduce the numbers of habitats available to bugs. In conjunction with this type of housing improvement, removal of litter and the identification of other places for bugs to conceal themselves are essential. Application of materials such as wall plaster by householders themselves could contribute to reducing costs and provide a means of permanently reducing levels of transmission.

TRYPANOSOMA RANGELI

Trypanosoma rangeli is found in man in Central and South America and is transmitted principally by *Rhodnius prolixus*. It is generally believed to be non-pathogenic as no recognized symptoms have been associated with the infection. Man and bugs are frequently infected with both *T. cruzi* and *T. rangeli*. *T. rangeli* belongs to the subgenus *Herpetosoma* and differs morphologically from *Schizotrypanum* trypanosomes (figures 68, p. 165 and 77). It measures in total length 25–37 μm from the pointed posterior tip of the body. The levels of parasitaemia in man and laboratory animals infected with *T. rangeli* are low, presenting diagnostic problems. Division of trypanosomes has not been seen in the mammalian host and there is still doubt as to whether or not multiplication takes place in mammals, although evidence of division in tissue cultures has been observed.

T. rangeli has been recorded from dogs, cats, monkeys (*Cebus*, *Ateles* and *Saimiri*), opossums, raccoons and anteaters. *T. rangeli* was initially observed in *Rhodnius prolixus*. It is important to distinguish this organism from *T. cruzi* if *R. prolixus* is being used in xenodiagnosis; this can be done as *T. rangeli* has a different morphology in bugs as well as a different cycle of development. *T. rangeli* develops in the gut, haemolymph and salivary glands and is transmitted not by contamination, as in *T. cruzi*, but by the bite of infected bugs. *T. rangeli* also develops in the posterior part of the gut of *Rhodnius* but the forms in the gut are not infective to mammals. Parasites, however, pass into the haemocoele from the midgut and then penetrate the salivary glands. *T. rangeli* produces epimastigotes and trypomastigotes in the vector, elongated by a long posterior extremity

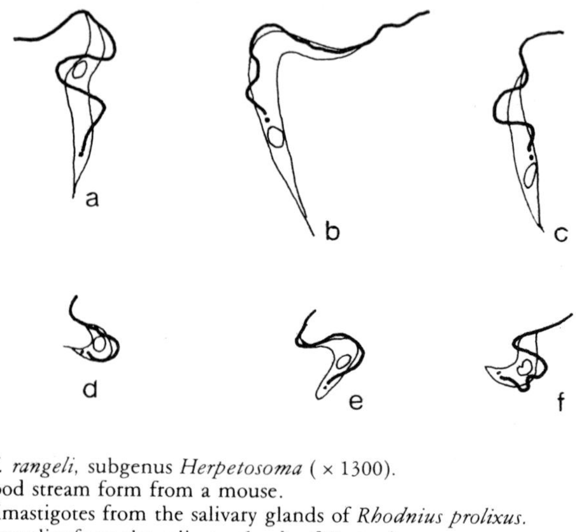

Figure 77. *T. rangeli*, subgenus *Herpetosoma* (× 1300).
a, Blood stream form from a mouse.
b–c, Epimastigotes from the salivary glands of *Rhodnius prolixus*.
d–f, Metacyclics from the salivary glands of *R. prolixus*.

up to 80 μm in length (figure 77).

Metacyclics are small C-shaped trypomastigotes 10—13 μm in length. *T. rangeli* can be grown satisfactorily in blood agar NNN culture media and the stages present mimic the forms observed in the vector. *R. prolixus* infected with *T. rangeli* also probe more frequently than control uninfected bugs, thus facilitating parasite transmission; infected bugs seem less able to fully engorge and this may be due to the effect of the parasite on pharyngeal musculature.

Other species of *Rhodnius*, *R. pallescens* (Panama) and *R. ecuadoriensis* (Peru) have been found infected with *T. rangeli*; *Triatoma* species have been infected but are not such efficient vectors as *Rhodnius prolixus*. *T. rangeli* is pathogenic to *R. prolixus*; this is caused by the penetration of *T. rangeli* into the haemolymph where subsequent invasion of gut musculature, fat body, Malpighian tubules, nervous and tracheal systems results in profound pathophysiological effects, particularly a decrease in excretion compared with uninfected bugs. Not all strains of *T. rangeli* cause such pathogenicity and different bug strains also respond differently to infection. *T. rangeli* has been implicated as a major factor in the control of *R. prolixus* populations.

OTHER HUMAN TRYPANOSOMIASES

Trypanosomiases in man have very rarely been found in Asia. The infections which have been described have been associated with organisms which are morphologically similar. The first observation of human trypanosomes in Asia was an infection described as *T. lewisi* discovered in a four-month-old male. Parasites were present in large numbers during bouts of irregular fever. The organisms were morphologically similar to *T. lewisi*. The child recovered spontaneously from the infection and the fever diminished when the parasites were no longer detectable. Some 35 years later the individual was found to be alive and healthy and free of any trypanosome associated changes in blood CSF and tissues; no parasites could be found by cultivation.

Two further cases of infection of *Herpetosoma* have been reported in India. A husband and wife were found infected and trypanosomes were observed during a short febrile period; the husband was otherwise healthy but the wife was anaemic and undernourished. The latest report was from two healthy Malaysian aborigines; the organism found in this case was smaller than those observed in the other two cases and the organism had a blunt rather than pointed posterior end. These individuals had no recent history of fever or anaemia.

These reports have promoted suggestions that human trypanosomiasis in Asia is widespread, although it is clear that it has little public health significance. However, it is likely that if it were widespread it would have been detected during malaria surveys.

It is believed that primates, particularly macaques, *Macaca*, are potential reservoir hosts in view of the finding of trypanosomes in these primates. However, the incidence of trypanosomiasis in *Macaca* is low(1–5 per cent) and the morphology variable; the parasitaemia in macaques is low and there is little or no pathogenicity. The relationships between these organisms and those found in man are unclear.

There is controversy in the literature regarding the possible occurrence of *T. cruzi* in Asia. The evidence suggests that those Old World monkeys which are found infected in European and American laboratories have acquired the infection elsewhere than in Asia. There is no evidence from primates caught in the wild or from man in Asia that *T. cruzi* exists there.

PART III

LEISHMANIASIS

Chapter 7. Introduction to the Leishmaniases

INTRODUCTION

Although leishmaniasis is not a household name like malaria or sleeping sickness, the diseases caused by infection with *Leishmania* species have had and continue to have significant impact on communities throughout much of the tropics. The impact is often localized, as is indicated by the vernacular names which often refer to foci of infection or to places where outbreaks occurred.

The six species which we accept as infecting man (see Tables 13 and 14) are very similar morphologically, but produce three strikingly different diseases and numerous varieties (figure 78). The infection may be predominantly visceral as in kala-azar or visceral leishmaniasis, it may be restricted to the skin, producing the chronic ulcer of oriental sore, or it is concentrated in the mucous membranes which are gradually eroded to produce the grossly disfiguring and often fatal condition known as espundia.

The parasites themselves are unusual in that they are almost entirely intracellular in the vertebrate host and live in mononuclear phagocytic cells (macrophages) which are precisely the cells whose main function is to ingest and eliminate foreign bodies. The disease produced is a combination of the direct effects of the parasites and the reaction of the body to their presence.

The majority of infections are zoonotic in origin, though there are important circumstances where man-to-man transmission has developed either ephemerally or long term, sometimes with devastating results.

Like the trypanosomes, *Leishmania* species are transmitted by a very limited range of vectors belonging to a single subfamily, the sandflies Phlebotominae. The dependence of the parasites on an insect vector and on animal reservoir hosts has the result that each species is usually associated with quite specific environmental conditions.

There is no absolute distinction between parasites causing visceral and

Table 13. The Old World *Leishmania* species parasitic in man.

Species	Main habitat	Main vertebrate host range	Main vectors	Disease spectrum
L. aethiopica	Tropical montane forest and gorges	Rock hyrax	*P. longipes*, *P. pedifer*	OS (chronic, dry) DCL
L. donovani	Temperate to tropical, mountains to plains, sylvatic to synanthropic, mostly sub-humid, warm summers, alluvial soil	Wild Canidae, savannah rodents (Africa), domestic dogs, man (India)	*P. (Larroussius)* spp., *P. argentipes*, *P. martini?*, *P. chinensis*	VL, MCL (Africa), CL, infantile VL, PKDL
L. major	Semi desert subtropics and tropics	Desert and savannah rodents: *Rhombomys*, *Psammomys*, *Arvicanthis*	*P. papatasi*, *P. (Paraphlebotomus)* spp.	OS (rural, wet)
L. tropica	Synanthropic in semi-arid subtropics	Man	*P. sergenti*	OS (urban, dry), Leishmaniasis recidivans, VL (rare)
L. sp. (Namibia)	Semi-desert, rocky areas	Hyrax?	*P. rossi*	OS (chronic)

DCL = Diffuse cutaneous leishmaniasis. Infantile VL = Infantile visceral leishmaniasis. MCL = Mucocutaneous leishmaniasis. OS = Oriental sore. PKDL = Post-kala-azar dermal leishmaniasis. VL = Visceral leishmaniasis.

Table 14. The New World *Leishmania* species parasitic in man.

Species	Main habitat	Main vertebrate host range	Main vectors	Disease spectrum
L. b. braziliensis	Tropical forest becoming synanthropic?	Edentates? Adapting to dog?	Many suspected vectors	OS, MCL (Espundia)
L. b. guyanensis	Tropical forest	Sloth and other edentates	*Lutzomyia umbratilis*	Pian bois
L. b. panamensis	Tropical forest	Sloths	5 spp. of *Lutzomyia*	OS
L. b. peruviana	Semi-arid highland valleys	Dog, man?	*Lu. verrucarum?* *Lu. peruensis*	OS
L. donovani	Mostly semi-arid tropical zone (expanding)	Domestic dog	*Lu. longipalpis*	Infantile VL
L. mexicana amazonensis	Wet tropical forest (Igapo)	Forest rodents, esp. *Oryzomys* sp., *Proechimys* sp. and opossum?	*Lu. flaviscutellata*	OS, DCL
L. m. garnhami	Cloud forest		*Lu. townsendi*	OS
L. m. mexicana	Humid tropical forest	Forest rodents	*Lu. olmeca*	OS, chiclero ulcer
L. m. pifanoi	?	?	?	DCL
L. sp. (Dominican Republic)	Forest?	?	?	DCL

DCL = Diffuse cutaneous leishmaniasis. Infantile VL = Infantile visceral leishmaniasis. MCL = Mucocutaneous leishmaniasis. OS = Oriental sore.

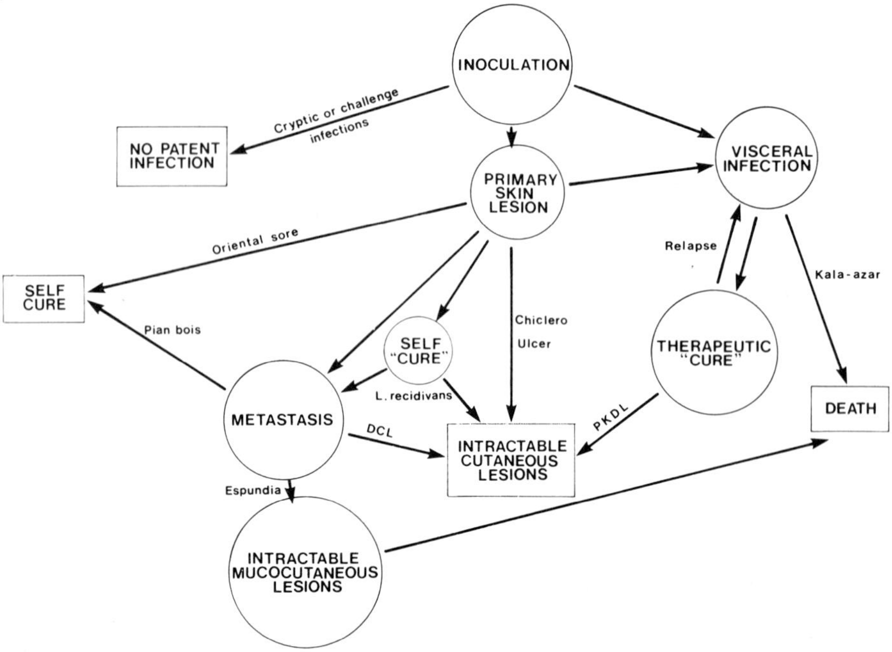

Figure 78. The 'Leishmaniasis Spectrum' or potential sequence of events following natural inoculation with *Leishmania* parasites. Each species of parasite may produce a limited section of the sequence, and most segments can be filled by more than one parasite species. The diseases named are only examples.
DCL = diffuse cutaneous leishmaniasis.
PKDL = post-kala-azar dermal leishmaniasis.

cutaneous infections in man. Thus, strains which are normally dermotropic may extend to the lymph nodes, and even visceralize, causing visceral leishmaniasis. This is the interpretation placed on recent findings using biochemical identification techniques of *L. tropica* strains isolated from visceral leishmaniasis cases from the Middle East. Conversely, normally visceralizing strains may be restricted to the skin, as cases described from Sudan and southern Europe demonstrate. Parasites causing cutaneous lesions in Spain and France are almost indistinguishable from those causing visceral leishmaniasis in infants and dogs. Subsequent to the curing of a visceral leishmaniasis infection, parasites may occur in large numbers in the skin, to which they are restricted, causing the condition post-kala-azar dermal leishmaniasis (PKDL).

Further, the behaviour of a parasite in animals in natural or experimental infections is not always the same as in man. From the practical point of view, however, it is useful to classify the parasites according to whether they normally visceralize or remain in the skin, and to examine Old World and New World cutaneous infections separately.

It is not intended to discuss in detail the systematic arguments which have attended the genus *Leishmania*, especially in a work concentrating on parasites which infect man. The scheme presented here is necessarily arbitrary and designed for simplicity and practicality. The main guiding factor is that to justify taxonomic distinction a parasite must be distinguishable by morphological, biochemical or experimental means. Ecological, epidemiological or zoogeographical features may indicate that taxonomic distinction is likely, but emphatically do not establish that it exists. Similarly, clinical features have little taxonomic significance.

PROGRESS OF INFECTION IN THE HUMAN HOST

In most cases man is incidental to the long-term survival of the parasite and the balance characteristic of well established host–parasite relationships has not yet been established. A spectrum of responses is therefore seen in man from complete refractivity to acute fatal susceptibility. The progress of infection with *Leishmania* is summarized in figure 78. The actual outcome of a given infection depends on the species or strain of parasite, on the immune status of the host, and on its immunological competence.

Parasites inoculated into an immune host are probably eliminated rapidly from the skin and do not establish an infection. There is evidence that immunity, or at least, positive immune response, may be acquired following a primary infection which never produced a clinical manifestation or even caused transient fever before being eliminated. It would be difficult to confirm this parasitologically today as one would have to detect infection in apparently unaffected people and leave them untreated; there is therefore considerable controversy over the clinical and epidemiological significance of these apparently cryptic infections.

The initial moments in an infection have recently been extrapolated from *in vitro* studies. Promastigotes (figure 79) are inoculated into the wound produced by the feeding sandfly. The cells broken by the sandfly's proboscis, and the saliva inoculated into the wound, attract mononuclear phagocytes (macrophages) and other white cells to the area. An important role of the macrophages is of course to identify and eliminate foreign matter, including parasites. There is a fine balance between the successful establishment of parasites in macrophages and their destruction. Certain macrophages are capable of killing parasites directly, while others need to be stimulated to do so. Only unstimulated, resident macrophages are suitable for the establishment of the infection. Promastigotes must transform to amastigotes (figure 80) within the macrophage in order to avoid being killed. Parasites which enter the circulation are probably eliminated rapidly, as normal human serum is lethal to both promastigotes and amastigotes. The effects of acquired immunity to the parasite or to the sandfly saliva at the initial moments in the infection remain to be fully studied.

Infected macrophages remain in the skin at the site of the sandfly bite and more macrophages develop from monocytes attracted to the site, where they also become fixed and infected. The earliest lesion is therefore manifested as an

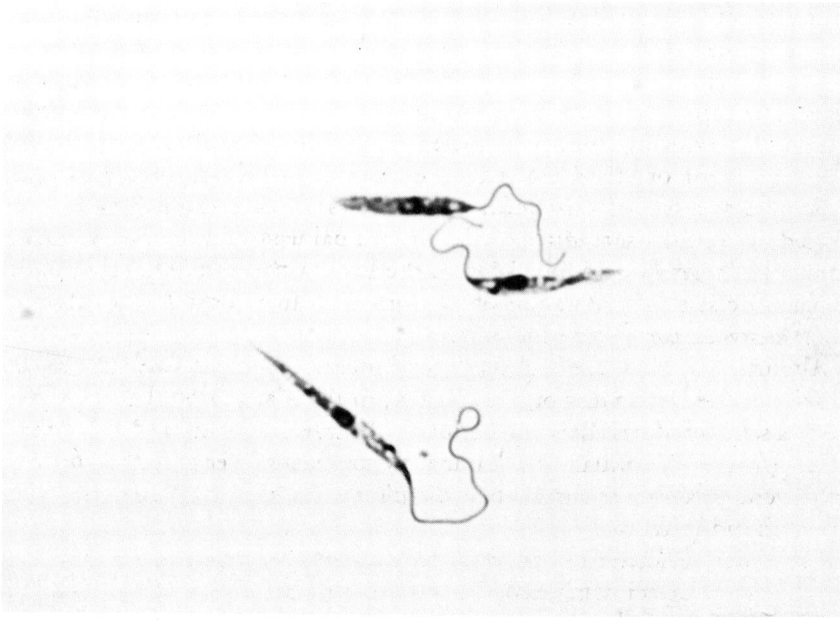

Figure 79. *Leishmania* sp. promastigotes in culture (× 1600).

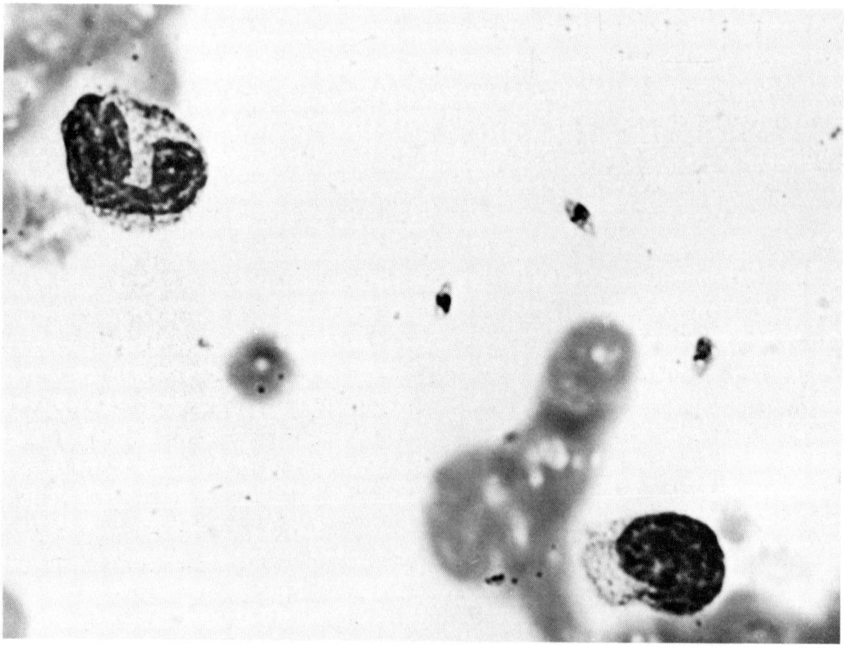

Figure 80. *L. donovani* amastigotes in a bone marrow smear. The parasites are often very scanty and extra-cellular (× 1600).

infiltration of macrophages in dermal tissue, a high proportion of which are infected. Transmission of the parasites from one macrophage to another occurs when an infected cell is broken and the parasites are released, to be engulfed by another macrophage. There is no evidence that, as has been suggested, infected cells divide producing clones of infected cells in the lesion.

At the point of initial infection the macrophage filled lesion may become surrounded by a lymphocytic infiltration which isolates it, causing necrosis of the infected tissue and a spreading, unsightly, but painless ulcer or oriental sore. This is followed by granuloma formation in the base of the ulcer and cure, leaving a characteristic scar. The duration of the infection, from exposure to self-cure, is usually between three and nine months.

Alternatively, from the initial point of infection the parasites may spread in the skin, in the lymphatics or, presumably, in the blood. Lymphatic spread may lead to a series of ulcers along the peripheral lymphatics, as in the South American disease 'pian bois'. In many predominantly cutaneous infections of *L. tropica* the lymph nodes draining the area where the ulcer is developing enlarge and parasites may be found in them.

Cutaneous diffusion of the parasites may be the consequence of a specific immunological defect combined with infection with the relatively non-immunogenic parasites *L. aethiopica*, *L. mexicana pifanoi* and *L. m. amazonensis*. The lesions do not become isolated by a wall of lymphocytes, as in oriental sore, and do not therefore ulcerate except by trauma. The parasites are then unrestricted, and may spread over much of the skin surface, particularly the cooler parts. The lesions are generally raised maculae whose exact conformation varies greatly according to the individual case. The spread of parasites in this diffuse cutaneous leishmaniasis, or pseudolepromatous leishmaniasis, is presumably assisted in part by macrophage motility, or lymphatic or blood movement as new lesions do not necessarily appear at the edge of the old lesions.

On the other hand, some chronic infections with *L. tropica* occur in which, subsequent to apparent cure and scarring of an oriental sore, satellite lesions appear on the rim of the scar. Again the lesions are usually non-ulcerating, often barely raised papules or maculae, and they are resistant to treatment. This condition is known as leishmaniasis recidivans, the variations of which have received many confusing terms, for example, tuberculoid and lupoid.

Visceralization is the rule with some species, particularly the *L. donovani* complex, though not all infections with these parasites proceed to the viscera. The route of visceralization is probably by means of macrophages circulating in the blood or lymph. The spleen and liver become heavily infected, as does the bone marrow. There is little if any necrosis of these organs, which become greatly enlarged with a massive infiltration of infected and uninfected mononuclear phagocytes. The infection is not focalized, but is diffuse throughout the organ, and there is usually remarkably little cellular host response. Following the diffusion of the infection in the viscera, some parasites of some strains are found in mononuclear phagocytes circulating in the blood. Indian strains freely infect people of all ages, producing a chronic but fatal illness, kala-azar, characterized by intermittent moderate fever, swollen abdomen due to hepatosplenomegaly, and general wasting, cachexia, the cause of which is unknown.

Visceral leishmaniasis in Africa is somewhat similar but there is a variable tendency to cutaneous manifestations as well. In the Mediterranean Basin and South America it is predominantly infants below two years of age who become sick, and the disease is termed infantile or Mediterranean visceral leishmaniasis.

As a sequel to kala-azar, the skin may become infected. The parasites then are quite numerous, but are apparently restricted to the skin, and respond poorly to chemotherapy. The infection often returns following apparent cure. This post-kala-azar dermal leishmaniasis does not occur in infantile visceral leishmaniasis, though dogs infected with the same parasite usually have heavily infected skin simultaneously with their visceral infection.

Metastasis of South American cutaneous leishmaniasis is characteristic of certain strains of *L. braziliensis*. Following apparent cure, the infection may reappear, up to 24 years later, usually in the mucocutaneous tissues of the mouth and nose, but also in the genital mucosa and even in the skin following trauma. The lesions are grossly destructive and disfiguring and are known as mucocutaneous leishmaniasis or espundia. In contrast to most forms of leishmaniasis described above, the parasites are extremely difficult to find in the lesions, which are mainly composed of granulomatous reaction tissue.

FACTORS AFFECTING HISTORY AND OUTCOME OF INFECTION

The outcome of infection in a given case depends on many factors, most of which are poorly understood and therefore controversial.

Parasite strain

Each species of parasite has the potential to produce a spectrum of diseases in man; to some extent this correlates with its behaviour in experimental animals. The potential of a given species may be unexpectedly wide, as is shown by the recent finding of *L. tropica* in occasional cases of visceral leishmaniasis and *L. major* in visceral leishmaniasis of West African rodents. The restriction of Mediterranean strains of *L. donovani* in man to the viscera of infants is possibly not caused by any lack of potential, as the age distribution of disease appears to be breaking down and, further, the parasites have been isolated from purely cutaneous lesions.

Size of inoculum

Most experimental infections are produced with an unrealistically large inoculum, but since the parasites from direct passage or culture may be very different from those in a natural infection, the *effective* size of the inoculum is unknown. Be that as it may, within wide limits the size of an experimental inoculum usually has little effect on the outcome of infection. The number of parasites in a natural inoculum is unknown, but is probably not more than several hundred and is likely to be less. In experimental infections the size of inoculum has an effect on the size of a cutaneous lesion and the incubation period.

Site of inoculum

This is an important factor in certain central American *L. mexicana* strains, which, if inoculated into the pinna of the ear or nasal septum, produce a chronic, eroding lesion, chiclero's ulcer. If inoculated elsewhere the outcome is a more rapidly curing ulcer of the oriental sore type. In other cases, however, cutaneous lesions will develop at the site of inoculation, and there is no evidence that lesions on any given part of the body are more, or less, likely to become chronic, to metastasize or to visceralize. The distribution of cutaneous lesions depends on sandfly biting habits, the clothing worn, and the time of day and activity at the time of infection.

The possibility that occasional infections of the pharynx, tonsils or nose may be the result of inhalation of an infected sandfly or even, for that matter, another insect infected with an insect flagellate should not be overlooked. In experimental infections the route of inoculation, for example, intraperitoneal, intradermal, intravenous, subcutaneous or intrasplenic, makes a considerable difference to the outcome; some normally cutaneous strains will readily infect the viscera if inoculated there; this however has little bearing on the outcome of natural infections.

Host genetics

It is usually very difficult to distinguish between genetically modulated response to the infection and acquired changes. Meticulous studies on the susceptibility of mice to *Leishmania* have demonstrated a close link with genetic make-up. The level of initial susceptibility to *L. donovani* is apparently governed by a single gene. The development of effective immunity and subsequent recovery is governed by a second gene located in the H_2 locus, where the genes responsible for transplant immunity are also found. The final outcome of *L. major* infection in mice may also be controlled by a single gene, but one not linked to the H_2 locus. In this case susceptibility is thought to be the result of suppressor T-lymphocytes. This is supported by the observation that irradiation, which disrupts lymphocyte production, may actually assist cure. However, in none of these systems has the actual mechanism of the resistance been worked out. The relevance of this work to human infection is demonstrated by an apparent difference in susceptibility of people of different ethnic origins to *L. braziliensis*. People of negroid stock suffer more severe infection with a greater tendency to develop espundia than those of Amerindian stock living in the same locality under similar conditions. Detailed genetic studies have not been carried out to determine whether or not susceptibility to DCL is genetically related. DCL patients in Ethiopia are from various tribal origins and blood groups, but there could well be genetic markers for susceptibility such as HLA (human lymphocyte antigen) type.

Acquired immunity

Previous homologous infection usually confers immunity, and there is cross immunity between certain strains. *L. major*, for example, protects against *L. tropica*, but the reverse is not true. Active infection is also thought to affect a secondary infection — secondary lesions will reach the stage of development of initial lesions very rapidly. This is Moshkovsky's rule, explaining the apparent synchronicity of multiple infections.

Nutritional state

Nutrition may be a factor in the outcome of *Leishmania* infection. In one instance healthy US servicemen in Sudan had only cutaneous lesions while Sudanese companions had visceral leishmaniasis. Kala-azar in India has been said to be associated with floods or famine, but it would be rash to suppose any direct causal relationship on the available evidence.

DEVELOPMENT OF *LEISHMANIA* SPECIES IN THE VECTOR

The factors which determine whether a particular sandfly is a good vector for a given *Leishmania* species are poorly known. A good vector must combine physical and physiological suitability for the development of the parasites with sufficient longevity for the completion of this stage. Some cyclic development was described by the early workers, but this was largely ignored until ultrastructural studies confirmed that, as with *Trypanosoma* species, *Leishmania* species undergo a series of morphological changes within the sandfly.

In the first moments of infection the blood and parasites are exposed to the anticoagulant saliva, to considerable pressure variations in the proboscis, to the mechanical action of the cibarial and pharyngeal teeth and, usually, to decreasing temperature. The ingested blood passes immediately to the midgut without being stored in the crop. This is in contrast to sugar meals which are usually stored in the crop. It may be assumed that in addition to blood the meal contains considerable tissue debris from the punctured epidermis and dermis, but the precise contents of the meal have not been determined. In some sandflies the cell structure of the

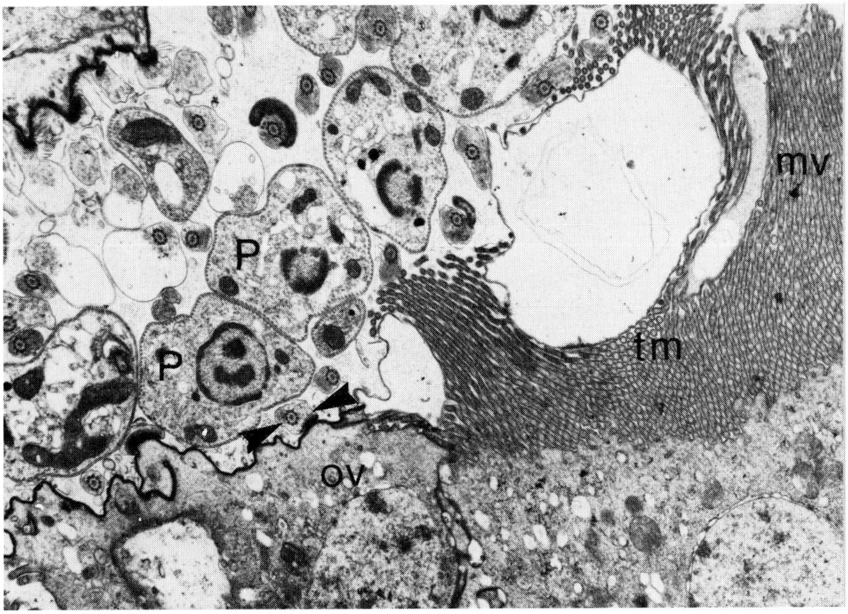

Figure 81. Electronmicrograph of the gut wall of a sandfly infected with *L. mexicana amazonensis* in the region of transition between the cuticular oesophageal valve, ov, and the microvillar lining, mv, of the thoracic midgut, tm; parasites, p, associated with the cuticle of the oesophageal valve have flagellar hemidesmosomes (flagellum arrowed) (× 7000).

Courtesy of Cambridge University Press and the Royal Society of London.

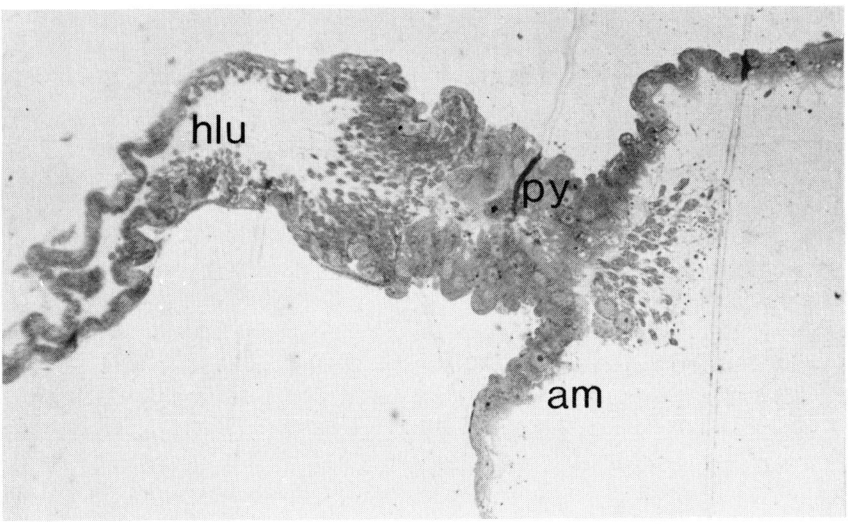

Figure 82. A light micrograph of a thick section of a *L. b. braziliensis* infected gut. am = abdominal midgut; py = pylorus; hlu = hindgut lumen (× 320).

Courtesy of Cambridge University Press and the Royal Society of London.

blood is destroyed and the haemoglobin crystallized within minutes of ingestion. This is true of lizard blood in *Sergentomyia* species and is said to be true of dog blood in various sandflies.

A mucilaginous 'peritrophic membrane' is secreted by the midgut epithelium, which encloses the blood meal. Digestion proceeds usually over 3–4 days, during which time the gut contents are largely absorbed, leaving a residue of faecal granules probably composed of partly digested haemoglobin. Defecation is a rapid process in which perhaps 20 spots of fluid are deposited which rapidly dry and appear as black spots. After defecation the midgut is empty and normally sterile, while a small residue may remain in the hindgut. Clear fluid may be found in the crop at all stages, but it is not known at what stage or at what rate this is released into the midgut.

While the blood is still fresh in the midgut the amastigotes transform into promastigotes, and grow and divide rapidly. At first the midgut becomes a seething mass of swimming promastigotes. As division slows down these become concentrated either at the anterior or posterior end of the midgut, where they may become attached in a palisade-like layer by inserting their flagellae between the microvilli of the midgut wall.

Suprapylarial parasites such as Old World mammalian parasites and *L. mexicana* become concentrated in the thoracic midgut, cease dividing, and attach to the cuticular lining of the proventricular valve. They are held in place by the flagellum, whose distal end expands to form a disc-like attachment organelle (figures 8, p. 21, and 81). These attached parasites or haptomonads conform to the pro- and paramastigote configuration. Further development may be dependent on succeeding blood meals, subsequent to which parasites may be found in the pharynx, where they are mostly attached to the cuticle, and in the proboscis, where they are swimming free in the lumen. The small swimming forms are again promastigotes, and are thought to complete the cycle.

The actual mechanism of transmission is in some doubt. It may be that the blockage of the proventricular valve causes regurgitation and inoculation of gut contents, including parasites, into the vertebrate host. Alternatively, the swimming forms in the proboscis may be carried in with the saliva. It is thought that infectivity to the vertebrate host is retained by all stages, in contrast to *Trypanosoma* species whose early, insect stages are not infective.

The development of peripylarian and hypopylarian *Leishmania* species in sandflies is less completely known. The former (*L. braziliensis* (*sensu lato*)) require a stage in the anterior part of the hindgut before eventually migrating forward to the thoracic midgut (figure 82) and foregut, where they become attached. In the case of the hypopylarian parasites of reptiles the midgut becomes sterile and the parasites attach to the cuticular lining of the rectum and rectal ampullae where they become rounded and immobile. It is assumed that hypopylarian *Leishmania* species are transmitted to the reptile host when the infected sandfly is eaten. However, there is doubt about the validity of reptilian *Leishmania*.

Chapter 8. New World Cutaneous and Mucocutaneous Leishmaniases

INTRODUCTION

It is probably wrong to talk of New World cutaneous leishmaniasis (NWCL), because one of the prominent features of the disease, in some parts of the distribution, is its tendency to metastasize to the mucous membranes of the oronasal region. This metastasis, which may be delayed until long after the cure of the initial lesion, clearly implies that the parasites survive for many years somewhere, but not necessarily in the skin.

There is evidence that mucocutaneous leishmaniasis was well known to Amerindians long before the European invasions as pre-Inca Peruvian, Mochica and Huaco pottery vases have been found in the form of figurines with grossly distorted oronasal regions. Although there are various interpretations of these, and although mucocutaneous destruction is commoner today in people of European and African origin than in indigenous Amerindians, many people think that some of these figurines depict mucocutaneous leishmaniasis. According to Hoeppli, cutaneous leishmaniasis was described by Pizzarro in 1571 from the cocoa-growing inhabitants of hot Andean valleys.

Parasitological interpretation of cutaneous leishmaniasis in the New World closely followed that in the Old World. Oriental sore containing Wright corpuscles was described from Bauru in the Sao Paulo Province of Brazil in 1909. An epidemic was affecting labourers on the Bauru–Matto Grosso railway, a foretaste no doubt of the problems connected recently with the Amazonas Highway and the Jari forest exploitation scheme. Shortly thereafter the great Brazilian pathologist Carini identified the insidious mucocutaneous lesions of espundia as being caused by *Leishmania*.

As long ago as 1764 Cosme Bueno attributed the transmission of uta (*L. peruviana*) in the Peruvian Andes to sandflies. Despite this and the convincing work in Europe and Asia incriminating sandflies as vectors and various wild animals as reservoir hosts, epidemiological study of *Leishmania* in South America proved intractable. Pioneer results were achieved in Peru, where it was demonstrated that dogs were reservoir hosts and sandfly transmission was postulated. Consequently, cutaneous leishmaniasis was almost eradicated from its mountain valley habitat. It is only in the past 20 years that a comprehensive picture has developed of the epidemiological situation in Belize, Panama and north-eastern Brazil. These findings, combined with more limited studies in other parts of South America, indicate clearly that there are many vector–reservoir–*Leishmania* combinations, which only intensive study of the whole of this vast area will elucidate.

GEOGRAPHICAL DISTRIBUTION AND PARASITES

The distribution of the organisms causing cutaneous leishmaniasis in the New World is much wider than simply as a disease in man as it is a zoonosis. Study of the distribution of the parasites in sandflies and animals has been hampered by the difficulty of identifying isolated strains, particularly those of some subspecies of *L. braziliensis* which are notoriously difficult to grow in culture. The disease sometimes appears in surprising circumstances which defy explanation, as it did in the 1970s in Texas and in the Dominican Republic. More frequently the presence of the parasite in an area is first indicated by an outbreak in labourers on pioneering projects such as railway- or road-building, mining operations or forest clearance in areas previously sparsely inhabited by a local population to whom medical services were not readily available. Forest clearance and agricultural development have led to environmental changes in which both vectors and, presumably, reservoir hosts have been eliminated. This has in turn led to the local elimination of cutaneous leishmaniasis.

It should therefore be recognized that the known distribution of NWCL is very labile due both to the changing state of knowledge and to real changes in distribution.

There were two related handicaps in the study of South American cutaneous leishmaniasis. The first was the assumption that the disease was imported from the Old World, and the second was the corollary that only one form of parasite was involved. Clinical differences became apparent which cast doubt on these assumptions, and these have now been followed by objective biological and biochemical differences which, fortunately, correspond well with the clinical and epidemiological information. It is now well established that there are two main groups of parasites which are, perhaps, best regarded as two polytypic species, *L. braziliensis* and *L. mexicana*. In addition a few other species have been described.

Peripylaria: *Leishmania braziliensis*

L. braziliensis is the most widespread species, extending south from Belize and Panama throughout the forested parts of South America (figure 83). It is characterized by peripylarial development in its vectors — that is that the hindgut triangle is occupied by parasites during their development. Most subspecies grow with difficulty in culture, but this is not true of the Panamanian subspecies. Cutaneous leishmaniasis has recently been found sporadically in northern Mexico, perhaps linking with the cases in Texas. Although the parasites have not yet been identified the habitat is so different from that in which *L. mexicana* is found that these are thought likely to be *L. braziliensis* parasites of unknown subspecies.

L. b. braziliensis is found in much of South America including Brazil and the Amazon regions of Peru, Colombia and Ecuador. Parasites from central and southern Brazil and Argentina belong to this subspecies by definition, but much remains to be worked out on the relationships between the different strains. In man, *L. b. braziliensis* produces a slow-healing often very extensive oriental sore which self-cures after a variable, sometimes extended time. Following the cure of the initial lesion the infection may metastasize, reappearing on the mucosal surfaces of the oronasal region, causing the disfiguring and eventually often fatal disease of espundia. While conclusive proof is lacking, it is now thought that espundia is always secondary, even though the primary lesion may not be remembered. The site of the cryptic hypobiotic parasites responsible for the secondary lesions is not known, though they have been isolated from the liver.

The host range of this parasite is not fully known, though it has rarely been isolated from forest rodents and marsupials. Parasites isolated from dogs in the Sao Paulo and Belo Horizonte regions of Southern Brazil are presumably of this subspecies. The vectors are members of the genus *Psychodopygus: Ps. wellcomei* is an identified vector.

L. b. guyanensis is mainly distinguished by its behaviour in man. It occurs in the Guyanas and neighbouring regions of Brazil, where its range probably overlaps with that of *L. b. braziliensis.*

The disease in man is known as 'pian bois' or forest yaws. There are one or multiple (sometimes hundreds) initial lesions, and there is a tendency for these to spread, often along the lymphatic ducts.

Little was known until very recently of the host range of this parasite, but recent studies indicate that the reservoir hosts are arboreal edentates, such as the sloth *Choloepus* and the anteater *Tamandua,* which inhabit the forest canopy. *Lutzomyia umbratilis* is the vector.

L. b. panamensis differs from the preceding forms in being relatively easy to grow in culture. It is found in Panama and presumably is the parasite isolated from the small proportion of the recent British military CL cases in Belize which were *L. braziliensis*. This subspecies has been extensively studied by the workers at the Gorgas Memorial Laboratory in Panama, and it is perhaps better known than any other New World form. The disease in man is usually a single slow-healing

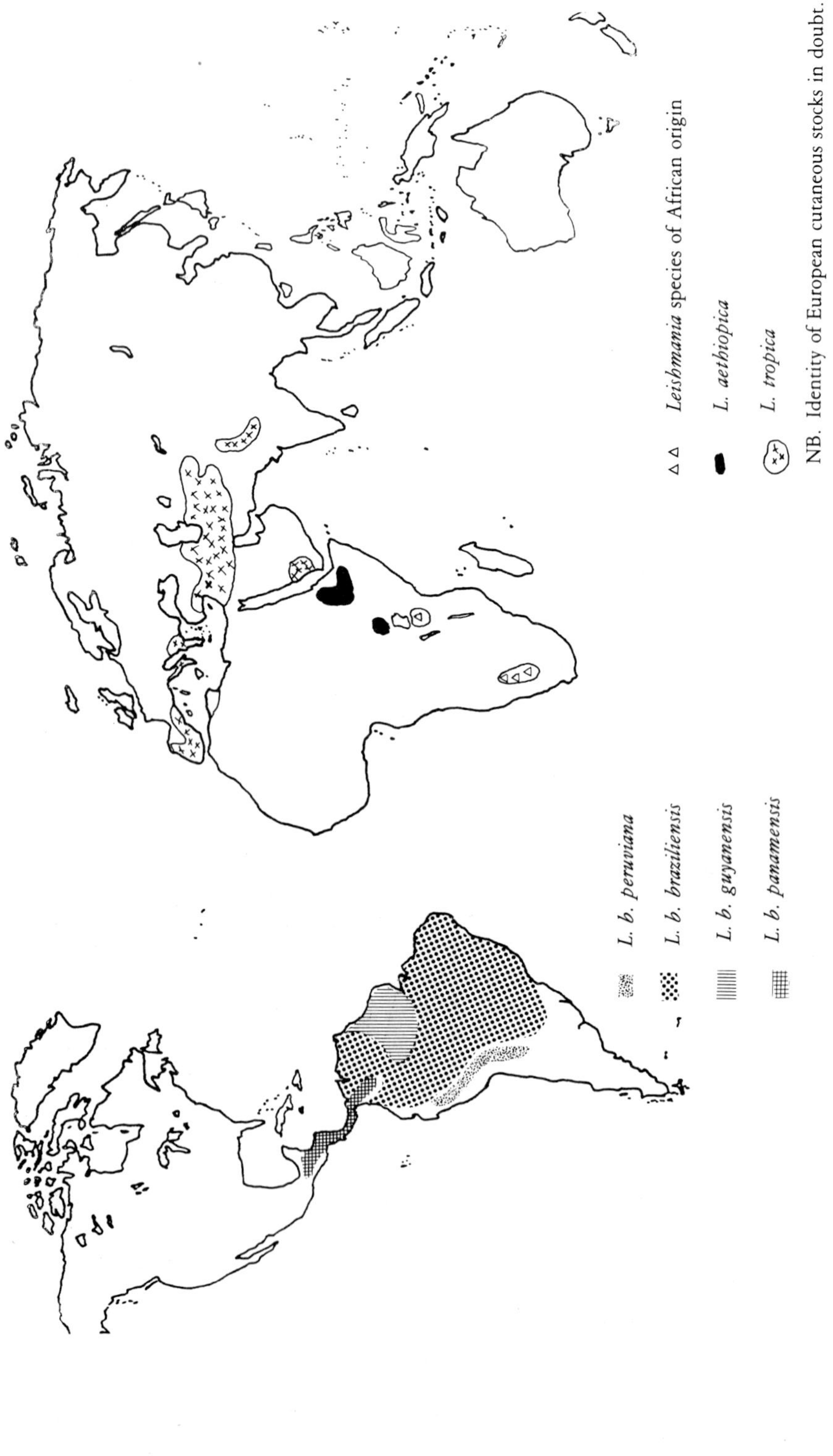

Figure 83. The geographical distribution of *Leishmania braziliensis*, *Leishmania tropica* and *Leishmania aethiopica*.

ulcer like that of *L. b. braziliensis*, but metastasis and espundia are not reliably reported in this subspecies.

The normal hosts of this parasite are the sloths, mainly *Choloepus hoffmanni*, of which a large proportion may be infected, and also *Bradypus infuscatus*. Occasionally other forest animals and even domestic dogs and equines have been found infected. The list includes marsupials, rodents and primates.

L. peruviana was the subject of pioneer studies by Hertig and Herrer, but has only recently become available for the application of modern methods of identification. The parasite was restricted to certain highland valleys of Peru, and possibly northern Argentina, between 1000 m and 3000 m in altitude. The human infection, known as uta, appears as one or several oriental sore-like lesions which heal without sequel. Similar parasites have also been isolated from domestic dogs which have sometimes had a much higher prevalence than man. With the advent of insecticides used in the control of bartonellosis which occurred in the same areas, the infection was apparently almost eradicated and has since been very difficult to find due to the household use of insecticides. It was therefore assumed that the peridomestic sandflies *Lutzomyia verrucarum* and *Lu. peruensis* were the vectors, and that there may have been no sylvatic reservoir host. Clinically and ecologically this parasite somewhat resembled *L. tropica* of the Old World, and it was suggested that it had been imported. However, recent isolates from Peru have been studied biochemically and in sandflies, in which they have peripylarian development; they thus resemble *L. braziliensis*: clear evidence that the Peruvian highland parasite is indigenous, and not imported.

Suprapylaria: *Leishmania mexicana*

Leishmania mexicana is typically characterized by rapid growth both in culture and in hamsters, and by suprapylarial development in the midgut of its sandfly vectors, without invasion of the hindgut triangle. The subspecific divisions of the species are perhaps less well established than for *L. braziliensis*. *L. m. pifanoi* is very close to *L. m. mexicana; L. m. amazonensis* and the recently described *L.m. aristedesi* from Panama are also very similar, and it is not clear that there are objective criteria for distinguishing the four subspecies of *L. mexicana*. The geographical distribution of *L. mexicana* is shown in figure 84.

L. m. mexicana is the name given to the parasite causing chiclero's ulcer in the chicle-producing rain forests of Yucatan and Belize. The infection in man usually causes a fairly insignificant self-healing ulcer, but if it occurs on the pinna of the ear, healing is long delayed, the cartilage is invaded and the entire ear may gradually be eroded. A variety of forest rodents (*Proechimys*, *Oryzomys*) are infected, but it is not clear whether any particular one is the main host; the vector is *Lutzomyia olmeca*.

L. m. pifanoi was named in Venezuela from cases of diffuse cutaneous leish-

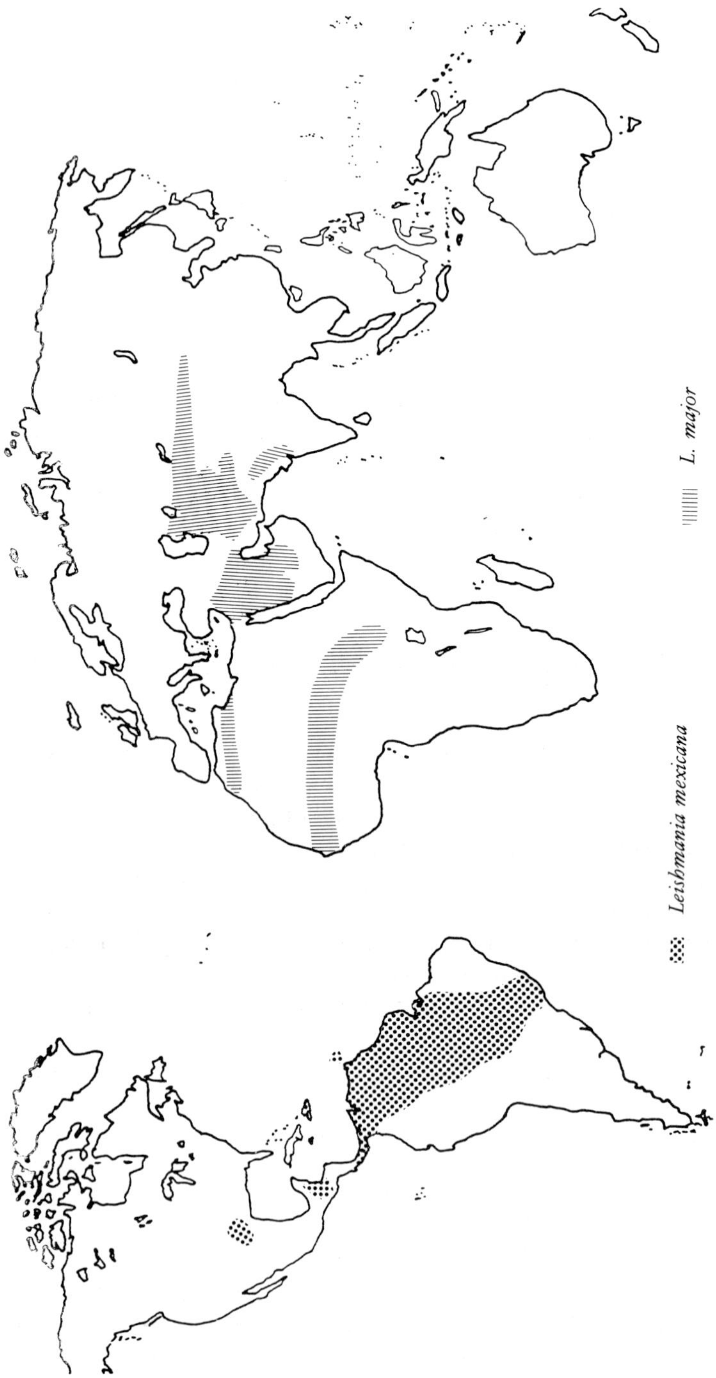

Figure 84. The geographical distribution of *Leishmania mexicana* and *L. major*.

maniasis. Simple *L. mexicana* cutaneous lesions in man are almost unknown from Venezuela, and little confirmed evidence exists on the natural hosts of the parasite. However, *L. m. amazonensis* described from the Amazon region of Brazil is much better known. The latter parasite is known from simple cutaneous lesions and DCL cases, and has been isolated from a wide variety of forest rodents and marsupials.

L. m. amazonensis has also been described from rodents in Trinidad, although human infections are almost unknown there. Further studies are required to determine whether the Venezuelan parasites are distinguishable from Amazonian strains.

Leishmania parasites have been seen, or even isolated, in many situations not included above, and doubtless both the host range and geographical range of *L. braziliensis* and *L. mexicana* are much wider than indicated. For example, *L. m. aristedesi* was named from Panama where it was isolated from animals in an area where human infection is unknown. However, now that biochemical methods are available for parasite identification, it is perhaps better to be conservative and await further results which will accurately define the limits of the above subspecies as well as the others which doubtless exist.

ECOLOGY AND EPIDEMIOLOGY

With the possible exception of southern Brazil and the probable exception of highland Peru, the cutaneous leishmaniases in South and Central America are sylvatic zoonoses. The parasites are maintained by vector–host systems entirely independent of man; transmission to man or his domestic animals is a relatively rare event, and transmission within the synanthropic environment is extremely rare. Therefore, in contrast to the Old World parasites, in large parts of their ranges the ecology of NWCL is largely independent of its epidemiology.

The NWCL parasites have a patchy distribution over the continent and isthmus; they are restricted to forested areas and, within the forest, to certain specialized habitats.

Unlike Old World cutaneous leishmaniasis foci, those of the New World seem to be 'diffuse' in Pavlovsky's terminology as opposed to 'elementary'. Elementary foci can be traced to an individual burrow or colony in which the infection may be transmitted indefinitely. All the elements of the cycle are found in a small, well defined area. The best examples in leishmaniasis are of course in the *Rhombomys* colonies of the southern USSR and in the hyrax colonies of highland Ethiopia. In diffuse foci the vertebrate hosts are not necessarily colonial, and do not provide the habitat of the sandfly vector. Vector and vertebrate host being less closely tied to each other ecologically, diffuse foci require a larger and more complex geographical area than elementary foci. Further, since the vertebrate host and vector are less strictly tied ecologically, there is a greater chance that the parasite will gain entry to abnormal hosts. Thus there is a tendency for parasites with 'diffuse foci' to be less dependent on a single vertebrate host or vector.

Our knowledge of the ecology of NWCL is dependent on a few intensive studies which have, of necessity, been localized. Nevertheless, a picture is emerging which seems more and more to be of wide application.

L. braziliensis has been extensively studied in Panama (*L. b. panamensis*). Although large numbers of forest animals were examined, the ecology remained poorly understood until it was discovered that a very large proportion (17 per cent) of sloths are infected. The two toed sloth *Choloepus hoffmanni* (figure 85), which was most commonly found infected, is a slow moving solitary arboreal animal which does not construct a nest, but wanders through the forest feeding on treetop vegetation. Populations have been estimated at around 12 per hectare. These features would seem to make these animals unsuitable as reservoir hosts of a parasite borne by a free-flying vector: the chances of a sandfly biting sloths twice in its life would seem to be very slim. Little is known about the specific habitat requirements of *Lu. trapidoi*, the main sandfly vector, but it is not a specific sloth-feeder. It would therefore seem that the high infection rates in sloths and sandflies must depend on some unknown ecological link between the two. For example, do the sandflies breed in the ants' nests in trees favoured by sloths?

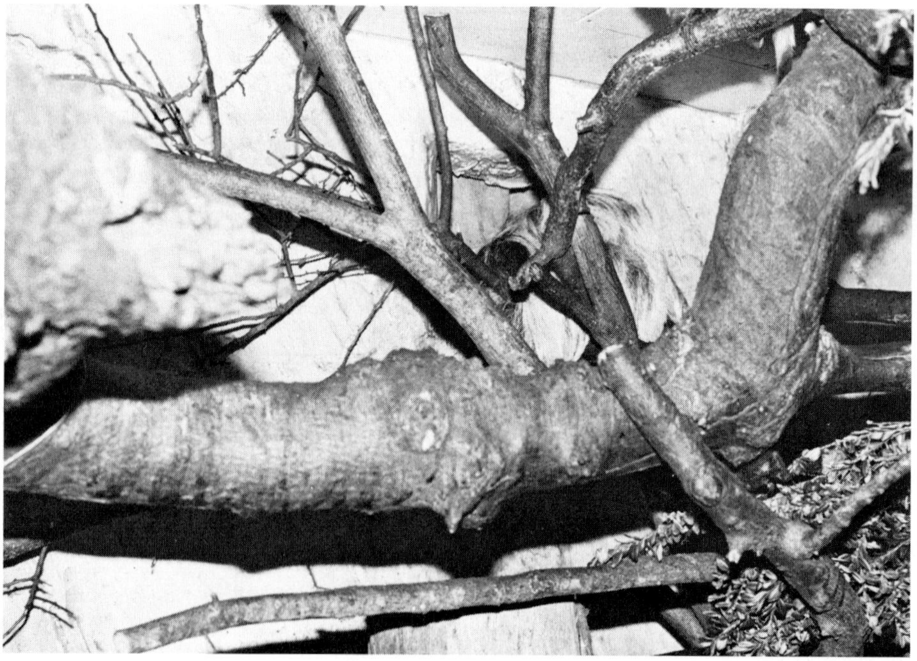

Figure 85. A sloth *Choloepus hoffmanni*. Difficult to see at rest in its zoo cage, this animal is almost invisible in a forest tree top.

A variety of other forest animals have been found infected, but in small numbers, and it is considered that these are more or less incidental hosts, the sloth being the only important one in the long-term maintenance of the parasite. Human infections occur when people enter the forest either visiting or for settlement. New settlements are afflicted with the disease for 2–3 years, but when the surrounding area is deforested the infection becomes restricted to the adult males, and their dogs, who hunt in the remaining bush.

Very similar situations have been described, though less completely, in areas of *L. b. guyanensis* infection. Early indications were that the infection was arboreal when a technician developed more than 100 lesions following a night's human bait catch in a tree top. This infection, and those of various scientists studying the disease both in Brazil and French Guyana, emphasize the risk involved in forest work or settlement. *L. b. guyanensis* is thought to be transmitted by *Lutzomyia umbratilis*, which may be found in great numbers, and which is frequently infected. The most recent work in Brazil has shown that like *L. b. panamensis, L. b. guyanensis* is a parsite of edentates; it has been found in a high proportion of sloths and in the anteater *Tamandua tetradactyla*. It is thought that the main hosts are the sloths but that the infection may be dispersed through the forest by the more mobile anteaters. At Manaus a high proportion of *Didelphys marsupialis*, an opossum, were infected. It is thought that this may have been due to disturbances in the forest and that opossums might bring the parasite right into the human environment.

The ecology of *L. b. braziliensis* is much less well known than the above. This is partly because of the difficulty of culturing the parasite. Strains have been isolated from dogs in southern and central Brazil, and rarely also from forest animals and domestic rats, but a true maintenance host remains to be discovered.

Human infections occur,like those of *L. b. panamensis*, in forest dwellers and immigrants. The rate of infection in indigenous Amerindians as indicated by skin testing is high, but these people suffer less severely than people of African or European racial origin.

The zoonotic origin of *L. mexicana* infection was first recognized in Belize, where variable numbers of forest rodents were found infected. *Ototylomys phyllotis*, the most frequently infected species, was restricted to forest habitat, where it was partially arboreal. In eastern Panama another forest rodent, *Oryzomys capito*, was infected at the very high rate of 36 per cent, and this species, along with *Proechimys guyanensis* (figure 86), is the main host in the Amazon region of Brazil. In this last region the infection is restricted to a certain type of forest between the regularly flooded forest along the river banks and dry forest in raised areas. The swamp or igapo forest is only infrequently visited by people collecting forest products. A large list of other rodents and marsupials have been found infected with *L. mexicana* subspecies, but none seems to play such a dominant role as *Proechimys, Oryzomys* and *Ototylomys*. The vectors throughout this range are *Lu. flaviscutellata* and its close relative *Lu. olmeca*. These species vary greatly in their attraction to man. In Belize, *Lu. olmeca* rarely feed on man except when disturbed during the day by his activities in the forest.

Human infection with *L. mexicana* has decreased in recent years with the reduction of chicle gathering and the increase in urbanization and forest destruction. The infection was characteristically found in the chicle collectors and other forest workers of Yucatan and Belize who nearly all became infected in their first year of work. The human disease is almost unknown in Panama despite the finding of infected rodents. In Trinidad also, human infections are rare or absent, although the animal reservoir exists in the forests. In Brazil, *L. mexicana* accounts for only some 10 per cent of the human leishmaniasis cases seen in Belém. In Belize, the disease has been contracted recently by British troops on jungle warfare training. As is usual with infections of military personnel, details of the localities

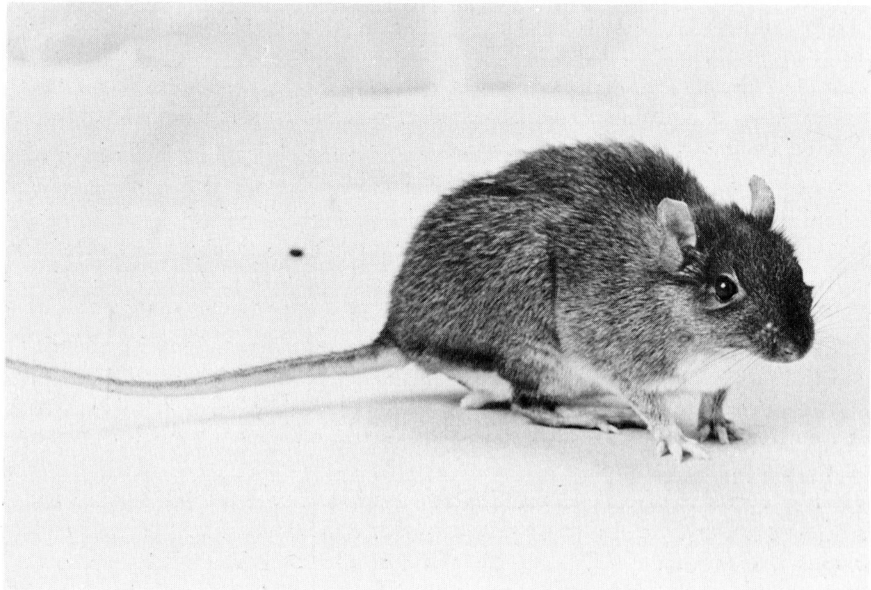

Figure 86. *Proechimys* sp., a reservoir host of *L. mexicana* in Central and South America.

and activities leading to infection are not readily available, but reports indicate that the infection is widespread in the forest, and that while some transmission may be diurnal, most is nocturnal. The parasites were mostly found to belong to the *L. mexicana* group, but a few were more similar to the *L. braziliensis* complex.

DISEASES

Clinical features

Cutaneous leishmaniasis in South America is normally sufficiently similar to that in the Old World that the two were not distinguished clinically by the first authors. As in oriental sore, the first indication of infection is a painless papule containing many parasites, which gradually expands, then ulcerates, eventually healing and leaving the characteristic scar. The lesions are commonly much more florid than in the Old World, and may be much more persistent. In *L. mexicana* infections on the cool cartilaginous tissues of the ear, self-healing is long delayed, and almost the entire pinna may be gradually eroded. Normally, however, *L. mexicana* lesions on the warmer skin surfaces are relatively benign and self-healing.

The main feature of the South American cutaneous leishmaniasis which is not shared by the main Old World forms is the fact that, sometimes following a long period of apparent cure, the infection may metastasize to areas of the body far removed from the site of the original lesion.

The factors which predispose the dissemination of the parasite are by no means fully understood. Metastasis in *L. mexicana* infection is associated with the incomplete development of the normal cell mediated immune response, though what causes this is unknown. On the other hand, metastasis in *L. braziliensis* is associated with excessive immune response, and possibly an autoimmune response as well. Thus, metastasizing *L. mexicana* infections are not accompanied by necrosis and ulceration, but by increasing areas of cutaneous tissue which become packed with infected macrophages, producing unsightly nodules over a wide area of the body, resembling the DCL cases described below in *L. aethiopica* infection, or the most severe manifestation of post-kala-azar dermal leishmaniasis.

Human experiments on this infection have only very rarely been performed, but confirm that the parasites isolated from one of these South American DCL patients produce a typical self-healing ulcer in the recipient. This was despite the fact that one recipient was a terminal cancer patient and was probably in a highly immunosuppressed state.

The proportion of *L. mexicana* infections which develop to DCL is difficult to assess, and varies from place to place. In northern Brazil about 25 per cent are thought to metastasize, while in Belize and Mexico DCL is virtually unknown. In Venezuela, where DCL was first described, simple OS-type infections with *L. mexicana* are almost unknown, and, although it is a rare disease, DCL is the predominant form.

L. b. guyanensis and *L. b. braziliensis* were first distinguished by the differences between their clinical manifestations. In the former case the infection spreads through the lymphatic system and nodules appear at intervals along the course of the ducts.

L. b. braziliensis lesions are usually apparently cured within two years of the initial infection. At any time, up to 30 years thereafter, the disease may reappear on the mucous membranes of the nose or mouth. These mucocutaneous lesions do not self-heal but continue to invade the tissues which become blocked with granulomatous infiltration, eventually necrotizing and eroding insidiously. An early indication is often the end of the nose, which becomes expanded with infiltrate and hyperplasia, producing the syndrome of 'tapir nose'. The tissues, including the septum, then become eroded. Similarly, the oral mucosa may be affected and eventually the face is effectively destroyed. Death frequently results as an indirect consequence, due to bacterial super-infection or obstruction of airways or the food passage. In addition to metastasis to the oronasal mucosa, the infection may reappear in other parts of the body, particularly at the site of a wound.

Diagnosis

Epidemiological information is of great importance in indicating cutaneous leishmaniasis, as the infection may occur in outbreaks or may be associated with specific geographical areas and habitats. Isolated cases or cases imported into non-endemic areas present considerable difficulties.

Differential diagnosis includes other chronic painless ulcerating or non-ulcerating cutaneous lesions such as lupus vulgaris, sarcoidosis, sporotrichosis, blastomycosis, donovanosis, syphilis and epitheliomas. DCL or the pseudolepromatous type of disease is clinically almost indistinguishable from lepromatous leprosy and can only be distinguished by finding the specific organisms. The chronicity of cutaneous leishmaniasis lesions is an important indication, but with improved access to medical services early lesions may be seen whose chronic nature may not yet be evident. Fortunately in early lesions the parasites are usually abundant and readily demonstrable.

During outbreaks or when there is other clear epidemiological supporting evidence clinical examination may be sufficient to indicate treatment. In general, however, it is desirable to demonstrate the parasites. Material is taken from the deep dermal tissue at the edge of the lesion by needle biopsy or by expressing tissue exudate from a blanched lancet wound. Some of the material should be cultured in NNN medium and inoculated into hamsters for eventual identification of the species of parasite, but for immediate diagnosis the rest of the material should be smeared onto a microscope slide, fixed and stained with Giemsa's or Wright's stain to demonstrate amastigotes. In some lesions there are innumerable parasites, while in others prolonged examination of the slide by a skilled microscopist may be necessary before amastigotes are seen.

Parasites are difficult to identify in sectioned biopsy material, though this may be valuable in indicating the pathological state of the lesion.

In old lesions, particularly those of mucocutaneous leishmaniasis, parasites are usually very scanty. Useful confirmatory evidence of the diagnosis is given by a positive Leishmanin or Montenegro test, in which 0·1 ml of a suspension of dead promastigotes is inoculated intradermally. A positive reaction is indicated by a delayed hypersensitivity reaction consisting of an indurated area 5 mm in diameter 48 hours after injection. Immediate and intermediate reactions have been demonstrated with an exo-antigen and this may be of value for differentiating the various pathological conditions in Brazil. Delayed hypersensitivity is retained following cure or healing, and can therefore be used for retrospective diagnosis for epidemiological purposes. Unfortunately there are frequent false positive reactions indicating inadequate specificity or a wide prevalence of self-cured cases. The Montenegro test remains negative in DCL and a negative test in the presence of confirmed parasitological diagnosis indicates this syndrome with its poor prognosis. Transformation from a negative to a positive reaction is required before treatment will be successful.

Serological diagnostic tests have been developed, for example, counter-current immune electrophoresis, IFA and ELISA. They are of great value, but specific antigens are still required.

Treatment

The treatment of NWCL presents various fascinating problems, though these are of little comfort to the sufferer. To begin with the number of sufferers in a given area is generally small and the development of effective treatment has not been a high priority within the pharmaceutical industry. Also, the factors determining the development of espundia are not understood and it is not clear to what extent treatment of early lesions will affect the incidence of espundia, but it is generally thought that intensive treatment of the initial lesion of *L. braziliensis* is desirable. This involves large doses of rather toxic antimonial drugs and it is therefore desirable that the parasite should first be identified to ensure that it is *L. braziliensis* and not one of the relatively benign strains of *L. mexicana*. Treatment of espundia is difficult and complex and, since so many of the sufferers are poor rural labourers, not generally available. Reconstructive surgery is often necessary, and in the initial stages non-specific treatment such as antibiotics and good diet may be beneficial.

In most cases of *L. mexicana* infection from Central America specific treatment is not indicated as the lesions will resolve naturally. For complicated *L. mexicana* cases which develop DCL, chemotherapy is rarely effective and the best that can usually be done is non-specific treatment such as radiant heat, hot baths or saunas, which relieve some of the unsightliness of the lesions. Pentavalent antimonials are the first line of attack and relieve many cases. Aromatic diamidines (Pentostam) are used for antimony-resistant cases. Pyrimethamine has been used recently with ambiguous results, and good results have been claimed for the antifungal antibiotic Amphotericin B. Cycloguanil pamoate may also be of value.

Chemotherapy of New World cutaneous leishmaniasis is a field where innovation and experiment are still urgently required.

Control

In general, NWCL is a sporadic zoonotic sylvatic infection for which control is not feasible. Transmission occurs diffusely in a massive area of primary and secondary forest in which the indiscriminate use of insecticides would be as impractical as it would be undesirable. Removal of the forest itself is being pursued all too actively and, far from controlling leishmaniasis, this may be causing *L. braziliensis* to be replaced by *L. mexicana* and *L. donovani*. Personal protection by prophylaxis or vaccination is not available. There are, however, specific groups of workers for whom protection is indicated and may be possible. Settlers, forestry workers, road builders and military personnel are the most at risk. It was found by the military in Belize that infection could be reduced by the avoidance of specific areas at night. Personal protection from sandfly bites at night by smoke, repellents and fine-mesh insect nets can be effective in reducing the transmission rate. Some transmission is thought to occur, however, when sandflies are disturbed during the day.

With the growing evidence that edentates are important reservoir hosts for *L. braziliensis* it is possible that specific control of sloths and anteaters in the vicinity of settlements may accelerate the disappearance of the disease.

Only in the Andean valleys of Peru has sandfly control been effective in reducing and almost eradicating cutaneous leishmaniasis in the New World. Even here, the main purpose of the control of peridomestic sandflies was the elimination of Oroya fever (bartonellosis) rather than leishmaniasis.

Chapter 9. Visceral Leishmaniasis

INTRODUCTION

Under this heading it is convenient to include all those leishmanial infections which regularly invade the internal organs, particularly the liver, spleen and reticulo-endothelial system of man. The distinction between cutaneous and visceral leishmaniasis is far from absolute, as already mentioned; recent evidence indicates that parasites resembling the normally dermotropic *L. tropica* (*sensu strictu*) may occassionally visceralize in man, and parasites isolated from the viscera of West African rodents resemble *L. major*. Further, parasites which normally visceralize in man may be restricted to the skin either subsequent to the visceral infection or in the absence of a preceding visceral infection.

Kala-azar or visceral leishmaniasis has many features in common with chronic malaria and it was not definitely distinguished as a disease entity until 1903. This was achieved by William Boog Leishman, the Scotsman whose name is now given to the disease. It was noted that there were indications that a disease distinct from pernicious malaria or other tropical fevers occurred in the notoriously unhealthy military station at Dum-Dum in the outskirts of Calcutta. Patients with Dum-Dum fever had a low grade fever with hepatosplenomegaly and severe, progressive cachexia (wasting) and this persisted despite antimalarial treatment. Leishman noticed distinctive structures in smears from the greatly enlarged spleen, but it was only two years later, when working with trypanosomes, that he recognized the similarity between the organisms in the spleen from Dum-Dum and degenerating trypanosomes in a dead rat. In fact he thought his parasites were degenerating trypanosomes, and that Dum-Dum fever was a trypanosomiasis. A modern international airport now stands at Dum-Dum and the fever is largely a thing of the past.

Donovan, working in Madras, on reading Leishman's work, recognized parasites which he had found in the spleens of patients dying of chronic malaria. He performed a spleen puncture on a patient, and found that the parasites were identical in fresh tissue, and were thus not degenerate forms. A short time later,

Rogers in 1904 cultured the organisms in citrated blood held at 22°C. He used material both from the "the endemic cachexial fever seen in Lower Bengal" and the "Assam epidemic form known as kala-azar" and demonstrated flagellated "trypanosomes" in both.

The parasites were found in Tunisia in children with anaemia and splenomegaly, and Nicolle, having first demonstrated similar parasites in dogs, was able to infect a dog with an extract from an infected spleen, which led him to suggest that the dog might be a reservoir of the infection.

With the aetiological agent known, it remained to determine the mechanism of infection. In that golden age of parasitological discovery it was easy to suppose that the infection was arthropod-borne, but which arthropod? Practically every blood-sucking arthropod was accused at one time or another — indeed, to this day occasional reports incriminate bed bugs or ticks. Slowly, however, evidence accumulated in favour of sandflies. Sinton showed a convincing coincidence between the distribution of visceral leishmaniasis and *Phlebotomus argentipes* (if Sinton's maps are compared with modern maps of the distribution of *P. argentipes*, one may be led to ask if he did not fit his data to a preconceived notion that this was the vector). It was not until 1931 that Shortt, Smith and Swaminath achieved their historic transmission to hamsters by bite, and sandflies could be formally incriminated. However, transmission to man was only achieved in 1942. It is remarkable how rarely transmission studies have been repeated. The main problem is the difficulty of rearing sandflies and persuading them to survive oviposition and to refeed. In spite of the paucity of experimental evidence, most workers are convinced that the usual mode of transmission is by sandflies, but there is also some evidence of transmission by other methods including transplacental and venereal, and by carnivory. However, there remain considerable problems in interpreting the epidemiology of visceral leishmaniasis on the basis of sandfly transmission alone.

The importance of dogs in the epidemiology of Mediterranean visceral leishmaniasis was recognized early, but was confused by the lack of correlation between the incidence of canine and human infection. Repeated attempts to find infected dogs in both Assam and southern India failed. There were persistent attempts to distinguish the dog parasite as *L. canis*. While the role of the dog has now been firmly established, as has the identity of the dog and human parasites, the reasons why canine and human infection have such different incidences in different areas and the importance of other reservoir hosts are the subject of active study, especially in South America and Africa. Extensive studies on the epidemiology of visceral leishmaniasis in Sudan had to be terminated prematurely and are tantalizingly inconclusive.

GEOGRAPHICAL DISTRIBUTION

The geographical distribution of *L. donovani* (including *L. infantum* and *L. chagasi*) is usually accepted as being coincident with that of visceral leishmaniasis in man or dogs (figure 87). This has largely been confirmed by biochemical taxonomic studies, but in a few localities visceral disease has been found to be caused by *L. tropica* (*s. str.*) and *L. donovani* infection is sometimes restricted to cutaneous lesions.

In the past, human visceral leishmaniasis was widespread in China between the Yangtse River and the northern borders, and sporadic elsewhere in that country, with a second important area of distribution in the west in Xinjiang (Sinkiang) Province. Occasional cases were reported from Mongolia, and the infection extended through southern USSR and into the west Asian countries to the Mediterranean, where it was common in southern Europe, particularly Greece, and the Mediterranean islands. Southern France and much of Spain are involved with occasional cases reported from Portugal. In North Africa, the coastal regions of Algeria and Tunisia are traditional areas of infection. The infection still has largely the same distribution but has become very uncommon in most of its range.

Within the area outlined above there seems to be a decreasing infectivity to man from east to west, so that in China people of all ages were infected but only infants are infected in Europe, and at the western extent of the range, in Senegal, the parasite is known in dogs, but human infection is almost unknown. However, a few recent reports from France indicate that the infections now occur more equally in all age groups and that perhaps the restriction to infants has to do with epidemiological factors rather than the infectivity of the parasite.

Human visceral leishmaniasis also occurs in the arid regions of north-east Brazil and in similar habitats in Venezuela. The parasites isolated from dogs and people in these areas are indistinguishable from *L. donovani*. In Para State, in the Amazonian rain forests, visceral leishmaniasis occurs much more rarely. Elsewhere in South and Central America, visceral leishmaniasis is very widespread but generally sporadic. Argentina, Chile, Ecuador, Peru and Uruguay are the only South American nations in which it appears not to be endemic.

Returning to the Old World we find visceral leishmaniasis in man, not associated with canine infection, and not restricted to infants, in a large part of north-west India, mainly in the alluvial plains of the Brahamputra and Ganges Rivers, but extending down the east coast to Orissa and Tamil Nadu with sporadic cases or outbreaks reported over a wide range including Bombay, Gujarat and Kashmir. Since 1950 the distribution of the disease has been largely restricted to northern Bihar State, where a major epidemic began around 1970. Epidemic visceral leishmaniasis occurs in Africa in the dry land of western Kenya and in southern Sudan. There are also areas where the infection is sporadic and

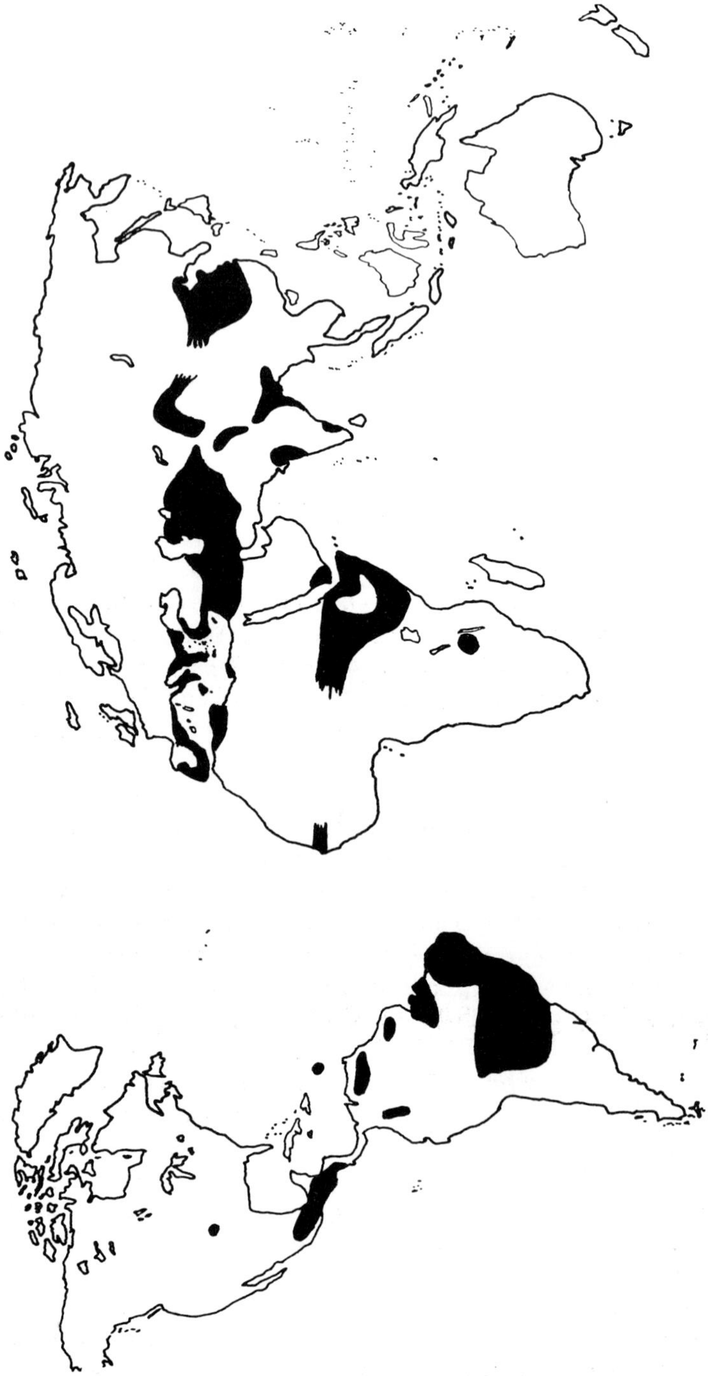

Figure 87. The world-wide distribution of *L. donovani* and visceral canine leishmaniasis.

presumably zoonotic in northern Kenya, southern Ethiopia and the Wabi Shebelli valley of Somalia. The Sudanese distribution consists mainly of the area between the White and Blue Nile, extending to the Ethiopian border in the east. In the west the disease is much less frequent, but has been reported from many localities, mainly in the semi-arid vegetation belt, as far west as Tanjdile in Chad. In the Nuba mountains of southern Sudan the infection used to resemble Mediterranean visceral leishmaniasis but there are no up-to-date studies in that area. Visceral cases further west are extremely rare, but have been reported from Gambia, northern Nigeria (possibly imported from Niger), northern Togo, and Upper Volta.

South of the subsahelian belt there have been apparently locally acquired individual cases in Gabon (a child whose brother had a cutaneous infection), Malawi, Zaire (two, one of which was possibly contracted in Rwanda) and Zambia.

PARASITES

With the exception of occasional aberrant strains from western Asia and India parasites from human visceral infections have not been consistently distinguishable from each other except on clinical or epidemiological grounds. Experimental infections in laboratory animals or sandflies, and quantitative comparison of DNA and isoenzyme patterns have failed to provide reliable distinctive features separating strains from any part of the range.

There is considerable clinical and epidemiological evidence that Mediterranean and South American parasites are likely to be different, and they have been named *L. infantum* and *L. chagasi* respectively. It is also possible that the East African and Sudanese parasites belong to distinguishable species: the name *L. archibaldi* is available for the latter. The validation of these three names must await objective methods of identifying isolated strains, though from recent evidence it seems that at the most they will be of subspecific rank. For the present, therefore, visceralizing strains from all major geographical localities should be termed *L. donovani*.

In Africa, visceral infection of man is commonly associated with one or numerous cutaneous lesions, and cutaneous lesions without visceral involvement may be produced by either *L. donovani* or *L. major*. Further, *L. major*-like parasites have been isolated from the viscera of rodents in Ethiopia, Kenya and Senegal. Thus the distribution of the different parasites is impossible to assess without critical identification of many isolates.

Infection with *L. donovani* by the above definition therefore occurs in three major clinico-epidemiological patterns: Mediterranean-type or infantile visceral leishmaniasis, Indian type visceral leishmaniasis or kala-azar and the African type which may be zoonotic as in Sudan or anthroponotic as in Kenya.

Natural mammalian hosts and reservoirs of infection

Canine visceral leishmaniasis more or less coincides with the human infection in northern China, the Middle East, the Mediterranean region and South America. The prevalence of infection in dogs is sometimes very high, and dog control has led to a reduction in human cases, indicating that the dog is an important reservoir of human infection. Other canids have been found infected in Brazil (*Dusicyon thous* and *Dusicyon vetulus*), in France (*Vulpes vulpes*), in Sudan (*Vulpes pallida*) and in the USSR (*Canis aureus*). Also, the bat-eared fox *Fennecus zarda* was found infected in a zoo in the USA. This animal presumably came from Saharan Africa. It is generally considered that the prevalence of parasites in these carnivores is probably insufficient for them to constitute a natural reservoir of the infection, except perhaps in the USSR.

In addition to canids, *L. donovani*-like parasites have occasionally been found in other carnivores, rodents, and even in ungulates. Cats are rarely infected but have been found in Brazil, and even Switzerland where the infection is almost unknown in dogs and quite unknown to man (however, the cat in question had been to Spain). Extensive work in Sudan showed infections in very small samples of the serval *Felis serval* and the genet *Genetta* and also in the grass rat *Arvicanthis niloticus*. Another rodent, *Acomys albigena*, was found infected in Sudan as well as the common rat *Rattus rattus*, which has subsequently been found infected in Yugoslavia and Italy. Most of the findings are difficult to interpret in epidemiological terms as the numbers involved are small and/or the feeding behaviour of the sandfly vectors is poorly known. Only in Sudan has it been possible to postulate with some conviction that the infection in man is normally a zoonosis, and that rodents are important reservoirs of infection.

On the other hand, in epidemic outbreaks in India and Kenya it is probable that no animals are involved, and that the parasites are transmitted regularly from man to man. In both these countries large numbers of dogs have been examined and, while two were found infected recently in Kenya, the proportion is so low that man must probably be regarded as the reservoir of canine infection. *Leishmania* isolated from the viscera of rodents in northern Kenya and various lowland localities in Ethiopia as well as Senegal are not *L. donovani*, and are probably not involved with human visceral disease.

In many parts of its range the prevalence of infection with *L. donovani* in all its hosts, including man, is apparently so low or so variable that the perpetuation of the parasite remains to be explained in ecological terms.

DISEASES

Clinical features

The clinical picture in visceral leishmaniasis varies considerably in different areas, but there is a fairly uniform basic pattern.

At the site of initial infection there may or may not develop a small leishmanioma, or papule which, unlike the chancre of initial *Trypanosoma* infection, usually regresses without ulcerating. The incubation period of both the initial papule and the visceral disease are variable and difficult to determine. Kala-azar has been known to develop within three weeks of exposure to infection, and an incubation period exceeding two years is not unknown. In some studies there is good correlation between the appearance of new cases and the seasonal distribution of sandflies with a six-month delay. Assuming that most transmission occurs towards the end of the sandfly season, 3–6 months is indicated as the commonest incubation period.

The first symptoms of visceralization are recurrent low grade fever, often with two daily peaks, which persists, with remissions, throughout the course of the disease. There is massive hyperplasia of the endothelial cells of the spleen, leading to splenomegaly (figure 88), and later of the liver, with hepatomegaly. Lymphatic involvement is indicated early by swollen lymph glands. Much of the parasite multiplication occurs in the bone marrow and there is disruption of its function leading to leucopaenia and thrombocytopaenia with relative monocytosis. The anaemia is not due to haemopoietic malfunction, but due to the destruction of erythrocytes in the grossly enlarged spleen and due to haemolysis, which may be immunologically mediated. Although the patient may be supporting enormous

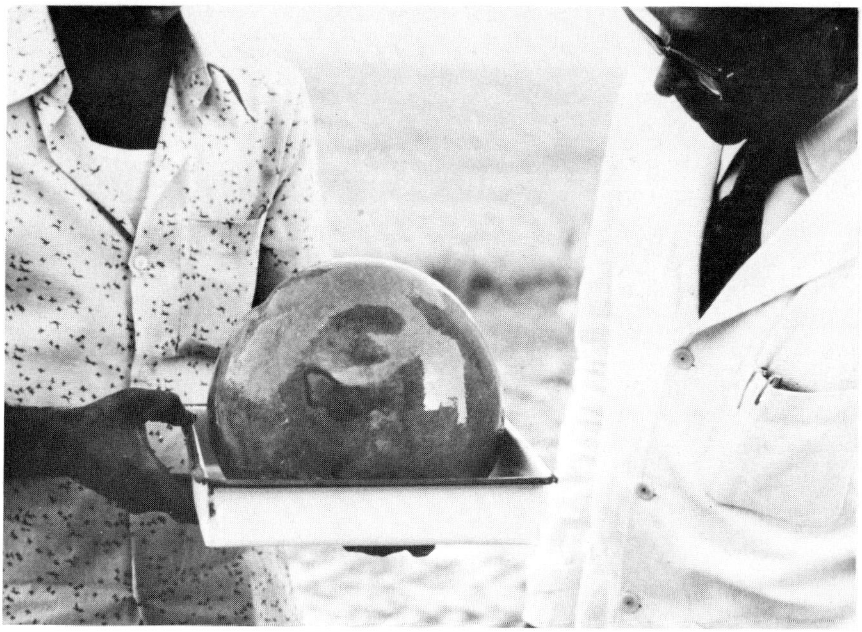

Figure 88. *L. donovani* spleen, Patna, India. Splenectomy is only practised in chronic cases persistently resistant to chemotherapy.

numbers of parasites he may feel comparatively well. There is no indication, other than the fever, of production of toxins and there is very little tissue necrosis or granulomatous reaction. Diarrhoea is frequent, but may be due to concommitant infection, as are many of the other features such as meningitis, cancrum oris, pneumonia and bronchitis. The fourth key feature, along with low-grade remittant fever, hepatosplenomegaly and leucopaenia, is cachexia. The cause of the cachexia is by no means clear, but is probably a combination of repeated diarrhoea, some loss of appetite, chronic fever and altered blood chemistry. The blood proteins are considerably modified by the production of enormous quantities of gamma globulin. Clearly these immunoglobulins are not effective in eliminating the parasites, and their stimulation must be a key factor in the survival mechanism of the parasites in the hostile environment of the host macrophages. Recent interpretations of pathogenesis in visceral leishmaniasis invoke immune complexes and autoimmune effects. This is an important area of current investigation.

In untreated patients, once the disease proceeds beyond the initial papule stage, death seems to be the outcome in as many as 90 per cent of cases, which is why kala-azar was so greatly feared in Assam and Bengal. The chronic disease is marked by progressive emaciation and general weakness with increasing susceptibility to other infections. The leucopaenia and thrombocytopaenia are associated with bleeding tendency and poor healing of minor cuts and abrasions. Weakness, anorexia, anaemia and general incapacity lead to vitamin deficiency and a chain reaction of increasing debility. Death is usually attributed to concommitant infections, often with normally inoffensive organisms, which become dangerous due to the debilitated state of the patient.

Recovery, whether natural or following treatment, may be complete, with rapid regression of the fever and of the swelling of the spleen and liver, and correction of the blood picture. However, in many cases the parasites are not completely eliminated, and may recrudesce in the skin giving rise to post-kala-azar dermal leishmaniasis, PKDL.

PKDL appears within two years of recovery, initially as a faint mottling of the skin. Parasites are present in much of the skin at this stage, but may become concentrated into hypo- or hyper-pigmented papules or macules which may swell and eventually ulcerate. PKDL may occur on much of the body surface, but is most prominent when the face is affected. Parasites may be numerous in the lesions and also in the unaltered skin, but bone marrow and organ biopsy is negative and there is no fever or other symptom of visceral involvement. Simultaneous visceral and cutaneous disease has only very rarely been recorded.

The proportion of patients developing PKDL is one of the factors in visceral leishmaniasis which varies geographically. PKDL is most frequent in Bengal and, perhaps, the southern part of the Chinese distribution. It is rarer in Assam; this was attributed to the virulent epidemic nature of the Assam outbreaks, with the expectation that PKDL would appear when the virulence of the parasites decreased. It is not clear that this prediction was justified as kala-azar has virtually disappeared from Assam. In Africa PKDL occurs infrequently in Kenya, while in Sudan it is more frequent, sometimes occurring simultaneously with the visceral disease, as happened also in one of the cases recorded from Zambia. Mediterranean, or infantile, visceral leishmaniasis rarely if ever develops into PKDL.

Immunological correlations

The enormous gamma globulin production leads to non-specific reactions such as a positive formol-gel test, which usually becomes positive when the infection enters a chronic phase after about three months of patency. Serological tests such as CFT and IFAT become strongly positive earlier in the infection (especially the latter) but suffer somewhat from lack of specificity. ELISA becomes positive very early, sometimes before the first symptoms have appeared. Unfortunately, however, this test is not much more specific than IFAT, cross-reacting with tuberculosis, lepromatous leprosy and Chagas' disease and probably many other conditions. At present specific antigens and monoclonal antibodies are being produced for use in these tests.

The ELISA reaction is lost soon after cure, and this loss is followed by the loss of IFAT and CFT positivity.

Cell mediated immune responses develop late in the disease and the Montenegro test is usually negative. This delayed dermal hypersensitivity reaction does not generally become positive until some months after cure. In contrast to the humoral immune correlates, delayed hypersensitivity remains for many years; this feature can be used epidemiologically for skin testing as evidence of previous exposure.

Diagnosis

That the signs and symptoms alone are far from pathognomonic for visceral leishmaniasis is indicated by the diversity of disorders which have been suspected and treated in patients returning to non-endemic areas where the correct diagnosis was not initially suspected.

Clinical indications include a chronic low-grade recurrent fever, with lymphatic involvement, splenomegaly and cachexia, combined with a history of residence in an endemic area. Diseases with which visceral leishmaniasis has been confused include malaria, brucellosis, toxoplasmosis and leukaemia.

In epidemics it is common practice to treat as visceral leishmaniasis those cases of chronic fever which do not respond to antimalarial therapy. Simple non-specific serological tests, particularly the formol-gel test, may be performed, but with improved access to medical services early cases are commonly seen, in which this test is negative, and treatment is given despite the negative test. This and other non-specific serological tests depend on the greatly increased serum protein levels. Of the more specific tests, IFAT is generally thought to be the most useful, but cannot be carried out at village clinics. Clearly, a sensitive specific serological test for visceral leishmaniasis which could be carried out at village clinics would contribute greatly both to the accurate diagnosis and treatment of patients as well as to our understanding of epidemics.

While indirect diagnosis may be sufficient to indicate treatment in areas of high incidence, reliance on indirect methods can lead to grave errors. Epidemics of malaria and visceral leishmaniasis may run concurrently, and it is important to carry out parasitological tests repeatedly. In areas of low incidence, differential diagnosis becomes much more difficult, and parasitological diagnosis is essential.

It was said in the Indian epidemics that parasites could be found in blood films of most patients. Films were specially prepared with a square tail in which the leucocytes, and therefore parasites, were concentrated. The detection of parasites required lengthy observation by a skilled microscopist. Circulating parasites have rarely been demonstrated in infantile visceral leishmaniasis, or in Kenya or Sudan.

Parasites may be demonstrated in cultures or smears taken from bone marrow, spleen or, less certainly, liver. Bone-marrow puncture combines safety with reliability and is the method of choice in most countries. For parasitological confirmation of numerous cases spleen puncture is practised in Kenya, and has been used elsewhere, and is said to be safe and reliable in expert hands. This procedure is far less painful and unpleasant than bone-marrow biopsy. Lymph-node biopsy is sometimes succesful in demonstrating parasites where other methods fail. This is especially true in Africa and the Mediterranean region.

Treatment

General debilitation may be so marked that good nursing and non-specific treatment with a high-protein, vitamin-rich diet and antibiotics may have dramatic, if temporary, effects and are vital factors in recovery. This is also true of canine visceral leishmaniasis, the symptoms of which can be obscured by good diet. Splenectomy is practised in China and India and is thought by some to speed recovery of old chronic cases in which the spleen reaches an enormous size (figure 88, p. 217). Following splenectomy the blood picture returns rapidly to normal.

Specific chemotherapy is, however, generally a prerequisite to recovery. Pentavalent antimony compounds were developed in India in the 1920s and have not yet been superseded. Pentostam or urea stibamine are universally used, though the response is very variable. Antimony-resistant cases are not infrequently reported from India, and doses required in Sudan are very much higher than those in India. The aromatic diamidines such as pentamidine are used in resistant cases if they remain positive following two or three courses of antimony. PKDL is notoriously difficult to clear completely, but usually responds dramatically, if temporarily, to antimony or the diamidines. Metronidazole (Flagyl), which is very effective in other protozoan infections (e.g., *Entamoeba* and *Trichomonas*), has been tried in visceral leishmaniasis with inconsistent results.

Cure is only confirmed when the bone marrow becomes negative, and PKDL is not seen for two years at least. If PKDL has not appeared in two years it is unlikely that it will.

Great promise is shown by the incorporation of drugs into microscopic lipid structures, liposomes, which are phagocytosed and carried to the lymphoid tissues where most of the parasites are. The drugs are thus concentrated at the site of infection and possibly in the very infected cells. Preliminary results indicate enormously enhanced activity in canine and laboratory infections. Human infections have yet to be treated with liposome entrapped drugs, but by this method the total dose of drug can be greatly reduced and this might prevent severe side effects.

ECOLOGY AND EPIDEMIOLOGY

Although the parasites causing visceral leishmaniasis show great uniformity over their wide geographical range, there is considerable variation in their ecology and epidemiology from area to area. In the southern part of its range in China, in India and probably in Kenya, the disease is thought to be maintained by inter-human transmission with no animal reservoir. In the rest of its range, except Sudan, it is zoonotic, with dogs as the main reservoir, though foxes have been found infected in France, Italy and Brazil, jackals in the USSR and rats in Yugoslavia and Italy. A third epidemiological pattern is found in Sudan, where the parasite does not occur in dogs, but has been found in rodents, mainly *Arvicanthis niloticus*, and in serval cats and genets which are carnivores. The infection rate in *Arvicanthis* is sufficient to indicate that this is probably a primary zoonotic system. Infection rates in dogs in the Mediterranean basin can be sufficiently high to account for the maintenance of the parasite in synanthropic surroundings, but it is clear that this is not a primary zoonosis. The following examples illustrate the complexity of the epidemiology of visceral leishmaniasis.

Sudanese visceral leishmaniasis

Certain patches of land, particularly the woodland with yellow 'azaza' soil have the reputation for harbouring visceral leishmaniasis. Later studies associated the infection with woodlands composed of *Acacia* and *Balanites* trees; these woodlands were slightly raised and less liable to flooding in the rains and were thus especially suitable for burrowing rodents. The US naval (NAMRU) teams found some one per cent of *Arvicanthis niloticus* in one of these woodland patches infected with parasites, which were identified as *L. donovani*. In addition, small numbers of other rodents and carnivores were infected, including a *Rattus rattus* in the town of Malakal, where transmission to man is not known. Isolation of the parasites was very difficult and the US workers think it likely that many infections were missed. There was thus convincing evidence of a primary zoonotic focus with definable landscape characteristics. The only problem is that parasites isolated subsequently from viscera of *Arvicanthis* and other rodents in Ethiopia, Kenya and Senegal turned out to be not *L. donovani* but *L. major* and an undescribed *Leishmania* species. It has therefore become necessary to reconfirm the identity of the Sudanese parasites.

The *Acacia–Balanites* woodlands supported large numbers of *Phlebotomus orientalis* which was shown to be an efficient vector: in certain areas almost four per cent of flies were found naturally infected with promastigotes. It was not posssible to demonstrate that *Arvicanthis* was a major blood-meal source for the sandflies nor, despite heroic efforts, to find the breeding places. Another tantalizing question was raised by the finding of infected carnivores. Are these in any way reservoir hosts? It seems unlikely that carnivores, with their low population density, could maintain the parasite, unless a sandfly population were maintained in the carnivore den. More probably, perhaps, as occurs with trypanosomes, the carnivores are infected by contamination when they eat infected rodents.

Human infections are clearly associated with certain areas, and occur in outbreaks, sometimes associated with famine or epidemics, and usually associated with population movements. There are great variations in the incidence, amounting to epidemic waves, but these have not been thoroughly documented. Unfortunately there is also no clear documentation of the cyclic fluctuations which doubtless occur in *Arvicanthis* populations and could be related to fluctuations in the human incidence. This is another question which was raised by the NAMRU team, but which could not be answered.

Around 1968, with the aid of the World Bank, an agricultural project was established on the Ethiopian side of the Ethiopia–Sudan border. Large numbers of peasants were attracted from the highlands, but there was wretched food and housing and almost non-existent health services. The main product, sesame seed, rapidly became an important export for Ethiopia, but the labourers suffered miserably from vitamin deficiency and malaria. Some of those with malaria were seen at Gondar, the nearest hospital, where many died despite treatment. Only after some time was it realized that those dying of 'malaria despite treatment' were in fact dying of visceral leishmaniasis.† Although the landscape in the area is similar to that in neighbouring Sudan, it has not been possible to confirm many of the Sudanese findings regarding reservoir hosts and vectors. The picture in that part of Africa is clearly complex.

† This experience may have been instrumental in causing the World Bank to insist on adequate provision of heath facilities on the projects supported by them.

Kenyan visceral leishmaniasis

Further south in Sudan, and in southern Ethiopia, northern Kenya and Somalia, visceral leishmaniasis occurs sporadically in the largely nomadic tribes. Health services in this area are minimal, and there are other causes of hepatosplenomegaly and fever, so accurate incidence figures are not available. Skin test surveys, if they are to be believed, indicate a great reservoir of cryptic human infection. An IFAT survey gives similar indications, but there is no parasitological confirmation in either case.

The epidemics which occurred in the 1950s and 1960s farther south, in central Kenya, are thought to have been introduced by soldiers returning from border actions in the north. The putative vector in the Kitui and Machacos areas is *Phlebotomus martini*, but only very few flies have been found infected, so the evidence is largely circumstantial. Despite considerable effort, vertebrate reservoir hosts have not been discovered. A small number of infected dogs were reported; not sufficient to constitute a reservoir. The epidemics themselves and simultaneous population movements radically altered the population of a wide area; it remains to be seen whether the parasite can become established in the long term, or whether it is incapable of maintaining itself indefinitely. With increasing movement of people in that part of Africa it is likely that the parasite will be repeatedly reintroduced, however, and further epidemics are likely if it does not become endemic. The most notable landscape feature associated with epidemic visceral leishmaniasis in Kenya is the presence of eroded termite hills produced by *Macrotermes bellicosus*. These are thought to provide a breeding site for *P. martini*, as well as shelter and a home for alternative blood sources.

Mediterranean infantile visceral leishmaniasis

In contrast to Africa, where the sandfly vectors are thought to breed in rodent burrows and termite hills, and the disease is associated with flat, moderately well watered country with fine-grained alluvial silt, or clay or laterite soil, in the Mediterranean basin the disease occurs in areas of fragmented limestone with high relief and little soil. These areas are quite unsuitable for burrowing rodents, which do not generally form colonies. The breeding places of the sandfly vectors, *P. major* in the east, *P. perniciosus* in most of the region, and *P. ariasi* in the Cévennes of southern France, must determine the distribution of the infection, as rodents are probably only involved incidentally, and dogs are distributed wherever there are people. The role of foxes in maintaining the parasite is not proven, but it is unlikely that foxes occur in sufficient numbers in most of the range of the infection to help significantly in the maintenance of the parasite. The role of man in maintaining the infection had been thought to be negligible, but recent immunoepidemiological evidence from the Italian mainland and Sicily suggests that cryptic infection in man may be of considerable significance. Once again we find immunoepidemiological evidence contrasting with parasitological information; the reconciliation of these discrepancies is vital to our understanding of the epidemiology of Mediterranean visceral leishmaniasis.

In both man and dogs the infection mostly occurs in the suburbs of towns and periurban areas, where gardens, walls and derelict buildings are thought to provide breeding sites for *P. perniciosus* and *P. major* and where there are relatively high concentrations of dogs. The more rural situations in the Cevennes and in Tuscany are different in that the infection is concentrated in foothill country with mixed woodland and widely dispersed people and dogs. While in the more typical areas the prevalence of infection in dogs may exceed ten per cent and human infection may be frequent, in the Cevennes and Tuscany no more than two per cent of dogs are infected and human infection is exceedingly rare.

The most conspicuous feature of human infection with Mediterranean visceral leishmaniasis is the restriction of the disease to infants. In most published accounts more than 90 per cent of cases occur in children aged between one and five years. This has never been fully explained; it is unlikely that only children are exposed to infection, indeed one would expect adults to be exposed to greater numbers of sandfly bites. The alternative suggestions are on the one hand that most adults are naturally refractive to infection, or alternatively that a large proportion of adults acquire immunity as a consequence of infection without disease. The immunoepidemiological evidence referred to above supports the second explanation, as would the apparent change in the age distribution of the disease in recent years. On the other hand, the age distribution of infection in visiting tourists is also biased toward infants; this and the rarity of transfusion visceral leishmaniasis in the endemic area argue in favour of natural refractiveness of adults. A fourth possible explanation is that people acquire resistance to infection by repeated exposure to sandfly bites. There is no direct evidence for this, but it would explain the apparent raised incidence in tourists and other short-term visitors.

The USSR and China

To the east of the Mediterranean, through Soviet Turkmenistan and Kazakhstan to Xinjiang (Sinkiang) in western China, and thence to the north-east of China, the pattern is, as far as is known, much the same. In many areas the territory affected is much more arid than in the Mediterranean foci. This is particularly true of the residual Kzyl Orda focus in Kazakhstan, which is thought to be one of the last remaining foci in the USSR, and where the infection is thought to be a sylvatic zoonosis. In the Soviet area of distribution information on the vector is largely circumstantial; a variety of apparently suitable sandflies occur, but none has been formally incriminated. In China, from around Beijing (Peking) northwards, the infection was largely infantile, though this was not as marked further west, and sometimes as many as 20 per cent of dogs were infected. Further south, few dogs were infected and the age distribution was less marked. *P. chinensis* was incriminated as the vector, and is the only likely vector in most of China. Following the mass destruction of dogs in the 1950s the disease almost disappeared. Recent reports suggest that the disease has not disappeared and that the racoon dog *Nyctereutes procyonoides* may be a reservoir host, as three infected individuals were found near Beijing.

The habitat range in China is much wider than in any other area, including the alluvial plain north of the Chang Jiang (Yangtse River), the enormous loess plateau of central northern China and the mountains to the west, to an altitude of more than 2000 m in Gansu Province. This is consistent with *P. chinensis* being the vector; this species or species complex has one of the widest geographical ranges of any sandfly (from eastern China to Ethiopia) and occupies a wide range of habitats.

India and epidemic kala-azar

The first epidemics of visceral leishmaniasis in India were confused with those of malaria, and their origin is therefore obscure. The disease has been concentrated in the alluvial plain of the Ganges and Brahmaputra rivers, particularly in lower Bengal. It has spread in epidemic waves up the Ganges as far as Uttar Pradesh and up the Brahmaputra almost to the limits of Assam. The spread of the infection to Assam coincided with the opening of the region to access from outside by the British. Thus the disease was dubbed 'Sarkari Bemari', British Government Disease! The interpretation of the epidemiological records is difficult. It has been said that there were waves lasting about five years and separated by ten years, but that the case numbers fell in the interepidemic period to about a quarter of the maximum. In the records from one of the Assam areas peaks can indeed be detected in 1885, 1897, 1913, 1925 and 1944, with a mean separation of almost exactly 15 years. At the same time, the epidemic waves were said to spread along lines of communication and infection was said to become focused on individual houses or villages, in which repeated infections occurred over a period of years. While the 15-year cycles were well marked in Assam, they were much less clear in Bengal and absent in Bihar and Madras. Predisposing factors such as floods, famine, and malaria epidemics have been blamed for the precipitation of epidemics. It is difficult to reconcile these views. For example, a wave is unlikely to move directionally if the infection is already present in the area. In the final analysis we know very little of the causes of the epidemics in India, though this has been a fertile field for speculation.

Throughout the range of Indian kala-azar, *Phlebotomus argentipes* is thought to be the vector. This is one of the very few sandflies whose breeding sites are reasonably well known. It is essentially a peridomestic synanthropic species in the affected areas, breeding in moist soil with high organic content in and close to houses. A particularly favoured site is in the shelter of the clay troughs which contain water and chopped vegetation for cattle feed. *P. argentipes* is largely restricted to alluvial soils with annual rainfall above 1000 mm and a minimum summer teperature of 27 °C. However, the sandfly has a much wider range than the parasite, occurring elsewhere in India and in South-east Asia. Whilst it is not generally thought to be a complex of species, its man-biting habits certainly vary from place to place.

Large numbers of dogs were examined parasitologically, mainly in Madras, with negative results. In the area affected by the recent outbreak in Bihar, some 20 per cent of dogs gave a positive ELISA reaction. From one of these promastigote parasites were cultured by workers at the kala-azar research unit at Patna, but they are not *L. donovani* and there remains no evidence that dogs play a role in the epidemiology of Indian visceral leishmaniasis.

The current outbreak in northern Bihar began in about 1970, following about 20 years in which the disease had become almost forgotten. Retrospective studies were attempted, but it was not found possible to determine a predisposing cause for the outbreak, to determine lines of communication along which it moved, to identify focal dwellings, or to identify the original source.

South American visceral leishmaniasis

The age of incidence of South American visceral leishmaniasis resembles that in the Mediterranean. Similarly, dogs have been found infected and the disease occurs mainly in small towns. The vector is the peridomestic sandfly *Lutzomyia longipalpis*. Many people consider that visceral leishmaniasis was introduced to South America by dogs imported from Europe with the Spanish and Portuguese settlers. Others have suggested that the infection is indigenous. This view is supported by the finding of four infected foxes *Dusicyon vetulus* in the main area of distribution in Ceara Province in Brazil and one *Dusicyon thous* in Para State. However, *L. donovani* strains from dogs infected in France will infect *Lu. longipalpis* of South American origin. This remains, therefore, an open question. Throughout the range in South America the infection is very sporadic in man. It is probably dependent on dogs for its maintenance, but it is also apparently dependent on *Lu. longipalpis*. This sandfly was apparently originally cavernicolous but has become adapted to living peridomestically. It sometimes occurs in enormous numbers with man-biting rates in excess of 100 per hour. It is astonishing that despite the abundance of the adults and intensive efforts, very few larvae have been discovered. There are indications that the infection is expanding into previously unaffected areas, notably in Colombia.

CONTROL

When kala-azar swept like a plague through Bengal and Assam, little could be done to control the spread and protect the people. The disease was known to be infectious and to spread along lines of communication. When infection appeared to concentrate in certain houses, these were burned, but without effect. In the Assam tea plantations some protection was gained by evacuating people and moving their residences as little as 200 m. But the first control method which proved to be effective in stemming epidemics was compulsory treatment of all cases. The same was done in the Bengal and Bihar epidemics, and this is thought to have controlled the disease prior to the introduction of malaria eradication, which almost eliminated visceral leishmaniasis from around 1950, until the recent Bihar epidemic started around 1970. Mass case detection and treatment was also effective in Kenya, but population movements were perhaps more important in stemming the epidemic.

So, although there were clear indications that *P. argentipes* was the vector in India, specific measures against this insect were not applied until the 1970s when the affected towns and villages in Bihar were sprayed twice annually with DDT.

Visceral leishmaniasis was largely eliminated from China following the revolution, by the elimination of dogs and the treatment of patients. Anti-rabies campaigns as well as malaria eradication and, occasionally, specific measures against sandflies have greatly reduced the incidence of visceral leishmaniasis, and eradicated it from many areas in the Mediterranean and Central Asia. However, *P. major* and *P. perniciosus* are less endophilic than *P. sergenti* or *P. papatasi*, so visceral leishmaniasis has not been as completely eliminated as urban cutaneous leishmaniasis.

Chapter 10. Old World Cutaneous Leishmaniasis

INTRODUCTION

Oriental sore was a well recognized disease long before anything was known of its cause.

Cutaneous leishmaniasis was once thought to have originated in Central Asia in zoonotic reservoirs, from which it emerged around the 14th century AD to spread south-east into north-west India, and south-west through Iran to western Asia and the Mediterranean basin, eventually reaching West Africa. The evidence for this story is based on the fact that cutaneous leishmaniasis was not mentioned in early texts from western Asia. The theory of spread assumes that the parasite causing leishmaniasis in man was recently derived from gerbils in Central Asia. The finding of sylvatic zoonotic reservoirs of cutaneous leishmaniasis in India, Israel, Libya and Senegal, quite apart from the biochemical taxonomic evidence, does not confirm this theory, which may have been counterproductive in reinforcing ideas about the transatlantic passage of cutaneous leishmaniasis to the New World. Nevertheless, there are anomalies in the distribution of cutaneous leishmaniasis. Its epidemic appearances and sudden disappearances often remain unexplained.

Aurangzeb, the Mogul emperor (1618–1707) apparently suffered from Delhi boil, which was known in Delhi as 'aurangzebi phora'. In the West it was known to 18th century travellers in western Asia (e.g., in Aleppo and Baghdad), but mainly came to attention in connection with military activities in outposts of empire such as Tashkent and Pendeh in Central Asia and Biskra and Gafsa in North Africa.

Among traditional interpretations of the disease, Ethiopians associate the infection with bats' urine — an interesting idea because we now know the reservoir in Ethiopia is the rock hyrax, which shares its habitat with bats. Moth scales, bad water and mosquito bites are alternative explanations in various countries. The infectious nature of the disease has been recognized for centuries in

Baghdad, where children were deliberately inoculated on the arm or buttock to protect them from facial lesions.

In the discovery of the parasite causing oriental sore and the elucidation of its life cycle there was a flood of new information around the turn of the century, followed by painfully slow piecemeal advance. The earliest descriptions of the pathology of Pendeh sore, 'bouton de Biskra' and Aleppo boil were confused by the numerous bacteria isolated from the sores. As early as 1885, the parasites causing Delhi boil were seen by Cunningham in a specimen preserved in absolute alcohol, transported to Calcutta and stained with picrocarmine, logwood, gentian violet, Spiller's purple, methyl blue, Bismark brown, fuschin, eosin and Gibbo's double staining fluid. Not surprisingly Cunningham misinterpreted the sections, thinking that the parasites were spores, and the infected macrophages the plasmodia of monadine Myxomycetes such as *Plasmodiophora*.

Coincidentally, *Plasmodiophora* has a motile myxoflagellate stage, generally resembling the flagellate stages of *Leishmania*!

In 1898 a Russian military surgeon, P. F. Borovsky, described in detail the clinical course of oriental sore, which he called Sart sore, and recognized the causative organism as a protozoan. (The Sarts live in the region of Fergana, in the Far west of Uzbekistan, at the head of the Syr Dar'ya river.) Borovsky's main success was that he looked at material from young sores in hanging drop and smear preparations as well as in tissue sections. Borovsky was of the opinion that the infection was spread through the respiratory tract like malaria (as was then still a widely held opinion). Only four years later, in 1902, the Russian physician Shulgin suggested that the infection was mosquito-borne, and quoted the seasonal incidence and protective effects of mosquito nets in support of this. According to Hoare, this was the first time that an insect vector had been postulated for oriental sore.

However, both these Russian studies, carried out in connection with military activities in Central Asia, were published so obscurely that they were largely ignored outside the USSR until they were brought to the notice of English-speaking people by Hoare in 1938.

In 1903 the American pathologist Wright, who gave his name to the stain, independently described the ulcer and parasites from a young girl who had developed skin lesions before emigrating from Armenia three months previously. The parasites were well illustrated and their protozoan affinities were recognized.

It was not until five years later that Nicolle cultured the parasites, thereby confirming their similarity to *Leishmania donovani*, cultures of which had previously been described by Rogers in 1904.

As for the insect vector, it was not until 1941 that this was conclusively demonstrated. The problem was similar to that described for visceral leishmaniasis. There were innumerable attempts to incriminate both *Phlebotomus* species and a wide variety of other arthropods. The problem centred mainly round the difficulty of persuading sandflies to feed, survive oviposition, and refeed in captivity, and this remains one of the most intransigent problems in laboratory studies on leishmaniasis.

The zoonotic origin of oriental sore in Baghdad and Aleppo was suggested by workers who found infected dogs and cats, but it was generally concluded that these were incidental hosts in these areas, and that man was the main host. Yakimov, however, demonstrated the zoonotic origin of oriental sore in Central Asia by finding infected gerbils and showing that outbreaks of human infection were the result of intrusion into the territory of the gerbils. It was possible to distinguish two quite different patterns of transmission in urban and rural foci in Central Asia and Transcaucasia. In urban foci the disease was transmitted from man to man with occasional infections in other animals. In rural areas the parasite 'belonged' in desert rodents, human infection being irrelevant to its long-term survival. It was even possible to distinguish the parasites morphologically, and they were named as subspecies of *Leishmania tropica, L. t. major* and *L. t. minor*. Extension of this pioneer work in the USSR to other parts of the Old World has demonstrated a variety of zoonotic patterns associated with sandflies of different groups, and parasites which can now be distinguished by objective biochemical studies. Ironically, some of the most recent work in the USSR calls into question some early assumptions, as many of the *Leishmania* strains isolated from desert gerbils are not infective to man.

Other very recent advances include the repeated discovery of the disease in Namibia, indicating that the sporadic reports from elsewhere in Africa may be the tip of an iceberg, and cutaneous leishmaniasis may be much more widespread in Africa than has been recognized so far. One of the problems, particularly in Sudan and West Africa, is the distinction between cutaneous leishmaniasis proper and the cutaneous manifestation of normally visceralizing parasites. Important outbreaks of cutaneous leishmaniasis in north-west India, Saudi Arabia and North Africa have allowed knowledge gained in the USSR and Iran to be applied over a very wide area, and in each case vectors and reservoir hosts have been tentatively identified.

In Ethiopia, as in Venezuela, diffuse cutaneous leishmaniasis was confused for many years with lepromatous leprosy (with which it sometimes occurs simultaneously). It was only in 1961 that patients in a leprosarium in Ethiopia were recognized as suffering from leishmaniasis, not leprosy. This led to an expansion of study in Africa and to the discovery of a hitherto unsuspected reservoir in the hyrax and the description of a new species, *L. aethiopica*.

Cutaneous leishmaniasis, like visceral leishmaniasis, was largely eradicated, partly as a spin-off from malaria control, following the widespread use of household insecticides. The disease remains rare in most of its urban foci, though there have been outbreaks as in the city of Bikaner in north-west India. However, with the increasing exploitation of semi-arid lands in North Africa and western Asia new rural foci have come to light, and there have been outbreaks of some importance.

GEOGRAPHICAL DISTRIBUTION

Cutaneous leishmaniasis is distributed in the Old World from Senegal to India and Mongolia, and from southern France to Namibia (figure 83, p. 200 and figure 84, p. 202). The traditional centres of distribution from which originated the vernacular names oriental sore, Delhi boil, Baghdad boil, Aleppo boil, 'clou de Gafsa', 'clou de Biskra,' Sart sore, Pendeh boil, have greatly reduced incidences today or are largely free from infection.

In most of these localities the disease was probably largely anthroponotic, caused by *L. tropica*, and has been reduced by insecticides. It has notably been largely eliminated from cities and towns in Georgia, Azerbaydzhan and Armenia in the southern USSR, but still occurs sporadically and sometimes in epidemics in north-west India (Bikaner), Pakistan, much of Afghanistan, Iran, Iraq, Israel (Jericho) and the Mediterranean countries of Europe, including France (rare), Greece, Italy (largely eliminated from the Abruzzo Region), Spain, Turkey and Yugoslavia.

Zoonotic cutaneous leishmaniasis caused by *L. major* still occurs in the semi-deserts of Turkmenistan and Uzbekistan, extending into northern Afghanistan, north-west India (Rajasthan) and much of Iran; it has recently been distinguished in Iraq, and extends to Israel. There is a discontinuity in Egypt and eastern Libya but important outbreaks occurred recently in western Libya. Cutaneous leishmaniasis elsewhere in North Africa has not been shown to be zoonotic; it occurs in Algeria, Morocco† and Tunisia, reappearing in West Africa in Senegal, where it is again clearly zoonotic. Sporadic cases occur in the Sahelian belt or Sudan savannah of West Africa, through Mali, Upper Volta, Niger, Nigeria, Cameroon and Chad to Sudan, where the distinction between cutaneous leishmaniasis and cutaneous manifestations of visceral leishmaniasis becomes very difficult. In the highlands of Ethiopia cutaneous leishmaniasis caused by *L. aethiopica* is found between 1500 m and 2500 m above sea level and is restricted to the wetter parts, with annual rainfall above 800 mm. This anomalous pattern is repeated in the geographically discontinuous distribution on the slopes of Mount Elgon in Kenya. Other cases of DCL have been seen in Tanzania, but attempts to identify transmission sites have been unsuccessful. Apart from Tanzania there is an enormous discontinuity between Kenya and Namibia, where cutaneous leishmaniasis has recently been discovered as a sporadic infection.

The Namibian parasites have yet to be fully described and identified. Whether or not these geographical discontinuities are more apparent than real remains to be seen, but the disease is unlikely to be common in the intervening areas.

---

†An outbreak occurred at Tata in S. Morocco in 1981, in old villages not associated with development or population movement, in stony hilly country, quite unlike other *L. major* habitats. *Meriones shawi*, in that area a peridomestic species, was found infected. This picture breaks all the 'rules', emphasizing the versatility and lability of *L. major*.

PARASITES

Leishmania tropica

It is assumed that the parasite originally named by Wright from an oriental sore, coming as it did from an Armenian immigrant in the USA, was of the urban endemic type found until recently in Armenia rather than the rural zoonotic type which was never found in Armenia. Thus the name *L. tropica* is correctly applied to this form. Some authors prefer to treat the different cutaneous parasites as subspecies, and call the urban endemic type *L. t. tropica* (of which *L. t. minor* is a synonym) while the zoonotic form is called *L. t. major*. We prefer to treat the different forms as full species. Parasites isolated from similar Middle-eastern localities have been shown to have similar morphological and biochemical features.

In humans, *L. tropica* (*s. str.*) normally produces a chronic lesion which ulcerates late, but which occasionally never completely heals, giving rise to the disease known as leishmaniasis recidivans. After healing, immunity to *L. tropica* is normally acquired. Man is the only known maintenance host for *L. tropica*.

Leishmania major

The name *L. tropica major* was given to the large parasites found in lesions in the ears of rodents and in the skin of settlers in the semi-desert steppes of south Central Asian USSR. Similar parasites have been isolated from Rajasthan in northwest India and from human and rodent lesions in Afghanistan, Iran and much of the Middle East and Libya and from viscera of rodents in Senegal. The visceral parasites isolated from rodents in southern Ethiopia and northern Kenya are biochemically similar, though they may not be associated with human disease in East Africa. This group of parasites is biochemically relatively uniform; the normal clinical picture is an acute, rapidly ulcerating lesion, commonly multiple, and giving rise to strong immunity against both *L. major* and *L. tropica*.

L. major is usually maintained by diurnal, colonial, herbivorous rodents: *Rhombomys opimus* in Afghanistan, Iran and the USSR; *Psammomys obesus* in Israel and probably Libya; and *Arvicanthis niloticus* in West Africa. In northwest India and parts of the southern USSR the maintenance hosts are the less colonial, more nocturnal, more granivorous *Meriones* species. At Hofuf in Saudi Arabia, *Meriones crassus*, a species highly adapted for desert life, is thought to be the reservoir host.

Leishmania aethiopica

Human infections in highland Ethiopia and Mount Elgon in Kenya somewhat resemble those caused by *L. tropica*, but are even longer lasting and more reluctant to ulcerate. *L. aethiopica* resembles *L. mexicana* in sometimes giving rise to diffuse cutaneous leishmaniasis. This, combined with the findings that the infection is zoonotic and that the vectors belong to the subgenus *Larroussius* normally associated with transmission of *L. donovani*, indicated that the parasite was very likely to be different from *L. tropica* or *L. major*. The original description was based on minor characters such as the infectivity in experimental animals, and a not very reliable cross-absorbed haemagglutination test. However, the naming of this species has been fully justified by subsequent biochemical results.

Maintenance hosts are the rock hyraxes *Procavia capensis* (*sensu* Corbet 1979) and *Heterohyrax brucei*.

Leishmania species

Cutaneous *Leishmania* parasites have been described from numerous anomalous situations, particularly in Africa. Diffuse cutaneous leishmaniasis has been described in Tanzania and a patient from Zambia had a combination of visceral and diffuse cutaneous leishmaniasis. The source of these infections must be wild animals, but details are unknown. In Namibia, where occasional human infections occur, a fascinating picture is emerging: parasites have been isolated from the rock hyrax *Procavia capensis* and from *Phlebotomus rossi*. The parasites are not, however, all the same and differ from those in Ethiopia.

DISEASES

The basic disease of cutaneous leishmaniasis begins as a papule which develops at the site of a sandfly bite. The papule enlarges slowly, then begins to necrotize centrally. The necrosis may either be acute, giving rise to the 'moist' ulcer characteristic of *L. major* infection, or slow in the case of the 'dry' lesion typical of *L. tropica* infection. Eventually the granulomatous swelling subsides, the ulceration heals and the patient is left with a permanent scar, which can be regarded as characteristic in highly endemic areas. Typically the lesion is painless and secondary infection is restricted to the dead tissue.

Variations from the above picture are frequent, and depend on the strain of parasite as well as, presumably, on the state of the patient. Each parasite species may produce a spectrum of disease, and these may overlap considerably.

The greatest uniformity is shown by *L. major* infection (figure 89). Here the main variation is in the size and number of lesions. It is not uncommon for more than 50 lesions to develop, each presumably at the site of a sandfly bite or probe (by analogy with *Trypanosoma* in tsetse flies, it may be that an infected sandfly tends to probe more frequently before feeding).

The time between infection and first appearance of the papule is usually a few weeks, and the ulcers usually appear 2–3 months after the sandfly biting season.

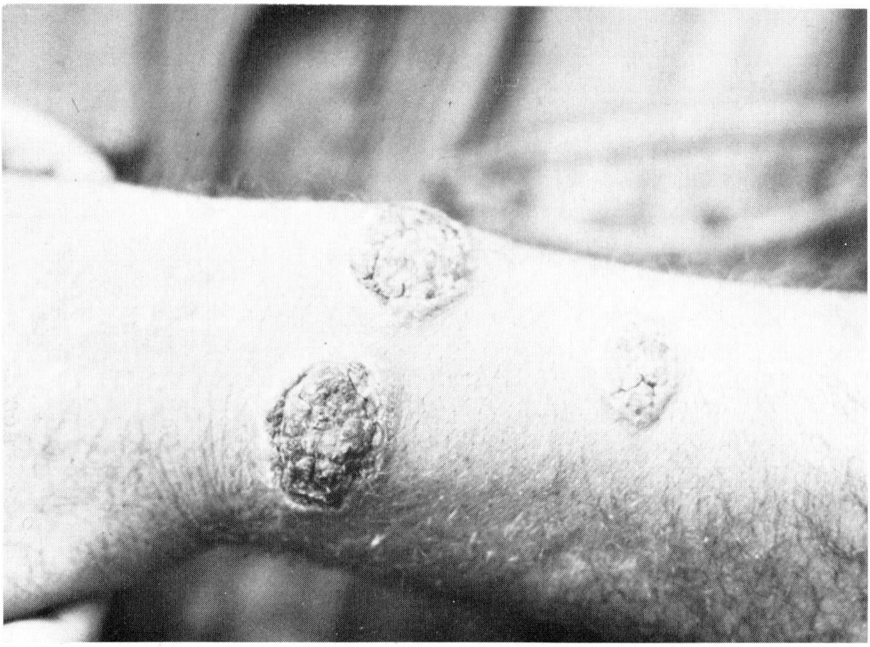

Figure 89. Healing ulcers of *L. major* on a forestry plantation labourer in Libya.

The majority of untreated ulcers have cured completely within nine months, and few survive more than one year.

Soviet workers have shown a great range of virulence of *L. major*. Many strains, especially from uninhabited deserts, either fail to infect man or produce a chronic lesion which ulcerates slowly, if at all, somewhat resembling that caused by *L. tropica*. Strains from areas where the parasite is transmitted among its rodent hosts and to man by *P. papatasi* cause the typical 'rural-type' oriental sore. Most further variation is probably associated with treatment, or with concomitant infection.

Urban cutaneous leishmaniasis is said by some to be clinically distinguishable from the rural zoonotic disease. Others have been unable to substantiate the differences between the 'acute wet' and 'chronic dry' forms. Clearly there is considerable overlap in the clinical disease, but there are also good differences. The incubation period in urban cutaneous leishmaniasis tends to be longer, the lesion takes longer to ulcerate, and often never fully ulcerates; likewise, self-cure is long delayed and while most cases resolve within a year, some last a lot longer.

In a small proportion of cases permanent cure is not achieved, and small lesions develop on or near the margin of the scar, extending the lesion insidiously over a wide area of skin rather like a fungal 'fairy ring'. These *recidivans* lesions are mainly on the face and can be grossly disfiguring.

Cutaneous leishmaniasis in Africa

Most of the cases of cutaneous leishmaniasis in Africa were until recently thought to be caused by parasites which usually visceralize. It was only after diffuse cutaneous leishmaniasis had been described that 'normal' cutaneous leishmaniasis was found to be common in Ethiopia; the disease normally resembling the 'dry' form characteristic of urban cutaneous leishmaniasis. There is considerable swelling of the affected area, followed by gradual necrosis associated with flaking of dry tissue and encrusted serous exudate (figure 90). Only rarely is there frank ulceration, which is one of the reasons why the disease was unrecognized in a country with poor rural medical services. The lesion is chronic, commonly lasting three years, but eventually resolves leaving an indistinct scar.

It is not possible to assess with any accuracy the proportion of patients who develop DCL, but it is small. DCL is characterized by a specific immunological inability to prevent the spread of the infection through the skin of the cooler parts of the body. Most of the lesions are raised papules covered with thin delicate skin which readily breaks with trauma, and the lesions as well as much of the surrounding apparently normal skin contain innumerable parasites. Apart from the gross disfigurement caused by the lesions and the susceptibility of the victim to superficial trauma, there are no signs or symptoms associated with this disease.

DCL is commonly associated with the other chronic scourges of the Ethiopian highlands, tuberculosis, leprosy and non-filarial elephantiasis.

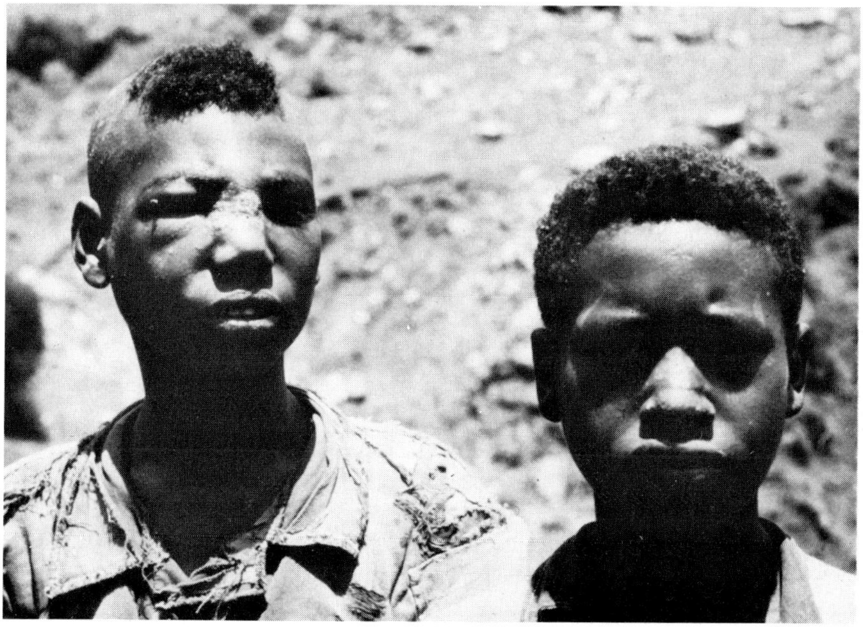

Figure 90. Typical chronic blind or encrusted lesions of *L. aethiopica*.

Treatment

Traditional treatments include mainly corrosive poultices prepared from plant juices (*Euphorbia* or *Ficus* species) or blister beetles (Meloidae). Later developments included a paste of sulphuric acid in charcoal and infra-red radiation with hot compresses. In Ethiopia, DCL was seen to regress during a superinfection of measles, and this was the rationale for an unsuccessful attempt to use malaria therapy. In Brazil the same condition is quite effectively controlled, though not cured, by repeated hot baths or sauna baths.

These treatments clearly indicate the unsatisfactory state of chemotherapy. As for VL, the drugs of choice are pentavalent antimonials, such as Pentostam, and aromatic diamidines, such as pentamidine. Both have serious toxicity problems and excessive pentamidine therapy has led to intractable diabetes mellitus in DCL patients. Both groups of drugs are also expensive. Controlled experiments in treatment of simple oriental sore are rare; it is difficult to assess the effect of chemotherapy on a lesion of variable incubation period and variable duration. Further, chemotherapy may only be justified in excessively severe cases, as the acquisition of immunity may be impaired.

Recent developments include a cellulose bandage impregnated with the antibiotic monomycin, which is at an advanced experimental stage in the USSR. Perhaps the most promising advance is the incorporation of drugs in microscopic lipid structures, liposomes. Although theoretically this method should be particularly good for visceral leishmaniasis and has indeed produced remarkable experimental results, it also shows considerable promise in experimental cutaneous infections.

ECOLOGY AND EPIDEMIOLOGY

There are three quite distinct epidemiological patterns in Old World cutaneous leishmaniasis, each associated with a given species of parasite. Each pattern shows considerable variation, however, and there are many endemic areas where the true pattern of transmission has not been established. In general, a given *Leishmania* parasite depends for its long-term survival on one or a small number of mammalian host species in which it causes a relatively benign, chronic infection. In each case the mammalian hosts are colonial, sedentary, and live in burrows, caves or houses. The second requirement for Old World cutaneous leishmaniasis parasites is one or a small number of species of sandfly vectors in which the parasites are able to establish a permanent infection, reaching the anterior portion of the alimentary canal. In every case which has been effectively evaluated the main reservoir host shares a microhabitat with the main vector, and foci of infection can be identified as places where the microhabitat of vector and host coincide, though each usually has a wider habitat range.

Zoonotic cutaneous leishmaniasis due to *Leishmania major* in the USSR

The most comprehensive studies on the epidemiology of any *Leishmania* are those carried out in Central Asia by Soviet workers. Many of these studies were carried out during summer scientific expeditions from Moscow institutions. More recently the independent institutes of the republics themselves have collaborated in the work and it has therefore been more comprehensive. These studies have accumulated an enormous amount of information, but what, a few years ago, looked like quite a simple situation has more recently been shown to be far more complex, and more needs to be learned.

The normal natural vertebrate host of *L. major* in Central Asia is the great gerbil *Rhombomys opimus*. This is a colonial rodent living in a wide variety of habitats in the arid and semi-arid steppes (figure 91). Only where the soil is too sandy to support its burrows or too rocky to be dug into, or on clay flood plains subject to complete inundation is *Rhombomys* absent. Its preferred habitat is in the semi-arid alluvial fans extending from the base of the mountains where the soil is composed of loess or silt, which is ideal for burrowing. The annual rainfall is generally below 25 cm, and the water table is usually between one and three metres deep.

The climate in these steppe regions is extreme. The limited precipitation is mainly in the winter, and may occur as snow. The winter temperatures are said to reach $-40\,^{\circ}C$ and the temperature during the hot dry summer months reaches $+45\,^{\circ}C$. For a few weeks in spring water is available and the temperature is

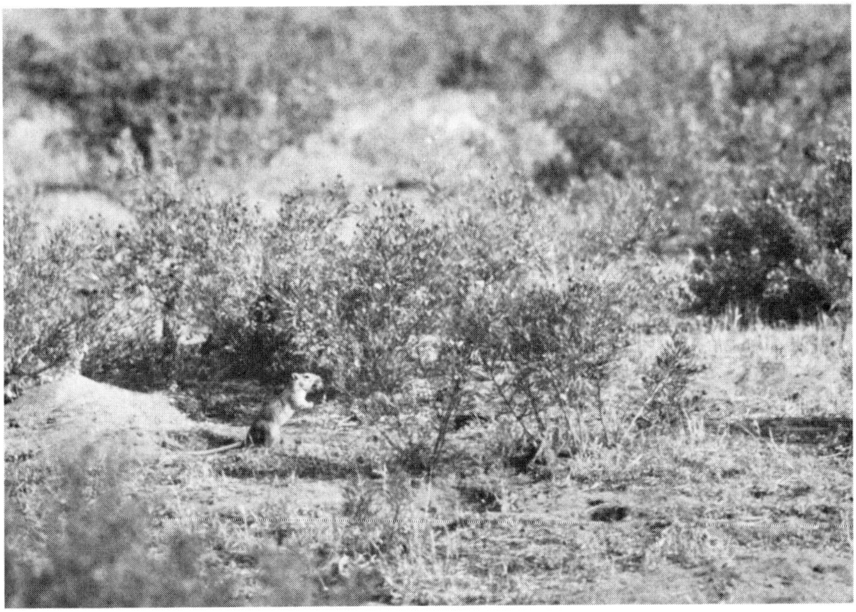

Figure 91. *Rhombomys opimus*, the main reservoir host of *L. major* in the USSR.

favourable for rapid plant growth.

A wide range of salinity is tolerated, in accordance with which available plant food materials vary. *Rhombomys* is unusual among rodents in being predominantly herbivorous as opposed to granivorous. While some 400 food plants have been recorded, it is probably dependent on certain grasses, for example, *Poa bulbosa*, and sedges, *Carex* species, which produce well developed rhizomes. These, with other foodstuffs, are gathered during the short spring growing season and are stored in underground chambers with a diameter of one metre.

A *Rhombomys* colony may measure 100 m in diameter and have several hundred burrow entrances. The extensive network of burrows and chambers may reach to three metres in depth. The same colony may be occupied for many generations, and gradually builds itself up into a mound above the surrounding landscape. The animals are sedentary, rarely moving outside the perimeter of the colony. The population of a given colony is usually reduced to one or two pairs in the winter, but may reach 20–25 animals at the peak, in late summer. Being relatively large rodents, *Rhombomys* are quite long-lived, and may reach an age of 18 months.

Being deep and permanent, with an accumulation of organic debris, *Rhombomys* colonies provide an ideal habitat for a wide variety of other vertebrates and invertebrates. While the evidence for sandflies breeding in gerbil burrows is largely indirect (emergence traps, etc.) it is well established that the adults, at least, make extensive use of the burrows, which provide an ideal microclimate for resting and breeding.

The sandfly species in a colony depend on the habitat, particularly on the nature of the soil and the depth of the water table. Of the three closely related *Phlebotomus* (*Paraphlebotomus*) species, *P. mongolensis* prefers the most arid zones and *P. caucasicus* and *P. andrejevi* require increasing humidity; *Phlebotomus (Phlebotomus) papatasi* is largely restricted to oases where water comes within a metre of the surface. This species has an unusual ability to exploit environmental change, and may occur in large numbers in recently constructed villages. Other sandflies in *Rhombomys* colonies are not thought to be involved in transmission either between rodents or to man.

The females of the *Paraphlebotomus* species are not readily separable, and much information on their comparative biology has to be based on their respective males. However, it is established that all three species feed preferentially on *Rhombomys*, and man is rarely bitten. Among all these sandflies, only *P. papatasi* feeds readily on man.

The sandfly season varies considerably in different parts of the range of *Rhombomys*. The northern limits, from the Aral Sea to Mongolia, are beyond the range of *P. papatasi*, and *P. mongolensis* maintains the parasite in gerbils. In the central parts of the range of *Rhombomys* the sandflies have a seasonal distribution, being commonest in midsummer. To the south the summer is too extreme and peaks occur in spring and autumn with very few sandflies in summer and none in winter. The variation in vector species has been used in the classification of zoonotic foci, from which the danger of human infection can be accurately predicted.

In *Rhombomys* the parasites are not acutely pathogenic. They concentrate in the margins of the ears which, as the animal is diurnal and less dependent on hearing, are relatively thick and fleshy. The infected margins do not ulcerate but become thicker and fleshier, and lose their hair covering (figure 92). Visceral infections have been found, but they have rarely been looked for and their significance is not clear, and the infection is not thought to reduce the life span of the rodents. The rodents remain infective for the duration of their life, and individuals infected in the autumn enable the parasites to survive until the following transmission season. All four species of sandfly mentioned are thought to be efficient vectors, though there is little experimental work to confirm this.

In nature the infection rate among gerbils is highest in the winter, when only adult animals are present, and lowest in the spring, when a large proportion of juveniles have not yet become infected. By late summer in many colonies the infection rate reaches 80 per cent or more. In any one area there is a variation in the infection rate among different colonies, those in the more rocky areas remaining relatively free. However, the parasite occurs almost throughout the range of the great gerbil with the exception of a small area to the north of the Aral Sea.

The infection rate in sandflies may reach 65 per cent, but is generally around

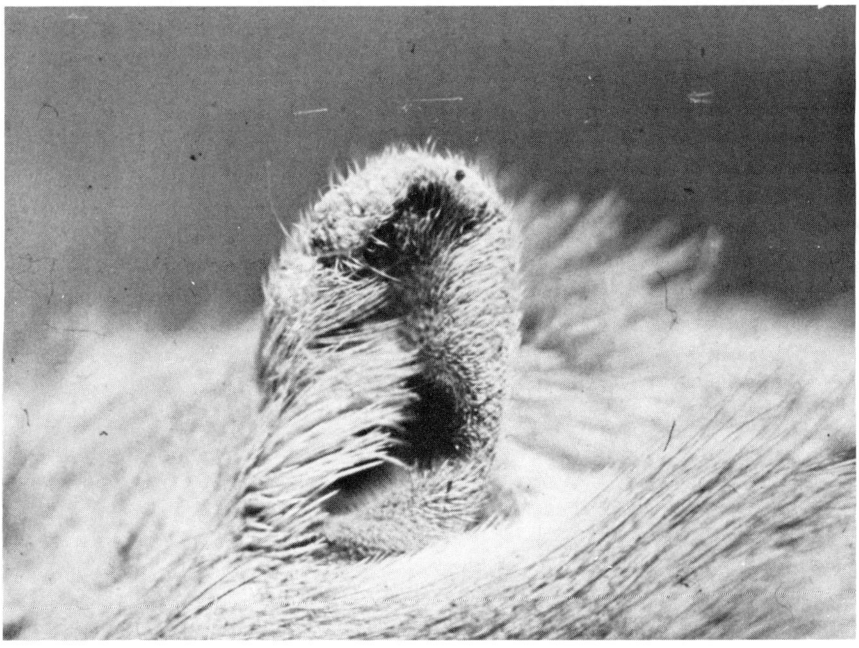

Figure 92. Ear of *Rhombomys opimus* infected with *L. major*, USSR. Courtesy of Yu. A. Dubrovsky.

one per cent.

Leishmania major in Central Asia can thus be seen to be intimately bound up with its main hosts which themselves are intimately related, the sandflies being dependent for food and habitat on the gerbils.

Various other animals have been found infected, but only *Meriones libycus* is thought to be able to maintain the parasite. Infection rates in *Meriones* are lower, the lesions are more severe and therefore less infective. In fact the main evidence that *Meriones* maintains the parasites is that there is a limited area of Turkmenistan where infected *Meriones* have been found where *Rhombomys* does not occur. None of the other animals found infected reach a rate above one per cent and they are all regarded as incidental hosts.

Human infection in the USSR

The great desert and semi-arid area occupied by *Rhombomys opimus* is a reservoir of *Leishmania major*. However, people entering virgin steppe in the height of the transmission season are rarely infected. It is usually one or two years following the start of development projects that people become infected, and then considerable epidemics can occur, disrupting severely the exploitation and colonization of these marginal areas.

The explanation for this is two-fold. Firstly, the dominant vectors in uninhabited areas are the *Paraphlebotomus* species which bite man very infrequently. It is only in the better watered areas with a water table around one metre deep that *P. papatasi* is common. And it is *P. papatasi* almost exclusively which transmits the infection to man. Where the habitat, originally unsuitable for *P. papatasi*, becomes occupied by man, in connection with irrigation and settlement, the changing environment seems to become particularly suitable for *P. papatasi*, whose populations increase greatly, transmitting the parasite from the relatively harmless reservoir to man.

The second important factor, which has not yet been fully evaluated, is the variation in infectivity of different strains. As mentioned above, strains isolated from gerbils or sandflies where *P. papatasi* does not occur are rarely infective to man, while a high proportion of those isolated in gerbil colonies where *P. papatasi* does exist are more infective and virulent.

The highly developed data on human infection has allowed a mathematical model to be produced estimating the probability of human infection in a given locality. In turn this has enabled the production of a detailed map which shows the distribution of human infection probability.

Zoonotic cutaneous leishmaniasis outside the USSR

We have concentrated on the epidemiology of *L. major* in Central Asia because of the wealth of data which is available. Soviet workers have concentrated their studies on cutaneous leishmaniasis hoping that it will serve as a model for other diseases with 'natural focality' in even less hospitable regions of the Union. Certainly the methods developed and data obtained have provided a very relevant base for studies on zoonotic cutaneous leishmaniasis in other parts of the world.

Foci of zoonotic cutaneous leishmaniasis with structures similar to that in the Central Asian USSR have been found in Mongolia (where human infections are not known), northern Afghanistan and north-eastern Iran. In north-western India and central Iran outside the range of *Rhombomys opimus* zoonotic foci exist in which *Meriones hurrianae* and *M. libycus* are thought to be the main vertebrate hosts and *Paraphlebotomus* species and *P. (Phlebotomus) salehi* are the vectors.

In south-western Iran and eastern Saudi Arabia presumed zoonotic foci exist, but while *Meriones crassus* is suspected in the latter country the main vertebrate hosts have not been confirmed.

L. major has recently been identified biochemically in Iraq, and ecological studies are in progress.

Further west, in Israel and Libya, the parasite has been found in the fat sand rat *Psammomys obesus*, another desert rodent which has many features in common with *Rhombomys*. *Psammomys* is a colonial, burrowing, diurnal, herbivorous rodent like *Rhombomys*, but its colonies and burrow systems are much smaller (figure 93), and its feeding requirements are much more specialized, consisting predominantly of succulent members of the Chenopodiaceae which require very salty soil. Thus, *Psammomys* is restricted to salt flats which occur at the edge of the desert near the coast, or where drainage is restricted, often as the result of failed irrigation schemes in the distant past (figure 94). Outbreaks of cutaneous leishmaniasis in desert labourers and soldiers have been associated with *Psammomys* and its role as a maintenance host is established. However, it remains to be shown whether *Psammomys* burrows are a major sandfly habitat: in some places they clearly are not. Further, large samples of *Psammomys* in Tunisia were uninfected, so there must be further conditions governing the association between *L. major* and *Psammomys*.

Elsewhere in North Africa, particularly Algeria, Morocco and Tunisia, cutaneous leishmaniasis exists which is probably zoonotic, but this has not yet been clearly established.

In West Africa recent work has shown that *L. major* occurs in rodents as a predominantly visceral infection, although the human infections in that region are typically cutaneous. The first rodent to be incriminated was the colonial, diurnal, herbivorous *Arvicanthis niloticus* in Senegal. Some four per cent of animals were found infected. *Arvicanthis* is said, in that area, to build nests in herbage, though in other parts of Africa it is a burrower. A second study carried out during a low point in the population cycle of *Arvicanthis* showed *Mastomys erythroleucus* and *Tatera gambiana* also to be infected. Among sandflies one closely related to *P. papatasi*, *P. duboscqi*, is the commonest mammal-biting species. Small numbers of *P. duboscqi* have been found naturally infected, and a

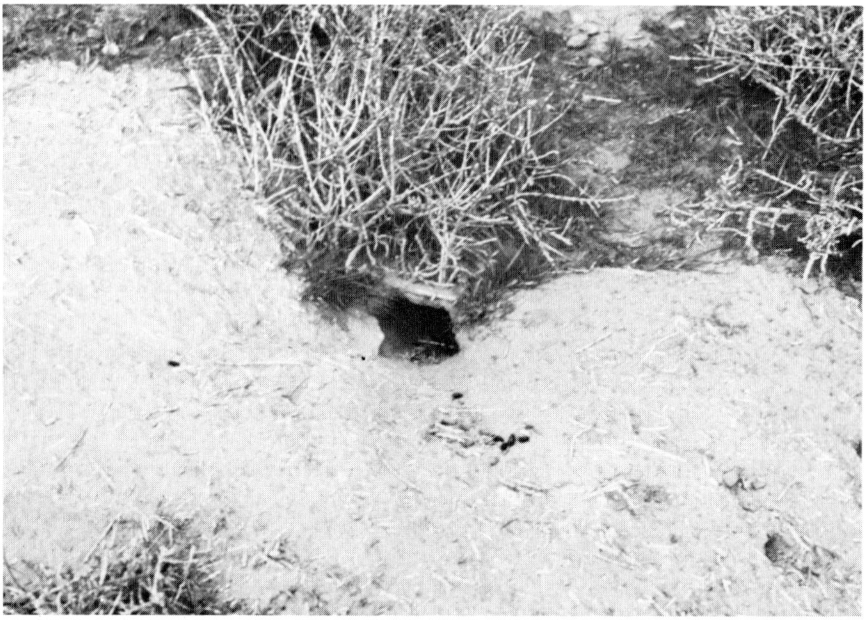

Figure 93. Characteristic entrance to a burrow of *Psammomys obesus*, a proven reservoir host of *L. major* in Libya.

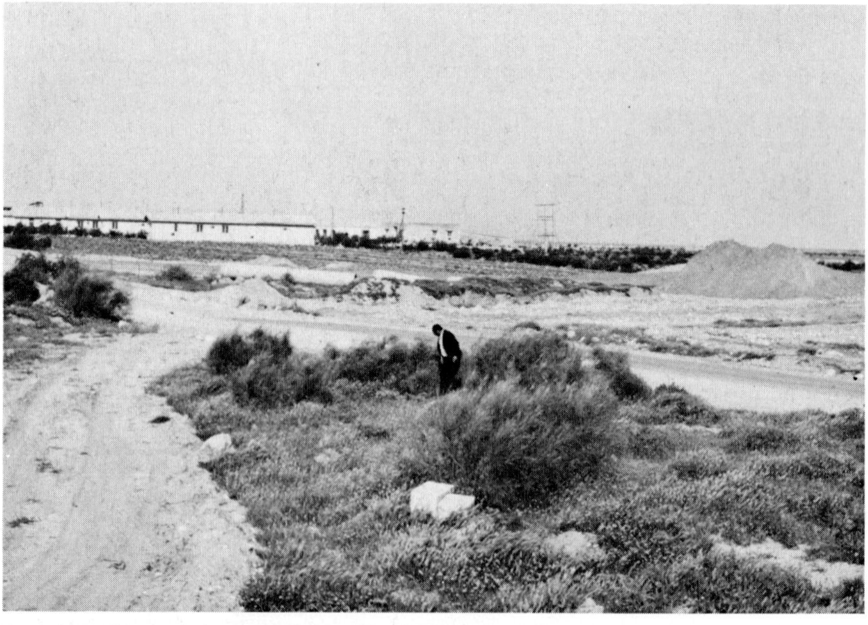

Figure 94. Lush growth in the wadi provides for abundant rodents, infected with *L. major*. Many labourers in this Libyan construction camp became infected.

reasonable picture of the ecology of the parasite in West Africa is being built up. The habitat in Senegal is very different from that of *L. major* in North Africa or Central Asia.

A few strains isolated from the viscera of rodents in southern Ethiopia and northern Kenya have been identified as *L. major*. One of these was shown to be infective to man, and was in fact used in an attempt to vaccinate people against *L. donovani* infection; but natural human infections are not known in the area.

Zoonotic cutaneous leishmaniasis due to *Leishmania aethiopica* infection

L. aethiopica has been identified from the Ethiopian highlands and from the slopes of Mount Elgon in Kenya. Parasites were isolated from human cases, from sandflies *P. longipes* and *P. pedifer*, and from the rock hyraxes *Procavia capensis* (figures 95) and *Heterohyrax brucei*.

Rock hyraxes, like *Rhombomys* and *Psammomys*, are colonial, herbivorous and diurnally active; they do not burrow, but live in deep rock crevices or in hollow trees which, like the colonies of *Rhombomys*, are rich in organic material, maintain constant temperature and humidity and provide a preferred habitat for the vectors.

The rock hyraxes have a much wider distribution than the parasites, being found in the arid lowlands and in the high mountains above the altitude limit for

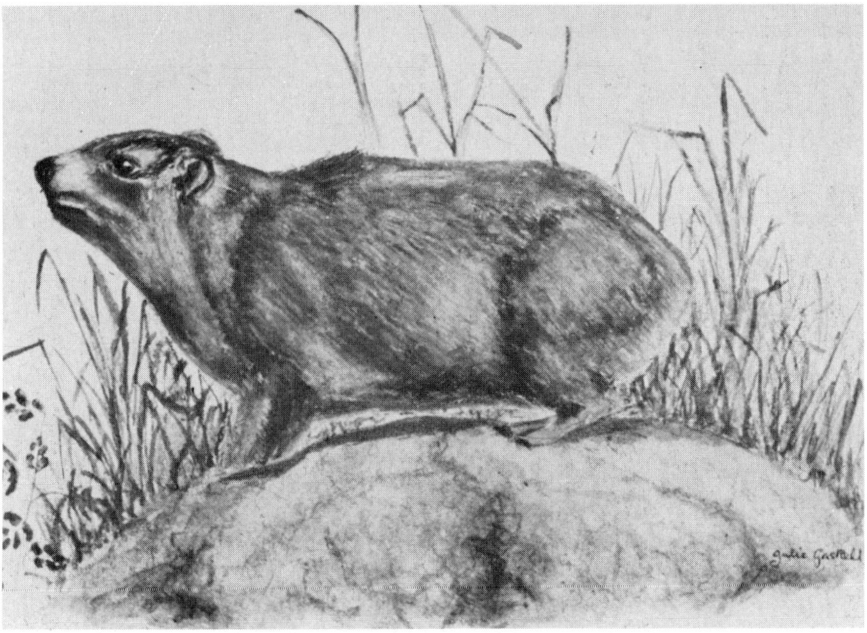

Figure 95. The rock hyrax *Procavia capensis*, the main reservoir host of *L. aethiopica* in Ethiopia and Kenya.

sandflies (2700 m). In the lowlands they are fed on by a wider variety of sandflies, but not *P. longipes* or *P. pedifer*. Similarly, the sandflies are more widely distributed than the parasite. *P. longipes* is common in towns and villages throughout the highlands between 1500 and 2600 m altitude. It has a wide food range, but prefers cows and man. Larvae have been found in shallow cavities in sandy banks which were not the home of any mammal or bird.

It is where the distribution of suitable vectors and vertebrate hosts overlap, in the cliffs and gorges of the highlands (figure 96) or in the relict forests with giant hollow fig trees in south-western Ethiopia, that *L. aethiopica* survives. Human infection is accidental and depends on living close to hyrax colonies. The sandflies living with hyraxes usually remain close to the colony, though movements of more than 200 m have been measured. In one town at 2600 m, people living within 50 m of hyraxes had the highest chance of infection, but lower down, at 2000 m, infection in people living almost one kilometre from the nearest colony showed microfocal clustering, indicating that transmission probably occurred in the houses.

In a third town, built defensively on a hilltop inhabited by many hyraxes, the incidence of human infection was so great that mainly children were infected, most adults being immune. Occasional cases of re-infection were seen in the oldest women.

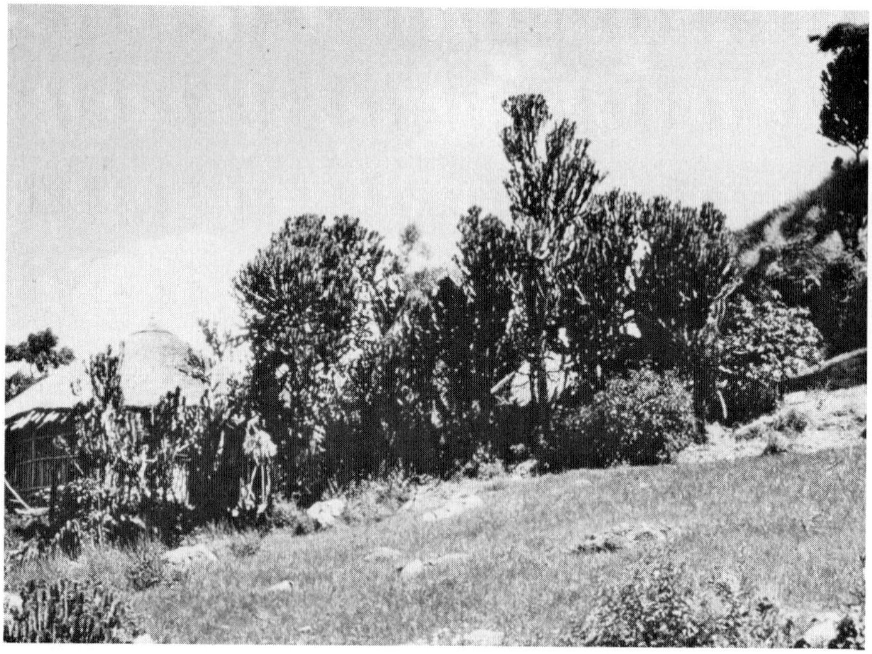

Figure 96. *L. aethiopica* habitat. The low cliffs were occupied by a hyrax *Procavia capensis* colony and three people living in the house became infected.

In Kenya a picture similar to that in Ethiopia has been described. In addition to two species of hyrax, a single giant rat *Cricetomys gambianus* was found to be infected.

The occasional human infections in Namibia have occurred in people who enjoy camping and other outdoor pursuits. The infected hyraxes were found in an area where people had been thought to contract the disease, as were the sandflies *P. rossi*, which were living closely with the hyraxes. However, as shown above, the hyrax parasites were different from the sandfly ones, which in turn were the same as the human ones. In Namibia there has been considerable destruction of predators, particularly hyaenas and jackals, which threatened sheep. This has led to an explosion in the hyrax population, which may be responsible for the spread of infection to man. Elsewhere in Africa occasional human infections occur, but little is known of their epidemiology.

Anthroponotic cutaneous leishmaniasis due to *Leishmania tropica* infection

With the finding of animal reservoir hosts for cutaneous and visceral leishmaniasis, workers were long reluctant to accept the existence of permanent non-zoonotic foci of cutaneous leishmaniasis. However, extensive unsuccessful attempts to discover animal reservoirs, and the success in control of methods assuming man–sandfly–man transmission have now convinced most people that man is the main host for *L. tropica*. It is thus an anthroponosis as opposed to a zoonosis.

Although *L. tropica* has been successfully eliminated in many parts of its range, less is known of its ecology than that of *L. major*. One problem is that there are some areas where *L. major* and *L. tropica* both occur, and the parasites have not always been differentiated.

The situation is further complicated by the finding that some cutaneous leishmaniasis ulcers in Europe are caused by *L. donovani*. It will be very interesting to see how much cutaneous leishmaniasis in Europe is due to each parasite. It can perhaps be assumed that in areas where the cutaneous disease is common and dominant, *L. tropica* is involved. This is the case in the cities of West Asia, such as Baghdad and Aleppo, in Crete and in the Abruzzo region of Italy. The identity of the parasites was confirmed in Crete and has recently been demonstrated in Tunisia.

Dogs are infected with cutaneous lesions resembling the human ones and the parasites have occasionally been identified as *L. tropica* (e.g., in Bikaner, north-west India). Adler was able to distinguish the two canine diseases caused by *L. tropica* and *L. donovani*. The clinical course and infection rate in dogs is similar to that in man, and most authors consider dogs to be alternative hosts, not true reservoirs. The finding of two tame brown bears infected in Baghdad is perhaps a mere curiosity, but the recent identification as *L. tropica* of a strain isolated from the viscera of a rat *Rattus rattus*, also from Baghdad, raises the question of a peridomestic rodent reservoir. Wherever anthroponotic cutaneous leishmaniasis occurs it is associated with *Phlebotomus sergenti*. Adler gave convincing evidence that this was the main vector in Crete.

P. papatasi has also been incriminated, as in Kabul, Afghanistan, but the picture is often confused as the parasites have not usually been convincingly identified. In Canea in Crete anthroponotic cutaneous leishmaniasis was endemic in the most densely populated parts of the old town, in contrast to visceral leishmaniasis, which was common in the suburbs with gardens. In Baghdad anthroponotic cutaneous leishmaniasis was also found mainly in the most crowded quarters. By contrast, epidemics of cutaneous leishmaniasis in Delhi and Kabul were at the edges of towns and were associated with major earth movements — the levelling of a refuse area in Delhi, and the construction of a new suburb in Kabul. Anthroponotic cutaneous leishmaniasis cannot consistently be associated with a particular type of housing or social class. Pringle tried, without success, to relate the infection in Baghdad to soil type and water table. While a lot of information is available on the habits and habitat of adult sandflies, there are no long-term prospective studies relating outbreaks of anthroponotic cutaneous leishmaniasis to sandfly population irruptions. Further, there is almost no information on differential larval habitats, without which the effective interpretation of epidemiological observations is severely limited.

DIAGNOSIS

Most of what has been said for NWCL diagnosis applies equally in the Old World. African cutaneous histoplasmosis is a further, though uncommon, differential diagnosis, but generally the same range of infections, including lepromatous leprosy for DCL in Ethiopia and Kenya, must be considered. The Montenegro test is of less value clinically as it only becomes positive when the lesions are almost resolved. Parasitological diagnosis requires the same procedures as in the New World, and is much more satisfactory in young lesions or those of DCL, in which parasites are very numerous. Cultivation of most Old World strains is easier than for *L. b. braziliensis*.

Retrospective diagnosis for epidemiological purposes may use the Montenegro test or examination for scars. The Montenegro test must be adjusted to suit the parasite being sought: the dose of antigen required to produce a positive reaction in cured *L. tropica* or *L. aethiopica* infection would produce an excessive reaction, with blistering and necrosis, in *L. major*. A significant proportion of positive reactors have no associated scar and it may either be that these are false positives or that the immunizing infection was ephemeral and passed unnoticed leaving no scar.

CONTROL

Vaccination

The traditional control of Old World cutaneous leishmaniasis, mentioned above, was by vaccination, or more accurately 'leishmanization', in which material from an active sore was inoculated into an area where the subsequent scar would be hidden by clothing. This method has been developed considerably, particularly in Israel and the USSR, where military and other personnel are involved in activities in desert areas enzootic for *L. major*, and in whom multiple lesions would seriously affect their efficiency. In general, satisfactory results are obtained when promastigotes of a recently isolated virulent strain are inoculated. The lesion and scar are not usually more than 2 cm in diameter (figure 97). However, there is a significant occurrence of large lesions which last a long time and are sufficiently

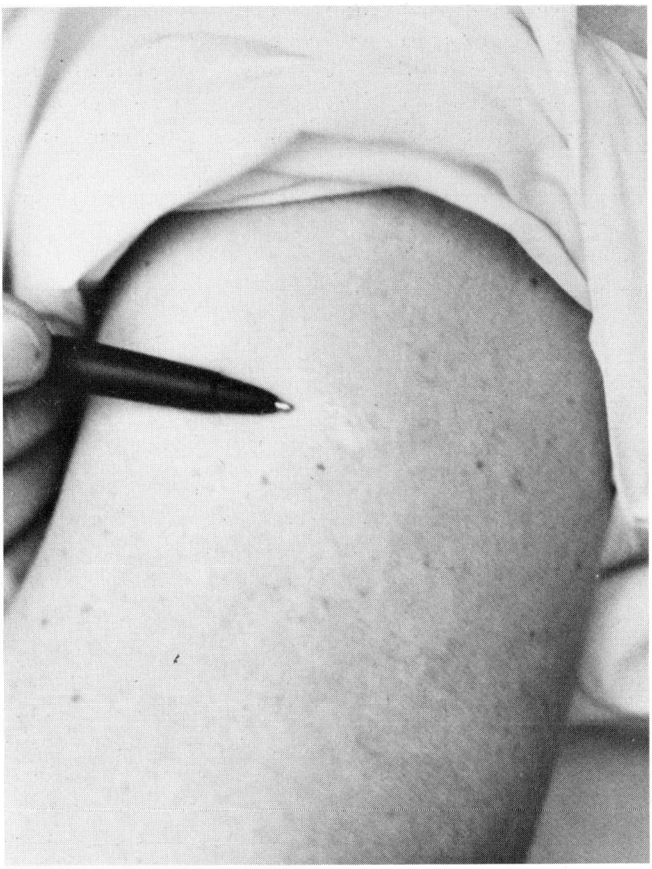

Figure 97. Typical vaccination scar for *L. major* in a Soviet scientific field worker.

unsightly that vaccination is not compulsory and is not carried out *en masse*. Further, immunity is not acquired until about three months after vaccination, so personnel must be identified and protected three or more months before being exposed in an enzootic area during the transmission season. The living promastigotes used must either be freshly extracted from cultures, or may be preserved in liquid nitrogen. These problems present serious logistic difficulties.

Sandfly and rodent control

As with most infections the most desirable control method is to prevent exposure. This has been achieved by control of sandflies and by control of reservoir hosts and their environment.

Sandfly control is hardly practical in the prevention of zoonotic cutaneous leishmaniasis infection. In Iran insecticide treatment of rodent burrows within 200 m of villages had little effect on the transmission rate to man. The agricultural use of insecticides has no doubt, along with other environmental changes, greatly reduced the prevalence of the parasite in previously unsettled areas. In many towns where anthroponotic cutaneous leishmaniasis was prevalent it has been eradicated by the combination of antimalarial campaigns and the use of household insecticides. Sandflies appear to be uniformly susceptible to DDT with

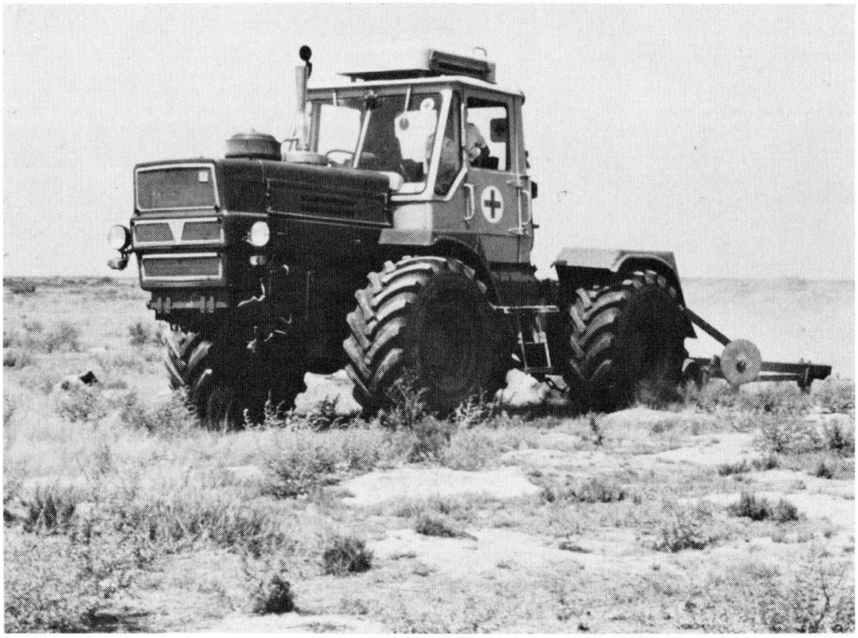

Figure 98. Use of a deep plough to destroy *Rhombomys opimus* colonies for the protection of an irrigation scheme in Uzbekistan, USSR against *L. major*.

the exception of *P. papatasi* in Bihar, which is moderately resistant.

Rodent control and environmental modification are required for the zoonotic infection. In settlements and agricultural projects in the steppes of Soviet Central Asia leishmaniasis assessment and control is integrated in the early planning stages. Colonies of *Rhombomys opimus* are mapped throughout the project area by aerial photography followed by ground survey. They are then systematically destroyed either by poisoning with zinc phosphide, or by ploughing to a depth of 50 cm (figure 98). The canals of irrigation projects are designed to form a barrier across which there will be no recolonization of *Rhombomys*. Elaborate control measures such as these have been restricted to the USSR, but could surely be adapted for areas where *Psammomys* is the reservoir. There are plans to control hyraxes in a very heavily infected Ethiopian town in an effort to control the disease.

Appendix I. *Trypanosoma* in Mammals and other Vertebrates

MAMMALIAN TRYPANOSOMES

Section	Stercoraria
Subgenus	*Herpetosoma*
Species	*Trypanosoma lewisi* (rat) cosmopolitan

Life cycle notes

1. Course of infection

Limited period of reproduction in blood and tissues, especially kidney medulla (vasa recta capillaries; placenta of pregnant mice, *T. musculi*) for the first 10 days after infection; reproduction ceases under influence of ablastin and parasites assume 'adult' form in blood; parasitaemia remains for variable period (possibly several weeks). Evidence of circadian rhythm in parasitaemia. Parasitaemia up to $2 \times 10^5\,mm^{-3}$.

2. Multiplication

Division in blood and tissues by multiple or binary unequal fission as epimastigotes; large rosettes of up to 16 parasites can be found.

3. Hosts

Members of genus *Rattus*; all uninfected rats susceptible; infection results in sterile immunity. Other rodents and lagomorphs.

4. Transmission

By contamination of mucous membranes or broken skin by metacyclic parasites in faeces of flea vector.

5. Vectors

Rat fleas *Xenopsylla cheopis* and *Nosopsyllus fasciatus*; up to 66 per cent of fleas can be infected experimentally; infection in flea remains for life; development in midgut, where intracellular forms occur in *N. fasciatus*, pylorus, hindgut and rectum; infective metacyclics in rectum in 5–7 days after the infective meal.

6. Pathology

Generally non-pathogenic, but pathological changes observed in liver, spleen, kidney and foetal absorption or abortion in females when pregnant.

7. Cultivation

Of vector forms on blood agar media; *Aedes aegypti* cell explants in hanging drop cultures and haematozoic forms in various tissue culture cell lines at 37 °C.

Other species of *Herpetosoma*

Parasite	Host	Vector	Distribution
T. grosi	*Apodemus*	*Ctenopthalmus agyrtes*	Europe
T. nabiasi	*Oryctolagus*	*Spilopsyllus cuniculi*	Europe
T. zapi	*Zapus*	*Megabothris abantis*	USA
T. microti	*Microtus*	*Nosopsyllus fasciatus* (exptl)	Europe/USA
T. tamiasi	*Tamias*	*M. acerbus*	Canada

1. Notes

The parasitaemia levels in other species do not rise as high as in *T. lewisi* itself. Reproduction in tissues as amastigotes is known to occur. Cultivation on blood agar media can be achieved but has variable results and passage may be difficult.

Section	Stercoraria
Subgenus	*Megatrypanum*
Species	*Trypanosoma theileri* (cattle) cosmopolitan

Life cycle notes

1. Course of infection

Very low parasitaemia means trypanosomes not readily detectable in smears; levels of one parasite per ml to levels detectable in blood smears can be found; seasonal changes in levels of parasitaemia highest in summer months; infections likely to remain for life of animal.

2. Multiplication

Reproduction in tissues as amastigotes or epimastigotes (unequal binary fission), occasional multiplication in blood associated with high parasitaemias in concurrent rinderpest infections, some species may not divide in mammal.

3. Hosts

T. theileri is solely a parasite of cattle but similar species ('*T. theileri*-like') occur in wild Bovidae, Ovidae and Cervidae.

4. Transmission

Likely to be by contamination of mucous membranes of mouth or of broken skin by metacyclic forms.

5. Vectors

Tabanidae, *Tabanus*, *Haematopota*; hindgut development; evidence for development of *T. theileri* in ticks where haemocoele reportedly infected; infection rates in vector variable; up to 27 per cent, possibly higher.

6. Pathology

Generally non-pathogenic. Pathogenicity associated with concurrent infections of bacteria, protozoa and viruses; parasites found in new-born calves causing heavy infections; febrile period after inoculation. Possible association between *T. theileri* and lymphocytosis and bovine lymphosarcoma. Central nervous system lesions sometimes observed.

7. Cultivation

On blood agar; also frequent contaminant in primary isolation of bovine cell lines (including foetal calf lines). Can be grown as bloodstream form at 37 °C in overlay of various monolayers (bovine foetal kidney, lymph node cells, chicken embryos at 37 °C).

Other species of *Megatrypanum*

Parasite	Host	Vector
T. melophagium	sheep	*Melophagus ovinus*
T. theodori	goat	*Lipoptena capreoli*
T. cervi	elk	unknown

FISH TRYPANOSOMES

Life cycle notes

1. Course of infection

Chronic infections usually with initial high parasitaemias with gradual decrease in numbers; no evidence of division in fish host. Pleomorphism in fish blood through growth of parasites.

2. Hosts

Found in freshwater and marine teleosts and elasmobranchs; distribution cosmopolitan; wide host range of several species, for example, *T. cobitis* in freshwater fish in Britain; *T. murmanensis* in marine teleosts off Newfoundland; *T. raiae* in elasmobranchs.

3. Transmission

By bite of leeches, for example, *T. cobitis* and *T. tincae* by *Hemiclepsis marginata*, *T. raiae* by *Pontobdella muricata*, *T. murmanensis* by *Johanssonia arctica*. Development in leech gut, crop and proboscis sheath as amastigotes, epimastigotes and sphaeromastigotes. Metacyclic trypomastigotes in proboscis sheath or crop. Infection can be lost after leech has fed or leech may remain infected for life.

4. Pathology

Generally non-pathogenic; haematological changes reportedly associated with infection in cod, plaice and freshwater fishes, decreased PCV and haemoglobin values, decrease in blood glucose, increase in globulin; histopathological changes in kidneys, spleen and liver in heavy trypanosome infection of carp.

5. Cultivation

Growth in blood agar media; carp trypanosomes can be grown on fish tissue culture media as trypomastigotes with MEM and ten per cent foetal bovine or calf serum.

Examples

Parasite	Host	Vector	Distribution
T. cobitis	*Cottus, Phoxinus Nemachielus, Gobio*	*Hemiclepsis marginata*	UK
T. raiae	*Raja* and other elasmobranchs	*Pontobdella muricata*	Temperate coastal waters
T. murmanensis	*Gadus* and pleuronectiform and perciform species	*Johanssonia* sp.	Atlantic coast of North America
T. danilewyski	Cyprinidae (carp)	*Piscicola geometra*	Europe
T. platessae	*Pleuronectes plattessa*	*Piscicola geometra*	European coastal waters

AMPHIBIAN TRYPANOSOMES

Life cycle notes

1. Course of infection

Infections are chronic with variable parasitaemias and usually with some evidence of reproduction in vertebrate hosts. Some reports of initial reproductive phase; reproduction when described is by binary or multiple fission. Cyclical changes in parasitaemia over 24 h period (and localization in kidney) in some Anura and over seasons (peak in spring).

2. Hosts and Distribution

Parasitic in Anura and Urodela; cosmopolitan distribution.

3. Transmission

Transmission by (a) bite of, leeches development in crop and proboscis sheath; (b) contamination in arthropod (sandfly and mosquito) transmitted species, development in hindgut.

4. Pathology

Reports of pathogenicity in *T. inopinatum* — anaemia haemorrhages and enlarged lymph glands — but generally believed trypanosomes non-pathogenic, although infections in tadpoles may be pathogenic.

5. Cultivation

Various blood-agar based media have been found satisfactory for growth of epimastigote stages of Amphibian trypanosomes. No attempts to grow haematozoic forms on tissue culture media have been made.

Examples

Parasite	Host	Vector
T. diemyctyli	Urodela—*Triturus v. viridescens*	*Batrachobdella picta*
T. pipientis	Anura—*Rana pipiens*	*Placobdella phalera*
T. rotatorium	Anura—*Rana clamitans*	*Culex territans*
T. bocagei	Anura—*Bufo* species	*Phlebotomus squamirostris*
T. bufophlebotomi	Anura—*B. boreas halophilus*	*Lutzomyia vexatrix occidentis*

REPTILIAN TRYPANOSOMES

Life cycle notes

1. Course of infection

Low grade parasitaemias sometimes only detectable by culture. Evidence suggests infections are long-lived in reptiles. No evidence of concentration of parasites in tissues. (Some reptiles can be infected with Salivarian trypanosomes experimentally).

2. Multiplication

Little evidence to date of division of reptiles or of concentrations of parasites in tissues. Morphology of parasites highly variable; usually large, up to 70–80 μm, with prominent undulating membrane, but also small, 20 μm; round or oval in shape and difficult to stain. No evidence of pathogenicity associated with infection.

3. Distribution

Worldwide distribution in lizards, snakes, turtles and crocodilians.

4. Transmission

By sandflies, *Glossina* and leeches (turtle trypanosomes), by bite and contamination.

5. Cultivation

Culture on blood agar type media.

6. Development

In some species in sandfly and culture as amastigotes promastigotes and sphaeromastgotes with no trypomastigote stage in the vector, although does occur in other species, for example, *T. grayi* in the crocodile.

Examples

Parasite	Host	Vector
T. grayi	Crocodylia—*Crocodilus niloticus*	*Glossina palpalis* *G. fuscipes*
T. boueti	Scincidae—*Mabuya striata*	*Sergentomyia bedfordi*
T. thecadactyli	Gekkoniae—*Thecadactylus rapicaudus*	*Lutzomyia trinidadensis*
T. platydactyli	*Tatentola mauretanica*	*S. minuta*
T. gerrhonoti	Lacertidae—*Gerrhonotus multicarinatus*	*Lu. vexatrix occidentis*
T. chrysemidis	Chelonia—*Chrysemys picta marginata*	*Placobdella parasitica*
T. brazili	Squamata (Ophidia)—*Helicopus modestus*	*Placobdella braziliensis*

AVIAN TRYPANOSOMES

Life cycle notes

1. Course of infection

Infection usually low grade, detectable sometimes only by culture. Chronic long-lived infections are frequent. Some species produce high parasitaemias, for example, *T. bouffardi* of African Ploceidae, but this is rare. *T. corvi* restricted to bone marrow in winter.

2. Multiplication

No evidence of division in most species, but two species, *T. avium bakeri* and *T. bouffardi*, do divide in birds. No cross-immunity between species.

3. Distribution

Worldwide distribution in many species of birds.

4. Transmission

Transmission by contamination of metacyclics developing in hindgut of vector. Salivary gland of mosquitoes and haemocoele of mites are other reported sites of development. Wide range of vector arthropods, for example, *Aedes*, *Simulium*, Hippoboscidae (*Ornithomyia*), mites (*Dermanyssus gallinae*).

5. Pathology

Generally no pathogenicity associated with infection. Splenomegaly and changes in lymphoid tissue in *T. bouffardi*.

6. Cultivation

In blood agar media (4N). Use of cultivation necessary as a technique for detecting trypanosomes from blood or from bone marrow. Examination of bone marrow a better indication of infection than peripheral blood.

Examples

Parasite	Host	Vector	Distribution
T. corvi	Corvidae	*Ornithomyia avicularia*	Europe
T. avium	Passerinae	*Simulium, Aedes*	Canada
T. bouffardi	Ploceidae	Unknown	Africa
T. macfiei	*Serinus canaria* (only found in laboratory)	*Dermanyssus gallinae*	UK

Appendix II. *Leishmania* Species of Animals other than Man

INTRODUCTION

Although many *Leishmania* species are capable of infecting a wide range of mammals, some are much more limited in their host range. The forms which are non-infective to humans are of little direct economic significance, but are important as experimental tools, models, and to complete the overall picture of the genus.

A single *Leishmania*-like infection was described from a blackbird *Turdus merula* many years ago, but avian infection has not been confirmed and the parasites of the genus remain restricted to lizards and mammals.

Lizard *Leishmania* species present anomalies and deserve much further study. As far as is known they are transmitted by sandflies, mainly *Sergentomyia* species, in which some species become established in the hind gut (hypopylarial development). It is supposed that the infection is transmitted when the sandfly is eaten by the lizard. The parasites are usually found as promastigotes in blood cultures, but amastigotes in circulating white cells have occasionally been seen. The identity of promastigote parasites attached in palisades to the cloaca of chameleons has yet to be established.

Lizard leishmaniasis is rarely reported from the New World, but has recently been discovered in Cuba. In the Old World it is common in East Africa, the Mediterranean region (in geckos) and Turkmenistan. Cryptic human infection with lizard leishmaniasis is thought to be responsible for positive skin tests in East Africa. *L. adleri*, the parasite implicated, is unusual among lizard *Leishmania* species in that it develops in the anterior 'station' in its sandfly vector *Sergentomyia clydei*. Studies indicate however that lizard '*Leishmania*' may in fact be trypanosomes.

LEISHMANIA ENRIETTII

This parasite was discovered in laboratory guinea-pigs at Parana, Brazil and has subsequently been rediscovered both in the same laboratory and in nearby domestic guinea-pigs. The guinea-pig *Cavia porcellus* is one of those domestic animals whose wild origins are unknown. The related wild form *Cavia aperea* was shown to be non-receptive, so the origins of this parasite are a mystery. The infection in the guinea-pig is cutaneous, and in many ways mimics human cutaneous leishmaniasis. It has therefore been extensively studied experimentally as a model of the human disease.

LEISHMANIA HERTIGI

This parasite was discovered during investigations on the epidemiology of *L. braziliensis* infection in Panama. It appears to be a specific parasite of the tree porcupines *Coendou* species, and is found in Brazil, Costa Rica and Panama. The organisms are morphologically distinct as they have large inclusions, visible with the light microscope. Ultrastructural studies show these structures to be distinctive virus-like particles described on p. 20.

Nearly all adult tree porcupines are infected. The infection is largely restricted to the skin, and there is no gross pathology at all.

L. herreri is a parasite of sloths in Costa Rica, and can be distinguished from *L. b. panamensis* mainly by its failure to infect hamsters.

LEISHMANIA GERBILLI

This species was described from Gansu and Xinjian (Sinkiang) provinces in north-western China. It is a parasite of *Rhombomys opimus*, in which it behaves exactly like *L. major*. The vector is *P. mongolensis*, one of the very few sandflies in these northern desert areas. Despite very high prevalence in *Rhombomys*, human infection is unknown.

Although this species was said to be morphologically distinctive, it is clearly very closely related to the parasites infecting *Rhombomys* in the northern steppes of the USSR. Like *L. gerbilli* these are transmitted by *P. (Paraphlebotomus)* species, and have limited infectivity to man.

Soviet workers insist that the 'non-virulent' strains transmitted by *Paraphlebotomus* species and the 'virulent' strains transmitted by *P. (Phlebotomus) papatasi* are not specifically distinct, as they cannot be distinguished by sero-taxonomic tests and their behaviour in gerbils is so similar. Further, many strains have intermediate virulence, so the true position of *L. gerbilli* with respect to the various forms of *L. major* in the USSR remains to be fully evaluated.

Bibliographies

A Bibliography of Chagas' Disease (1909–1969). Index Catalogue of Medical and Veterinary Zoology Special Publication No. 2, by M. Olivier, L.J. Olivier and D.B. Segal (United States Department of Agriculture).

Chagas' Disease (South American Trypanosomiasis). A Bibliography. By M.A. Miles and Jean E. Rowe, 1970. *Supplement to Tropical Diseases Bulletin* vol. 67.

Bibliography of Leishmania and Leishmanial Diseases, Vols. I and II. By D. Heyneman, K. Hoogstraal and A. Djigounian. (Special Publication US Naval Medical Research Unit Number Three Cairo, Egypt).

A Partly Annotated Bibliography on Infections, Parasites, and Diseases of African Wild Animals. L. Karstad, 1979, IDRC-135e (Ottawa: International Development Research Centre).

World Health Organization. Leishmaniasis Reference List 1890–1963. Mimeographed documents by D. Heyneman and H. Hoogstraal, WHO/Leish/67/3 and *1960–1966* WHO/Leish/67.4.

Phlebotomine Sandflies 1973–1981. Annotated Bibliography. Commonwealth Agricultural Bureaux. ISSN 0141-593X. 684 references prepared by Commonwealth Institute of Entomology, 56 Queens Gate, London SW7 5JR.

Trypanosomiasis Bibliography January 1978. US Department of Agriculture, Veterinary Services, 1978 (Hyattsville, MD: USDA Veterinary Services), 182 pp., 27 000 references.

Selected Texts for Further Reading

Adler, S., 1964, *Leishmania. Advances in Parasitology* **2**, 35–96.

Adler, S. and Theodor, O., 1957, Transmission of disease agents by Phlebotomine sandflies. *Annual Review of Entomology* **2**, 203–226.

Apted, F. I. C., 1980, Present status of chemotherapy and chemoprophylaxis of human trypanosomiasis in the eastern hemisphere. *Pharmacology and Therapeutics* **11**, 391–413.

Ashcroft, M. T., 1959, The importance of African wild mammals as reservoirs of trypanosomiasis. *East African Medical Journal* **36**, 289–297.

Baker, J. R. (ed.), 1982, *Perspectives in Trypanosomiasis Research* (New York: John Wiley, Research Studies Press).

Bardsley, J. E. and Harmsen, R., 1973, The trypanosomes of Anura. *Advances in Parasitology* **11**, 1–72.

Barker, D. C., 1980, The ultrastructure of kinetoplast DNA with particular reference to the interpretation of dark field electron microscopy images of isolated purified networks. *Micron* **11**, 26–62.

Bray, R., 1974, *Leishmania. Annual Review of Microbiology* **28**, 189–217.

Brener, Z., 1979, Present status of chemotherapy and chemoprophylaxis of human trypanosomiasis in the Western hemisphere. *Pharmacology and Therapeutics* **7**, 71–90.

Buxton, P. A., 1955, The natural history of tsetse flies. *Memoirs of the London School of Hygiene and Tropical Medicine*, No. 10 (London: H. K. Lewis).

Chance, M., 1979, The identification of *Leishmania*. In *Problems in the Identification of Parasites and their Vectors*, edited by A. E. R. Taylor and R. Muller (Oxford: Blackwell Scientific Publications), pp. 55–74.

Chance, M. and Walton, B. C. (eds), 1982, *Biochemical Characterisation of Leishmania.* Proceedings of a Workshop held in Washington, 9–11 December 1980 (Geneva: UNDP/World Bank/WHO Special Programme for Research and Training in Tropical Diseases).

De Raadt, P. and Seed, J. R., 1977, Trypanosomes causing disease in man in Africa. In *Parasitic Protozoa*, edited by J. Kreier (London: Academic Press), Vol. 1, pp. 175–237.

Epidemiology of Trypanosomiasis. 1980. *Insect Science and its Application* **1**, 1–121. Collection of papers on epidemiology of trypanosomiasis and *Glossina* ecology.

FAO, 1980, *Trypanotolerant Livestock in West and Central Africa.* FAO Animal Health and Production Paper 20/1 and 20/2 (Rome: FAO), Vol. I. A general study; Vol. II. Country studies produced in collaboration with the International Livestock Commission for Africa and the United Nations Environment Programme.

FAO, 1980, *The Environmental Impact of Tsetse Control Operations*. FAO Animal Health and Production Paper Rev. 1 (Rome: FAO).

FAO, 1980, *Insecticides and Application Equipment for Tsetse Control.* FAO Animal

Health and Production Paper 3 (Rome: FAO).
Finelle, P., 1974, *Chemotherapy and Chemoprophylaxis against Animal Trypanosomiasis. Recent Advances Present Situation.* World Health Organisation Mimeographed Document TRYP/INF/74.55 (Geneva: World Health Organisation).
Ford, J., 1971, *The Role of the Trypanosomiases in African Ecology. A Study of the Tsetse Fly Problem* (Oxford: Clarendon Press).
Gardener, P.J., 1977, Taxonomy of the genus *Leishmania*: A review of nomenclature and classification. *Tropical Diseases Bulletin* **74**, 1069–1088.
Gibson, W., Marshall, T. de D. and Godfrey, D. G., 1980, Numerical analysis of enzyme polymorphism: New approaches to the epidemiology and taxonomy of trypanosomes of the subgenus *Trypanozoon. Advances in Parasitology* **18**, 175–246.
Glover, P. E., 1965, *The Tsetse Problem in Northern Nigeria*, 2nd edition (Nairobi: Patwa New Agency (E. A.) Ltd).
Godfrey, D. G., 1979, The zymodemes of trypanosomes. In *Problems in the Identification of Parasites and their Vectors.* Edited by A. E. R. Taylor and R. Muller (Oxford: Blackwell Scientific Publications), pp. 31–53.
Greathead, D.J., 1980, Biological control of tsetse flies an assessment of insect parasitoids as control agents. *Biocontrol News and Information* **1**, 111–123.
Hoare, C. A., 1972, *The Trypanosomes of Mammals, A Zoological Monograph* (Oxford: Blackwell Scientific Publications).
Hommel, M., 1978, The genus *Leishmania*: Biology of the parasites and clinical aspects. *Bulletin de l'Institut Pasteur* **75**, 5–102.
Hargrove, J. W., 1977, Some advances in the trapping of tsetse and other flies. *Ecological Entomology* **2**, 123–137.
Hoogstraal, H. and Heyneman, D., 1969, Leishmaniasis in the Sudan Republic. 30. Final epidemiologic report. *American Journal of Tropical Medicine and Hygiene* **18**, 1091–1210.
Human African Trypanosomiasis. Proceedings of a Symposium, 10–12 December, 1976, Antwerp 1977, *Annales de la Société belge de Médecine tropical* **57**, 191–542.
Jordan, A. M., 1974, Recent developments in the ecology and methods of control of tsetse flies — (*Glossina* spp) (Dipt. Glossinidae) — a review. *Bulletin of Entomological Research* **63**, 361–399.
Jordan, A. M., 1976, Tsetse flies as vectors of trypanosomes. *Veterinary Parasitology* **2**, 143–152.
Keymer, I. F., 1969, Investigation on the duiker (*Sylvicapra grimmia*) and its blood protozoa in Central Africa. *Philosophical Transactions of the Royal Society of London* **B255**, 33–108.
Kilgour, V., 1980, *Trypanosoma*: intricacies of biochemistry, morphology and environment. *International Journal of Biochemistry* **12**, 325–332.
Killick-Kendrick, R., 1978, Recent advances in outstanding problems in the biology of Phlebotomine sandflies. *Acta Tropica* **35**, 297–313.
Kreier, J. P. (ed.), 1977, *Parasitic Protozoa. Vol. I. Taxonomy, Kinetoplastids and Flagellates of Fish* (London: Academic Press).
Lainson, R., 1982. Leishmanial parasites of mammals in relation to human disease. In *Animal Disease in Relation to Animal Conservation. Symposia of the Zoological Society of London*, No. **50**, 137–179.
Laird, M. (ed.), 1977, *Tsetse, The Future for Biological Methods in Integrated Control.* IDRC-077e (Ottawa: International Development Research Centre).
Langley, P. A., 1977, Physiology of tsetse flies (*Glossina* spp) (Diptera: Glossinidae): A review. *Bulletin of Entomological Research* **67**, 523–574.
Leach, T. M. and Roberts, C.J., 1981, Present status of chemotherapy and chemoprophylaxis of animal trypanosomiasis in the eastern hemisphere. *Pharmacology and Therapeutics* **13**, 91–147.

Lewis, D.J., 1982, A taxonomic review of the genus *Phlebotomus*. *Bulletin of the British Museum (Natural History) Entomology Series* **45**, 121–209.

Lumsden, W. H. R. and Evans, D. A. (eds.), 1976 and 1979, *Biology of the Kinetoplastida. Vols. 1 & 2*. (London: Academic Press).

Lumsden, W.H.R., Herbert, W.J. and McNeillage, G.J.C., 1973, *Techniques with Trypanosomes* (Edinburgh: Churchill Livingstone).

Mahmoud, M.M. and Gray, A.R., 1980, Trypanosomiasis due to *Trypanosoma evansi* (Steel, 1885) Balbiani, 1888. A review of recent research. *Tropical Animal Health and Production* **12**, 35–47.

McGhee, R.B. and Cosgrove, W.B., 1980, Biology and physiology of the lower Trypanosomatidae. *Microbiological Reviews* **44**, 140–173.

Molyneux, D.H., 1975, Diagnostic methods in animal trypanosomiasis. *Veterinary Parasitology* **1**, 5–17.

Molyneux, D.H., 1977, Vector relationships in the Trypanosomatidae. *Advances in Parasitology* **15**, 1–82.

Molyneux, D.H., 1982, Trypanosomes, trypanosomiasis and tsetse control: impact on wildlife and its conservation. In *Animal Disease in Relation to Animal Conservation. Symposia of the Zoological Society of London*, No.**50**, 29–55.

Mulligan, H.W. (ed.), 1970, *The African Trypanosomiases* (London: George Allen & Unwin; Ministry of Overseas Development).

Ormerod, W.E., 1979, Human and animal trypanosomiasis as world public health problems. *Pharmacology and Therapeutics* **6**, 1–40.

Pan American Health Organization, 1975, *New Approaches in American Trypanosomiasis Research*. Scientific Publication No. 318 (Washington: Pan American Health Organization).

Pan American Health Organization (eds.), 1977, *Symposium on Chagas Disease* (Washington: Pan American Health Organization).

Schofield, C.J., 1979, The behaviour of Triatominae (Hemiptera: Reduviidae): A review. *Bulletin of Entomological Research* **69**, 363–379.

Service, M.W., 1980, *A Guide to Medical Entomology*. Macmillan Tropical and Sub-Tropical Medical Texts (London: Macmillan).

Shaw, J.J., 1969, *The Haemoflagellates of Sloths*. London School of Tropical Medicine Memoir No. 13 (London: H.K. Lewis).

Steck, E.A., 1971, *Chemotherapy of Protozoan Diseases* (Portland, Or.: Division of Medicinal Chemistry, Walter Reed Army Institute of Research), 4 Volumes.

Taylor, A.E.R. and Baker, J.R., 1978, *Methods of Cultivating Parasites* in vitro (London: Academic Press).

Tobe, S.S. and Langley, P.A., 1978, Reproductive physiology of *Glossina*. *Annual Review of Entomology* **23**, 283–307.

Trypanosomiasis and Leishmaniasis with Special Reference to Chagas' Disease. 1974, Ciba Foundation Symposium 20 (New Series). (Amsterdam: Elsevier–North Holland).

Wallace, F.G., 1966, The trypanosomatid parasites of insects and arachnids. *Experimental Parasitology* **18**, 124–193.

Wells, E.A., 1972, *Infection of Cattle with Trypanosomes of the Subgenus Megatrypanum (Hoare, 1964)* (Slough, UK: Commonwealth Agricultural Bureau).

Williams, P. and Coelho M. de V., 1978, Taxonomy and transmission of *Leishmania*. *Advances in Parasitology* **16**, 1–42.

Williamson, J., 1979, Effects of trypanocides on the fine structure of target organisms. *Pharmacology and Therapeutics* **7**, 445–512.

World Health Organization, 1972, Trypanosomiasis. *Bulletin of the World Health Organization* **47(b)**. A collection of papers on human trypanosomiasis in the Lambwe Valley, Kenya.

World Health Organization, 1979, *The African Trypanosomiases*. Report of a Joint WHO Expert Committee and FAO Expert Consultation. Technical Report Series, No. 635 (Geneva: WHO).

World Health Organization, 1980, *Studies on Leishmaniasis*. VBC Circulars (prepared by Dr. A. T. Zahar) Nos. WHO/VBC 80.749, WHO/VBC 80.776, WHO/VBC 80.786, WHO/VBC 80.825.

Zeledon, R. and Rabinowich, J. E., 1981, Chagas Disease: An ecological appraisal with special emphasis on its insect vectors. *Annual Review of Entomology* **26**, 101–133.

Zuckerman, A. and Lainson, R., 1977. In Leishmania *in Parasitic Protozoa*, edited by J. Kreier (London: Academic press), Vol. 1, pp. 57–133.

Zwart, D., 1979, A review of studies on three mouse infective *T. vivax* strains. *Veterinary Science Communications* **3**, 187–206.

Index

Page numbers in italics refer to illustrations.